Kindly presented January 1983

by Janssen Pharmaceuticals.

To: LX LIBRARY

ANAESTHETIC DEPT.

P.D.H.

Relief of Pain in
Clinical Practice

Relief of Pain in Clinical Practice

SAMPSON LIPTON

Director, The Centre for Pain Relief,
Department of Medical and Surgical Neurology,
Mersey Regional Health Authority,
Walton Hospital,
Liverpool 9, Great Britain;

Clinical Lecturer,
Department of Anaesthesia,
Liverpool University Medical School,
Liverpool;

Visiting Fellow,
The Bio-Engineering Unit,
Faculty of Aeronautics and
Mechanical Engineering,
University of Salford,
Greater Manchester,
Great Britain.

BLACKWELL
SCIENTIFIC PUBLICATIONS
OXFORD LONDON EDINBURGH
MELBOURNE

© 1979 Blackwell Scientific Publications
Osney Mead, Oxford, OX2 0EL
8 John Street, London, WC1N 2ES
9 Forrest Road, Edinburgh, EH1 2QH
214 Berkeley Street, Carlton, Victoria 3053

First published 1979

Distributed in U.S.A. by
Blackwell Mosby Book Distributors
11830 Westline Industrial Drive
St Louis, Missouri 63141,
in Canada by
Blackwell Mosby Book Distributors
86 Northline Road, Toronto
Ontario, M4B 3E5,
and in Australia by
Blackwell Scientific Book Distributors
214 Berkeley Street, Carlton
Victoria 3053

British Library Cataloguing in Publication Data

Lipton, Sampson
    Relief of pain in clinical practice.
    1. Anesthesia   2. Pain
    1. Title
    616′.047   RD81

ISBN 0 632 00362 6

Printed in Great Britain
at the University Press, Oxford
by Eric Buckley
Printer to the University

This book is dedicated to
Gloria Patricia Lipton

As pain constitutes the career of 'L'homme douloureux' so its diagnosis and relief constitute the career of many physicians. The passion of patients trying to persuade physicians to engage in this or that pain-relieving intervention is matched only by the passion of physicians recommending this or that pain-allaying treatment. Just as the 'seriousness' of the patient's devotion to suffering is measured by his resistance to relinquishing his chosen career, so the 'seriousness' of the physician's devotion to relieving pain is measured by his resistance to admitting defeat in his struggle against 'pain'

T. S. Szasz in
Soulairac, A. (ed.) (1968) *Pain Symposium*, p. 98

Contents

Contents

Preface

There has been no complete textbook on the treatment of pain for many years. There are two reasons for this. First, the material which should go into such a volume is so vast that several years are needed to assemble it; and second, by the time it has been assembled large portions are out of date. There is no easy solution to this problem and that is why I have been careful to limit the contents of this volume by reducing them, on the one hand, to those useful practical measures which in my opinion are not described in sufficient detail elsewhere; and on the other to cover in fair detail some of the more common chronic pains. In this way some useful information can be transmitted before it is superseded by newer material.

This book is designed for the specialist and in particular for those who are likely to make active use of the information it contains. It will also be of value to those medical practitioners, and indeed to ancillary workers, who are really interested in modern methods and what they offer the patient.

In my own practice I use methods acquired from the many clinics that I have visited and the many clinicians who have been kind enough to demonstrate their techniques to me. These methods are now often carried out by me in a somewhat different fashion from that seen originally. In this book I describe what I do now and I have no doubt that other clinicians starting with these methods will speedily develop their own variations, and this is how it should be. One can only hope that clinicians developing useful variations and new methods will publish them speedily in the medical press so that all can benefit, which is my principal reason for writing this book.

Pain relief medicine is now in a most interesting phase as the recent discovery of the endogenous opiate substances and their receptor sites is bound to open up new methods of treatment. Ideally if the cause-producing pain cannot be removed then a non-addictive analgesic drug with no side-effects should be given. So far nothing remotely approaching this ideal has been produced. One can only hope that activity by the western world drug companies and our pharmacologists, stimulated by new discoveries, will bear fruit.

Books require references and bibliographies, and I have tried to limit these to essentials. For any particular author the references tend to be the most recent ones, as these contain details of earlier works. The bibliography will form a practical and useful 'pain library'.

I am indebted to Mrs R.Filbin, the medical illustrator, and Mr J.W. Stammers A I I P, the Principal of the Central Photographic Department, The University of Liverpool, for their help in preparing the diagrams, films, and line drawings; to Miss Norah Brown and Miss Carol Mayes for the preparation of the manuscript; to Dr D. Harty, Consultant Radiologist, Walton Hospital, Liverpool, for providing Fig. 12; and to my wife as without her encouragement and smoothing of my path this book would still be on the typewriter ribbon.

Introduction

All patients in pain are treated by analgesic or narcotic drugs long before they arrive at a Pain Relief Centre. If they have become addicted or habituated to their drugs these must be contolled before proper assessment and treatment can be instituted. Often psychiatric help is necessary to carry this out.

Many patients do not take their analgesic drugs regularly and thus patients suffering from chronic pain should have their drug regime examined. Often they wait until their pain recurs before taking the next dose. They should be instructed to take a following dose of drug at such a time that absorption occurs before the previous effect wears off.

In the treatment of chronic-pain patients a distinction must be drawn very clearly between those with a short expectation of life, from say cancer, and those with a normal or approximately normal expectation of life, such as those suffering from migraine. In general when the pain of patients with a short expectation of life is no longer controlled by drugs, then the ablative methods of pain control can be used justifiably. There is a proviso that the patient and their relatives have been informed clearly about the potential complications of such methods as cordotomy, pituitary injection of alcohol, and destructive nerve blocks. The reason these techniques should only be used on patients with a short expectation of life is that the patient will die before the inevitable return of pain occurs and the recurrence of pain may be accompanied by dysaesthesiae, hyperpathia, and anaesthesia of the affected dermatomes.

In all patients before undertaking any active measure for relieving chronic pain it is imperative that a careful medical history is taken and physical examination made. Any nerve deficits or other abnormalities are noted and if possible these deficits and abnormalities are demonstrated to the patient and their relatives.

Patients with a normal expectation of life have to be treated in somewhat different fashion from those with a short one. They must not be prescribed addictive drugs as they will inevitably become drug addicts. The

I

ablative methods of treatment are to be avoided for the reasons previously mentioned and therefore these patients are often treated with non-specific methods such as external electrical stimulation; acupuncture; repeated nerve blocks using simple anaesthetic solutions; alpha feedback and so on. Often these methods are used in combination with each other and with mild analgesics, but only after the normal traditional methods of mobilisation; immobilisation; physiotherapy; release of scar tissue surgically; corrective operations and the like have been tried.

Sometimes the method of treatment is obvious as when subcostal nerve blocks with neurolytic agents are used for a solitary secondary tumour in a rib, or a percutaneous cordotomy for unilateral inoperable cancer pain below the C_5 dermatome. Often, and this particularly applies with pain in patients with a normal expectation of life, the treatment is not obvious and then a series of diagnostic investigations are necessary. These can include X-rays; isotope scans; haematological and electrolyte measurements; lung function and many, many others. These may be followed by diagnostic blocks of one kind or another which can indicate the origin of the pain and thus how to treat it. These investigations may not point to one specific treatment method but suggest further diagnostic measures. Throughout the investigation and subsequent treatment there should be a constant awareness on the part of the physician in charge of the patient that there must be a reasonable relation between the time chronic pain is suffered, its degree, whether the cause of the pain is threatening to life, and the complexity and dangers involved in diagnosis and treatment. As an example, pain in the chest should not have cardiac catheterisation performed as a preliminary investigation. Similarly, undue persistence in investigation or treatment should be avoided as, for instance, in a patient who has had several spinal operations for chronic pain without much benefit, it would be unwise to undertake another such operation.

Often the patient is referred to the pain-relief clinic because all the simple and usual methods of pain control in non-specialised units have been tried and have failed to help. Any simple measure of treatment that has inadvertently been omitted should be tried before drawing up a diagnostic regimen. The simpler portions of this regimen will be tried first and as each of these may be followed up for a few weeks, some time may elapse before completion. There is no avoiding this. The diagnosis and treatment of chronic and painful conditions, when they are refractive enough to reach a pain-relief centre, is a time-consuming business and cannot be hurried. For instance in an atypical facial pain after the neurological and other examinations prove normal; after the skull X-rays and other investigations, and the psychological profile shows no gross abnormality; then specific measures can be carried out. These may involve trials of ergot preparations, of clonidine, and of methysergide. Then nerve blocks of the stellate ganglion, the infraorbital nerve, or the sphenopalatine region, may be performed. The whole procedure may take many months to complete. Many patients referred to a pain-relief centre are not of this complexity and the time involved will be much less than this. It also depends on whether the centre is equipped to deal with this type of case, in other words whether it is a multi-disciplinary pain-relief referral centre or a relatively simple 'blocking clinic'. It can, of course, be a mixture of the two.

In the succeeding pages some conditions in which there is difficulty of both diagnosis and treatment are mentioned. No individual lists of investigations and treatment are given for each of these conditions, as these will depend on the facilities the individual physician has available and the personal preferences of this physician. It must be emphasised that there is no single method of treating a particular patient and therefore no 'correct' method is available, rather there is a series of treatments or methods and it is up to the individual physician to carry out first the one which is thought most suitable by him. Another physician will not necessarily be of the same opinion. They can be equally correct.

It must be mentioned that always there are some patients suffering from chronic pain who cannot be cured or even helped. The physician can only treat them symptomatically and sympathetically. He will have to tell them that at the present time there is no satisfactory method of treatment for their condition and that if they persist in seeking active treatment they may finish up much worse than when they started. They must be advised to live with their pain using whatever simple help can be provided, however difficult it is to do this. At the Liverpool Centre for Pain Relief these patients in addition are given some hope for the future by being told that new methods are constantly being developed and although there is nothing for them now there may be in a year or two. Their names are placed on a special list which is reviewed regularly to see if the newer methods are applicable to any of the old patients. They are also asked to write in once a year asking if anything new is available for them. This double-check method ensures that they are not forgotten.

Chapter 1
Basic Treatments

DRUG THERAPY

Analgesic drugs are available of varying potency and it is not proposed to produce a list of these here. The principles have already been mentioned. The drug is given regularly at intervals related to its half-life in the blood stream. This type of drug, as in any other, has its effect either locally on the tissues at peripheral nerve endings, or at various levels in the central nervous system.

It is important to avoid producing narcotic drug addiction in patients with a normal expectation of life. Similarly it is indefensible to avoid giving narcotic drugs to patients with a short expectation of life if this is the only immediate method of giving them some relief.

There are other problems with these drugs that must be kept in mind, especially for patients with a normal expectation of life. Some of them have complications occurring with prolonged use. The danger of kidney damage with phenacetin and aspirin is well known. As phenacetin is altered to paracetamol in the body this drug also should be avoided for long-term use. It would appear that the danger of kidney damage is greatest in the case of phenacetin and is present to a lesser extent with the others mentioned. It is, however, present in these and therefore other drugs should be used instead if possible.

Apart from the complications occurring with prolonged use there are side-effects which can be so unpleasant that the particular drug must be withdrawn. There was high hope that Fortral (Pentazocine) would prove to be the non-addictive narcotic that has been desired for so long. Unfortunately such has not proved to be the case. It is for practical purposes non-addictive in oral doses but there is a high level of unpleasant side-effects in ambulant patients. However, such are the benefits of using this drug that it should be given a trial in all severe pains in patients with a normal expectation of life. If side-effects occur the dose should be halved. If at this reduced level the side-effects are still marked the use of this drug is abandoned.

4

It would appear from these few remarks that if Pentazocine cannot be used then drugs such as DF 118 (Dihydocodeine) is the strongest that can be used in the patient needing a narcotic, and Brufen (Ibuprofen) and Naprosyn (Naproxen) can be used instead of aspirin and the other anti-rheumatic agents. Brufen and Naprosyn are also useful analgesic agents in their own right without much in the way of gastric effects, though these can be severe on occasion.

There are other non-analgesic drugs which can be used in certain of the painful conditions which find their way into pain-relieving centres. A commonly used one is Deseril (Methysergide) which can be most effective in migraine, some of the atypical facial pains, and in cluster headaches. It is always worthwhile trying this drug in this particular group of conditions when ergot has failed. There is one very unpleasant effect that may be produced by Methysergide, namely that in prolonged and high doses pleural, retroperitoneal, and cardiac fibrosis occurs. For this reason it is wise to give no more than 4 mg of the drug daily and to stop using it for one month every five or six months. If these precautions are adhered to there is little danger of fibrosis occurring. At the Liverpool Centre for Pain Relief the dose of this drug is kept to 3 mg daily for three monthly periods only. Such drugs as the beta-blocking agents are useful as a last resort in migraine and allied conditions but their effect on cardiac rate must be monitored with care. Another substance which may be used under these circumstances is the monoamineoxidase inhibitors. These, acting in the same fashion as a beta blocker, prevent adrenaline effects on peripheral blood vessels and vaso-dilatation does not occur. When the monoamineoxidase group of drugs are used the diet of the patient has to be controlled to avoid amines, and this presents problems. They should therefore only be used when the patient has been fully briefed in their dangers and when the physician is prepared to give continuous and close supervision.

These two drugs can be used empirically in other chronic painful conditions which have not responded to any other drug therapy and where the primary condition causing the pain precludes more active treatment. Such a condition as the Thalamic Pain Syndrome would fall into this category; and in similar fashion an alpha blocker, such as chlorpromazine, can be used empirically in conditions of this kind. When a sympathetic block of one of the limbs is required intravenous guanethidine can be used to produce a long-lasting block for days. Guanethidine produces a non-specific sympathetic block and if a more definite alpha block is required this can be obtained with thymoxamine. When used for sympathetic block of a limb a tourniquet is used round the upper portion of the limb and 10-20 mg

Guanethidine Sulphate B.P. is injected into the peripheral portion of the limb. The tourniquet is deflated in 5–10 minutes but care is needed in case there is a fall in blood-pressure (Hannington-Kiff).

Trigger-point injections

In many painful conditions not specifically rheumatic there are small nodules present which are painful to touch or pressure. The pain produced by these nodules may not be in the same dermatomes as the nodules and may be at a distance. If these painful nodules are injected or have an acupuncture needle inserted into them, the pain is often relieved. In many conditions there may be painful areas rather than nodules and these must be sought out meticulously (Travell). In one form of acupuncture the acupuncturist searches the whole body very carefully for sensitive places and when found uses these places as acupuncture needle insertion points.

Sympathetic block

The three main blocks of this type are detailed in the nerve-block section of this book. When pain is limited or mainly limited to one side of the body or limbs and is of a diffuse type with some element of heat or discomfort in the pain (discomfort meaning unpleasantness), then it is worthwhile carrying out a sympathetic block related to the involved portion of the body. This type of block is particularly useful in causalgia, and it is important in that case to be persistent (Fig. 1a). Daily stellate blocks can be carried out, as can lumbar sympathetic ones though with more difficulty. It is possible to insert long-term catheters near the stellate ganglion or lumbar sympathetic chain and inject regularly through this as advocated by Bonica. For limbs the method of Hannington-Kiff previously mentioned is exceedingly useful.

Somatic nerve blocks

These are of two types. First, the diagnostic block where the procedure is designed to give information as to the origin of the pain. This information can be positive or negative as a block which ablates the pain indicates the site of development, while a block which has no effect equally indicates where it is not arising. The accuracy of this method varies with the mental processes of the patient, and with the well-known placebo effect. For this reason if irreversible procedures are going to be carried out on the strength of a diagnostic block then the block must be repeated at least once and preferably twice.

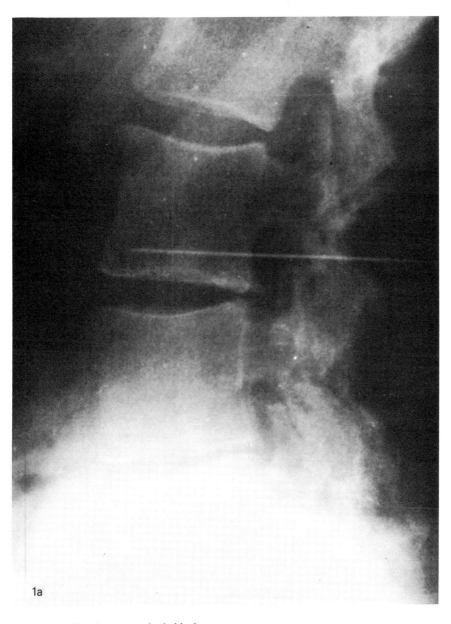

FIGURE 1*a*. Lumbar sympathetic block.

If there is still doubt after these blocks have been carried out on more than one occasion then the differential spinal block may be helpful.

Secondly are the blocks used for treatment and these are of two types, short- and long-acting ones. The short-acting blocks use simple anaesthetic solutions such as lignocaine or marcaine and will give up to five or six hours of anaesthesia. These solutions may have other substances added to them such as one of the long-acting steroid compounds. These blocks may be repeated as in subachromial bursa injection, as usually there is residual benefit from the first block and this benefit is increased after the second. If the benefit on a number of occasions lasts only the expected time that the anaesthetic solution used is expected to produce then thought will have to be given to a long-acting local block. These are either alcohol or phenol solutions. Alcohol is not much used except for gasserian ganglion block because it tends to produce neuritis so that various solutions of phenol are usually used (Fig. 1*b*). These are 2 per cent and 6 per cent when the solutions are at room temperature, but a stronger solution of phenol can be obtained by warming the solution while it is in contact with phenol crystals. An 8 per cent solution of phenol is the strongest solution that can be conveniently obtained at room temperature but a 6 per cent solution is the one

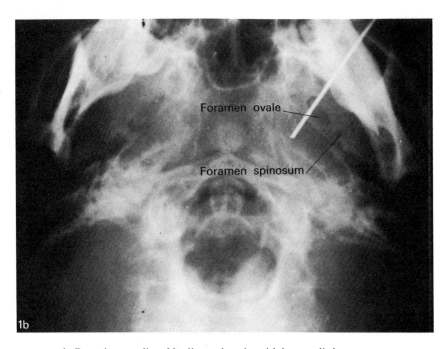

FIGURE 1*b*. Gasserian ganglion. Needle needs to be withdrawn a little.

used in the Liverpool Centre. There has been no obvious lack in effect when this solution has been used.

There is another block in which two solutions are used together and which have proved useful. This is the mixture of 2 per cent Benzocaine in Arachis Oil with 6 per cent Urethane solution. The needle is inserted into the tissues to the required depth and 2 per cent Benzocaine in Oil is injected followed by twice the quantity of 6 per cent Urethane without (and this is the important part of the procedure) moving the needle at all. The benzocaine and the urethane must mix in the tissues. When used for, say, subcostal nerves the analgesia produced by this block lasts from a few weeks to six months depending on the reaction of the patient. Presumably as in all long-acting blocks the length of time the block lasts depends on how close to the nerves the solution is deposited and how quickly the tissues recover.

It must be remembered in all these blocks that sooner or later the block wears off and if the condition for which the block is carried out is not improving, the pain will recur. It is common experience that long-acting blocks do not produce complete pain relief for more than six weeks. They will, of course, give satisfactory pain relief for a much longer period than this.

Spinal Blocks

These are of three types. First, the subarachnoid injection when the anaesthetic solution is placed in contact with the cerebrospinal fluid. In this situation the nerve roots are at their most vulnerable to injected material as there are no coverings to them at all. It is most important to know exactly where the injected solution is moving within the cerebrospinal fluid when long-lasting effects are required. If this is known then the nerve roots which are being affected by the injection are also known. It is for this reason that substances injected into the cerebrospinal fluid are made up into light or heavy solutions compared to the specific gravity of the cerebrospinal fluid itself. The light solution normally used is 100 per cent alcohol and this is particularly suitable when it is desired to affect the mid dorsal spinal nerve roots. A spinal puncture is made at the upper or lower dorsal spine (or lower cervical or upper lumbar if necessary) and the alcohol is floated in the required direction by positioning the patient. Except when anterior nerve roots are to be affected to relieve spasticity it is the posterior roots which are affected for pain relief, and therefore the patient is positioned in such a way that the posterior nerve roots will be bathed by the injected alcohol. In the case of a light solution such as alcohol the patient is placed on the painless

side with the painful side uppermost and tilted forwards 45° to bring the
posterior nerve roots to the highest point of the spinal canal. The lengthwise
tilt of the patient will also need to be adjusted so that the required root or
roots carrying the stimulation it is desired to block, are at the highest point
of the cerebrospinal fluid (Fig. 1c).

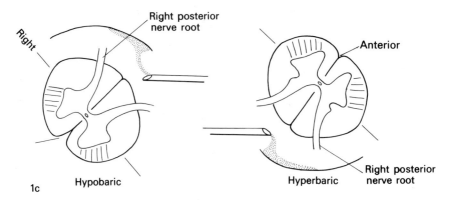

FIGURE 1c. Subarachnoid block, light and heavy solutions.

When the solutions used are heavy ones the patient is positioned in
reverse fashion to that just mentioned. The patient lies on the painful side,
is tilted posteriorly and the body is arranged so that the roots to be affected
are at the most dependent part of the cerebrospinal fluid. The usual heavy
solutions are 1 in 20, or 1 in 15, phenol in glycerine. Sometimes the phenol
is made up in Myodil (Iophendylate B.P.) which is radio-opaque and can
be seen on X-ray plates. Phenol in myodil appears to behave as a weaker
solution than the same strength made up in glycerine. The glycerine solutions are viscid and therefore do not move up and down the spinal theca as
rapidly when the patient's position is altered and for this reason many
operators prefer them to alcohol in all positions of the spinal theca except
the mid dorsal region. In this region the imbrication of the vertebral spines
make it difficult to perform spinal puncture at the level of the nerve root to
be affected.

Diagnostic subarachnoid blocks can be used to predict the value of
a subsequent long-lasting phenol block, but the author has not found them
of much value and they do subject the patient to an extra procedure. If
phenol and alcohol subarachnoid blocks are confined to patients with
inoperable cancer pain then there is no need for a preliminary diagnostic
subarachnoid block (in the author's opinion).

The diagnostic subarachnoid block which is likely to give most useful information in those patients where it is uncertain whether their pain is produced from an organic cause, is the differential spinal block. Here a spinal needle is inserted subarachnoid and first saline is injected, followed by varying and increasing concentrations of local anaesthetic solution designed to block successively sympathetic, sensory, and motor nerve fibres. The procedure finishes with a total spinal block. Theoretically this differential spinal block will distinguish pain produced mentally from that produced somatically. In the latter case some indication can be given as to whether the pain arises in the sympathetic system, or not. The results of this investigation must be interpreted with care as they cannot always be taken at face value.

There are two other spinal methods of injection which are of value in chronic pain relief. The epidural or extradural block is particularly well known in midwifery but long-acting anaesthetic solutions can be injected in this way. Phenol in glycerine can be used in this region but it will not have such a profound effect on the nerve fibres in the roots because they are covered with a layer of dura which the nerve root carries with it when it penetrates the dura. One very valuable way in which this block can be used for long-lasting effects using short-acting local anaesthetic agents is by inserting an epidural catheter in the usual sterile fashion, placing a sterile microfilter in its outer end and then using it as a long-term implant. In this way relief can be given to patients with pain in spinal dermatomes over many weeks and, on occasion, months. Patients with inoperable cancer who are too ill to be treated in any other way can be managed in this fashion. Similarly patients who do not have pain from a malignant condition can have relief of their pain for a period. Often a simple continuous block of this kind enables patients to recover their poise and increase their threshold to pain.

The third method of spinal injection is not commonly used and is much more difficult to carry out than either of the two blocks already mentioned. This is the subdural injection which is made between the arachnoid and the dura. Injected solutions made in this position travel out along the nerve roots and as the solution lies underneath the dura it will have more effect on the nerve fibres than an epidural block. The injected solution travels bilaterally along both nerve roots at a given level though the patient lies on the painful side and more of the phenol in glycerine solution travels to the lowermost side than to the upper. Another very useful feature of this injection is that the injected substance travels up the spinal cord against gravity. The patient is usually placed on the painful side with the head and shoulders raised about 30° when the cervical nerve roots are to be injected. It is a very useful block in this region and spread over all the cervical nerve roots can be obtained with a series of these injections. It might be thought that the placing of the spinal needle subdurally requires great expertise but while not easy the technique is rendered much simpler with the use of an image intensifier. This particular technique was devised by Maher and its use now advocated by Mehta.

Local spinal injections are used in some of the various methods which attempt to relieve pain arising from the apophyseal joints. It has been noticed for a long time that many patients thought to have pain in the lumbar region, or a sciatica, or both, due to a retropulsed vertebral disc, have had no relief after exploration of their lumbar disc spaces and often no retropulsed disc was found. It seemed logical that the pain these patients suffered must be arising elsewhere. Skyrme-Rees believed this pain to arise in the posterior spinal joints and devised a method of cutting the nerves carrying sensation from these joints. The Skyrme-Rees method was said to produce severe blood loss on occasion and therefore a similar result was obtained by other operators using a heat lesion produced by a radiofrequency current (diathermy current). The anatomy of the nerve supply to this joint has been elucidated in detail by Bradley and also by Mehta and Sluijter and a scheme of coagulating this nerve supply has been worked out both for the lumbar and for the cervical region.

The Cordotomy

Nowadays when one refers to cordotomy in pain-relief clinics the percutaneous cervical cordotomy (PCC) is the method that is being discussed. This is not to say that there is no place for the surgical cordotomy but the PCC can be carried out by any medical practitioner who cares to spend the time to learn the technique (not forgetting the related anatomy and physiology) and thus leave the neurosurgeon free of the thousands of patients with inoperable cancer pain who would benefit from the PCC. At the Liverpool Centre surgical cordotomies are carried out only on those patients where the PCC method has failed or where a thoracic cordotomy is particularly required.

There are two varieties of PCC (Fig. 2). A high C1–C2 lateral approach PCC and a lower anterior C5–C6 percutaneous cordotomy (Fig. 3). The latter has advantages when the patient has either had a C1–C2 PCC on one side, producing a high analgesic level and requires a bilateral procedure, or has very poor lung function. Either of these two methods gives good

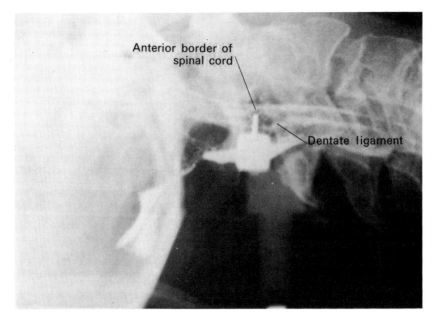

FIGURE 2. C1–C2 Lateral percutaneous cervical cordotomy.

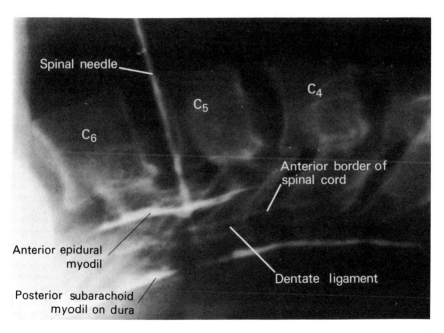

FIGURE 3. C5–C6 Anterior percutaneous cervical cordotomy.

analgesia on the opposite side of the body and limbs to that on which the cordotomy is performed. This being due to the normal cross-over of fibres forming the antero-lateral quadrant of the spinal cord. It is this portion of the spinal cord which is sectioned in the surgical cordotomy and coagulated in the PCC.

The great value of the cordotomies over all other types of pain-relieving procedures is the high percentage success rate achieved and the quality of the pain relief obtained.

Because in the opinion of the author this method of pain relief is not sufficiently used and because not enough detailed instruction has been written about it, the method has been given in considerable detail in this book.

Pituitary Injection of Alcohol (Moricca's Operation)

This operation is used in the relief of inoperable cancer pain (Fig. 4). It is particularly suited for trial in those patients where either the primary condition is widespread and bilateral and the patient is in severe pain only controlled by large doses of narcotic drugs, or where the primary cancer is hormone dependent. The percentage success rate for relief of pain in this method does not approach that of the cordotomies as only 40 per cent become completely pain free as opposed to 85 per cent in the cordotomy. Indeed of this 40 per cent half of the patients have complete pain relief which lasts more than four months, a much lower proportion than in the cordotomies. Also in the cordotomy of the 15 per cent of patients who do not get complete pain relief about half get considerable relief, enough to allow a reduction in the quantity or strength of their analgesic drugs. In the pituitary injection of alcohol for pain a further 30 per cent obtain some relief after the procedure. Thus the total of patients benefited is 70 per cent. It would be much more satisfactory if the method produced more than this but until another method appears with more satisfactory results the pituitary injection of alcohol will continue to be used. It is a very simple operation to perform and it can be carried out on patients in very poor condition indeed.

In those patients in whom it is used for tumour regression a number of pituitary injections of alcohol are needed over a period of time.

Carefully carried out there are few complications to the technique. When there is, it is the consequence of destruction of the pituitary in part or occasionally in whole. Fortunately pituitary function tends to recover in time and in any case the principal deficit produces a diabetes insipidus and this is easily controlled.

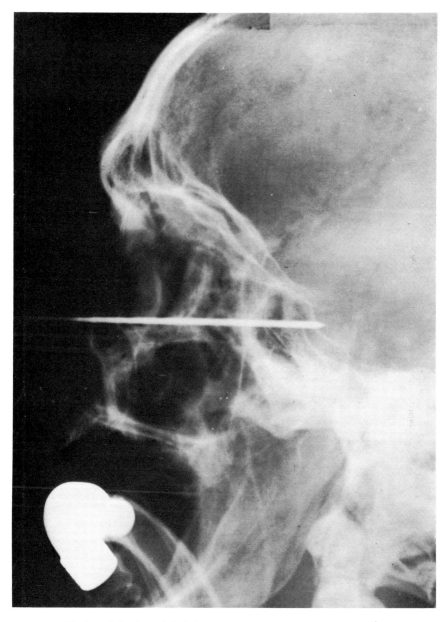

FIGURE 4. Pituitary injection of alcohol.

Electrical stimulation

This technique is based on the Gate Control Theory of Melzack and Wall. There is considerable controversy over how modulation of nervous stimulation produced by noxious stimuli is effected in the central nervous system and whether the theory provides an accurate picture. However, it does not matter in practice whether the theory is 100 per cent correct or not, it suffices if the theory can be tested and produces a method which can be used in clinical practice for the relief of pain. The Gate Control postulates that by increasing stimulation through the larger nerve fibres, modulation, i.e. suppression, will occur in nerve conduction along small nerve fibres. As pain is transmitted over small nerve fibres or rather the nervous stimulation produced as a result of noxious stimulation is transmitted over small nerve fibres it is this type of stimulation which is modulated. If it is reduced to the extent that it is insufficient to produce the psychic phenomenon known as pain, then pain relief occurs.

There are two types of electrical stimulation. One is known as transcutaneous stimulation where an electric current is passed in or near the skin of the painful region and in a proportion of patients produces a greater or lesser degree of pain relief. The method is of use in chronic painful conditions where the amount of pain is not severe or where a non-surgical method is required. There is a vogue for this method at present as there is for acupuncture. It stems from the same requirement to have a method of pain relief which does not involve destruction of the central or peripheral nervous system and therefore can be used on patients with a normal expectation of life.

The second type is to have the stimulating electrodes in close proximity to either the spinal cord (usually the posterior columns) or near the aqueduct or internal capsule. For this second type a temporary electrode can be placed epidurally in the spinal column and tested over a period of days or even weeks (Fig. 5). To some extent a similar system can be applied to the brain. Although surgery may be used to implant these electrodes permanently it does not involve destruction of the central nervous system and therefore there is the possibility of long-lasting relief without recurrence of the pain.

It is rather interesting that stimulation of brain electrodes for relief of pain have produced corresponding high levels of Encephalin-like substances in the spinal cerebrospinal fluid (unpublished data, Miles and Lipton). Naloxone, a narcotic antagonist, will abolish for the period of its action any pain-relieving effects produced by electrical stimulation and is

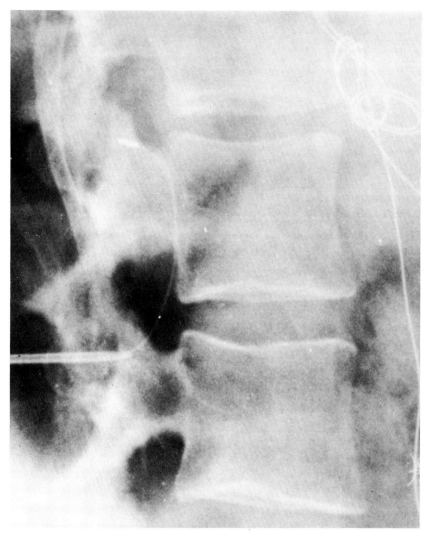

FIGURE 5. Epidural electrodes.

a known antagonist to Encephalin. Thus there is some evidence that the pain-relieving effect of electrical stimulation may be due to the production of an intrinsic morphine-like substance. A similar effect is believed to be present in acupuncture pain relief but not in pain relief produced by the pituitary injection of alcohol (unpublished data, Miles, Lipton, and Williams).

Multiple Sclerosis

A similar technique of implanting an epidural electrode as mentioned above has been used in patients suffering from multiple sclerosis. It is said to be particularly effective in those patients whose problems are due to spasticity.

Acupuncture

This is a form of peripheral nerve stimulation. It is effective in some varieties of pain and because it is a non-invasive method with negligible risk it can be used freely. The author has produced benefit in some patients suffering from sciatica and has found it useful in intractable migraine where it seems to reduce the frequency and severity of the attacks. It does not appear to relieve the condition in its entirety.

The author has found that he obtains as much benefit for his patients from acupuncture peripheral nerve stimulation when any point in the dermatomal region of the pain is used as when the classical acupuncture points are used.

There is an undoubted useful phenomenon present in acupuncture which can be used for pain relief. Much research is being carried out at the present time and a useful simple technique may eventually appear. As has just been mentioned acupuncture effects can be removed by injecting the patient with the narcotic antagonist naloxone and this suggests that acupuncture stimulation may produce its effect through the mediation of an intrinsic morphine-like transmitter agent.

Operant Conditioning

It is obvious that patients with chronic pain do receive some benefits from their pain behaviour. A patient who does not complain or show signs of suffering, who does not cry out with pain, and who lies quietly in bed, tends to be ignored. If the same patient does all of these things then immediately they receive attention. It comes from nurse or doctor or family, and is accompanied by sympathy and medication. Thus the pain patient's behaviour is positively reinforced. Painful behaviour will tend to be repeated on other occasions and may be increased in its expression. Operant conditioning is designed to reverse this procedure. It must be emphasised that operant conditioning is to be used only in chronic pain patients. It must not be used in patients suffering acute pain.

The basic technique used in operant conditioning is to ignore the patient's pain behaviour. This means that if the patient is in a hospital ward he or she is ignored when they complain of pain, and are drawn into social activity and conversation when they do not do this. An important part of the treatment is to give sufficient analgesics on a regular (timed) basis so that the patient has no need to go into their pain behaviour routine to obtain medication. This medication is given as a coloured fluid with a distinctive taste. After a suitable initial period the quantity of medication can be reduced without the knowledge of the patient.

The success of the treatment can be assessed by the activity shown by the patient. A log of activity can be made by the patient who can see his progress day by day.

Added on to the above programme of operant conditioning there may be group therapy sessions. There is nobody more capable in showing one pain patient the pain games he is playing than another pain patient who knows them all.

A miscellaneous group

These treatments include hypnosis and various forms of relaxation. The relaxation methods may be developed by artificial means such as Alpha feedback, or form part of a philosophy such as Yoga or Zen Buddhism. If a patient who has chronic pain obtains satisfactory relief or even partial benefit from one of these methods then it is a useful and valuable method for that patient.

FURTHER READING

BRADLEY K.C. (1974) The Anatomy of Backache. *Aust. N-Z. J. Surg.* Vol. **44**, Number **3**, pp. 227.

HANNINGTON-KIFF J.G. (1974) *Pain Relief*, p. 69, Intravenous Regional Sympathetic Block. Heinemann, London.

LIPTON S. (1977) *Persistent Pain.* Academic Press, London and New York.

MEHTA M. (1973) Spinal Analgesia. In *Intractable Pain.* Chapter **15**. Saunders, London.

MEHTA M. & SLUIJTER M. (1977) *Paper given to the joint meeting of the British and Dutch Intractable Pain Societies.* Leiden, Netherlands.

SLUIJTER M. (1977) Blocks in the Head and Neck region. Proceedings: *Anaesthetists and Pain Relief*. Boerhaave meeting, Leiden, Netherlands.

STERNBACH R.A. (1974), Ed. *Pain Patients, Traits and Treatment*. Academic Press, New York.

SWERDLOW, M. (1974), Ed. *Relief of Intractable Pain*. Excerpta Medica, Amsterdam.

Chapter 2
Operant Conditioning

It is important to assume that all pain is real. It is certainly real to the sufferer. The normal method of classifying pain into organic, which implies that the pain is real and present, and psychogenic, which implies that the pain is imaginary and therefore not present, is unrealistic and does not help treatment. An assessment of the patient should be made at as early a stage as possible, to decide whether the presence of pain reflects emotional stress or actual tissue damage. This can be a relatively easy decision at a multidisciplinary pain clinic where suitable psychiatric referrals are easily obtained but in small blocking clinics the physician in charge of the patient must keep this possibility in mind. Certainly if a given patient does not respond to treatment in a normal fashion a psychiatric opinion should be obtained.

It is a common experience that pain of a given intensity produces very different responses in two different patients. Pain regarded as a minor evil by one is the continuous agony of the other. Also pain response in a given patient will vary from time to time, depending on their attitude and attention to their pain. How often does one hear a patient remark 'I was feeling low that day and the pain was bad'? Pain is affected by suggestion, by the expectations of the patient, their level of anxiety, and the benefit (or otherwise) they get from the situation. Certain sensations are present when pain is perceived and they vary with the amount of pain present. Pain produces discomfort and fear, and motivates the patient into activity to remove the affected part from the noxious stimuli if that is possible, or to such motor activity as rubbing the part. Autonomic phenomena are also produced such as sweating, a rapid pulse, alteration in blood-pressure, and nausea. If these phenomena appear when there is organic cause for the pain this can be readily understood.

The patient with pain from inoperable cancer for instance, becomes withdrawn, cannot be bothered to take part in the usual family give and take, does not read, or even watch television. Eventually their whole life revolves round their pain. At night they usually get a few hours sleep after taking some medication, only to wake again in a few hours. Further medication is taken, a cup of tea or coffee, a walk round the house if they are ambulant or a restless period if they are not, and eventually a further short period of sleep. This night history is so typical that it can almost be taken as diagnostic in cases where doubt exists as to recurrence of the disease or presence of a secondary tumour. Pain is influenced by the state of mind of the patient —the degree of anxiety for himself, his family, and for the future, for the prognosis, for the unpleasantness of the condition, and other complications apart from pain. These are all what may be called 'legitimate' responses to pain but what of those patients whose responses to pain appear exaggerated in relation to the amount of pain experienced, and has some or all of the phenomena already mentioned. Are these then to be considered 'illegitimate' responses to pain? Are they to be ignored and how is the patient to be treated?

If these responses are produced not from an initial tissue-damaging noxious influence but arise from anxiety, i.e. a variety of fear, the patient will nevertheless feel them in full intensity. The patient will lay these at the door of any concomitant painful state or strong sensation or discomfort. Pain is normally taken to be a sign of physical disease but it is common in psychological disorders. Pain is a conscious experience and if the patient is anxious, the pain is made worse. Waters distinguished three types of pain affected by psychological causes. These were psychogenic magnification of physical pain, tension-producing psychogenic muscular pain, and hysterical pain which he called psychogenic regional pain. Merskey found that the commonest association of persistent pain in psychiatric illness was with hysteria, anxiety neurosis, and neurotic depression. In addition he found that these patients tended to be married, to come from large families, to do relatively unskilled work, and to be very persistent in seeking additional consultations.

It must be recognised that chronic pain may be a symptom of depression and occasionally it is the only symptom. In this type of condition the expertise of a psychiatrist is essential. Some pain-relief clinics put all or most of their patients through the Minnesota Multiphasic Personality Inventory test (MMPI), which distinguishes levels of depression, anxiety, hypochondriasis, and other parameters compared to the normal.

Most patients with chronic pain—certainly those limited in their activity or even invalided by pain—are rarely successful, or have well-adjusted personalities. The life of these patients is centred on and around their pain. No human activity is free of motive so it must be asked what motive have these patients in organising their lives in this fashion? In other words, what rewards do they get? Life is a series of actions and reactions. If the action is followed by a reaction that a person finds rewarding or satisfying it is more than likely that if the given situation recurs again the action which produced the satisfying reaction will be used. In this way a behavioural pattern emerges. This type of conditioning, i.e. alteration of behaviour by rewards, is known as operant conditioning.

A patient who is unsuccessful, anxious, and dissatisfied may find that an illness produces more response from those around him than under normal conditions. A painful state may give much more attention and pleasant treatment than experienced under any other condition. Further, the patient is relieved of the necessity for difficult decisions, for work, and for facing up to the unpleasant facts of life.

Such a patient is quite content to let the situation remain at this level. He adopts the career of being sick and in pain. Relief is not required. As Szasz states, 'Whose pain should the Physician control: the patients? That of his relatives, tortured by the patient's complaints? Or his own, generated by his inability to help the patient?'

Operant conditioning produces this chronic invalid and by suitable manoeuvres operant conditioning can remove it. The basis of using operant conditioning to improve and modify pain behaviour is to ignore pain and complaints of pain in such a way as not to reinforce the pain. At the same time desired behaviour is reinforced with attention. Pain-relieving medication is not dependent on the presence of pain but is given at fixed times whether pain is present or not.

However, first, it is necessary to go a little deeper into the process by which a patient suffering from chronic pain has the pain behaviour reinforced. Initially it has to be recognised that as chronic pain lasts for some time the patient's behaviour to the pain can be modified by learning. The patient signals that he has pain by actions which are called operants. For instance, the painful limb is protected, a face is pulled and a low moan emitted. If the result of this operant is that somebody rushes up with a soothing hand, expressions of sympathy, and other comforting behaviour one can say that the operant has been reinforced and therefore it is likely that the operant will be used again in the future. Conversely, if the operant is not followed by a reinforcer or pleasant consequence then it is likely to diminish in frequency and eventually disappear. If the operant is followed by what is known as an aversive consequence, i.e. a punishment, there is usually a diminution in the frequency of the operant but this reverts to the pre-punishment rate when the punishment stops.

It is not difficult to see benefits which can accrue to patients and how these positively reinforce pain. These are very fully dealt with by Fordyce in many papers but a few examples can be given here. A husband or wife receives little or no attention from the spouse but the presence of a chronic pain (i.e. a sciatica or back pain) produces a wife or husband who is concerned and helpful. In these cases pain means concern and helpfulness and the pain is powerfully reinforced. Conversely there is little reinforcement to normal fit behaviour. Again it is common experience that if pain has been produced by an accident, and litigation is in process, there is usually little benefit obtained by treatment until the litigation is resolved one way or the other. Here the potential reward of litigation is a positive reinforcer of pain behaviour.

There are many operants but one of the most potent is provided by the physician in the method of prescribing pain-relieving drugs. Usually these are prescribed to be given as required (P.R.N.)—in other words, give when pain is present. This means no pain, no drugs, and it is more than likely that there will be exaggeration of pain behaviour with consequent dependency on the drugs or even addiction.

It is now easier to see how operant conditioning works. It will include identifying and removing reinforcers of pain behaviour; increasing physical activity; decreasing medication and eventually eliminating it. It will be necessary to remove the patient from his or her normal environment otherwise control cannot be obtained over the relevant operants. Further, before returning the patient to normal life again (i.e. outside the hospital) the family of the patient must be instructed in the method, or conditions will revert to the pre-operant conditioning period. It is preferable that some attempt be made to do the same to the patient's immediate workmates. This tends to apply more to men than women as more men than women go out to work. The housewife tends to remain within the confines of a knowledgeable circle.

It will be obvious that the medical and nursing staff of the operant conditioning team will need to be highly trained, and what is more, trained in ways which are rather foreign to the normal image of medical and nursing personnel. For instance, instead of lavishing attention and care on the patient when he or she is apparently suffering pain (and thus reinforcing chronic pain behaviour), an opposite system must be used. They are trained to be unresponsive under these conditions and to give attention when the patient's activity follows socially useful ways. Thus pain behaviour is not reinforced and activity is.

A different system is also used for medication. There is an initial period when the patient's requirement of drugs is evaluated and these form the base line. After this assessment these quantities of drugs are spread over the twenty-four hours on a fixed-time schedule, without regard to pain or activity. In the initial period the total dose is greater than base line to make sure the patient is adequately treated. This medication is given in liquid form in such a way that the patients can have no knowledge of quantity of drugs by taste or colour. As the medication is given without regard to pain, it is no longer a pain reinforcer. Eventually the dose of drug is reduced, ultimately to zero, over a time-scale of many weeks. This is not done without the patient's knowledge who is informed that this will be done before entering on the treatment. The patient is not told, while treatment is in progress, that progressive reduction of the drugs is occurring.

A most important feature of operant conditioning is the record that the patient keeps of his daily activity. As the whole purpose of operant conditioning is to increase these activities and in particular to bring the patient back to normal, or reasonably normal, social activity, it is useful to have a record of it. The patient keeps an hour by hour record of what they do and also a corresponding record of their pain level. They will record whether they sit, walk, or lie down; when they go for lunch and where they have it and for how long.

These records are available to the ward staff at the bedside and they can comment and reinforce this part of the operant-conditioning process. This will involve praise for steady progress, suggestions that perhaps they are attempting to do too much too quickly or on the contrary are not going fast enough. Gradually over a period of two to three weeks a change occurs until they are carrying out a full or almost full day of activities. They realise that they are able to behave in a reasonably normal way in spite of pain.

The above is the 'pure' operant conditioning method as described and advocated by Fordyce. Some workers add group treatment sessions to this programme (Sternbach) so that there can be a more positive feedback to the patient from the staff and from the other patients. One of the most valuable advantages of group therapy in this way is that it allows the patient to realise that there are others similar to themselves and that they are not alone.

FURTHER READING

BERNE E. (1964) *The Games People Play*. Grove Press, New York.
BOND M.R. (1971) The relation of pain to the Eysenck Personality Inventory. Cornell Medical Index and Whiteley Index of Hypochondriasis. *Brit. J. Psychiat.* **119,** 671.

DAHLSTROM W.G., WELSH G.S. & DAHLSTROM L.E. (1972) *An MMPI Handbook. Vol.* I. Clinical Interpretation (rev. ed.). Minneapolis, Minn. University of Minnesota Press.

FORDYCE W.E., FOWLER R.S., LEHMANN J.F., DE LATOUR R.I., SAND P.L. & TRIESCHMANN R.B. (1973) Operant conditioning in the treatment of chronic pain. *Arch. Phys. Med. and Rehab.* **54**, 399.

STERNBACH R.A. (1974) 'Varieties of Pain Games'. In *Advances in Neurology.* Vol. 4. Ed. J.J. Bonica. Raven Press, New York.

SZASZ T.S. (1968) *The psychology of persistent pain: A portrait of l'homme douloureux.* In *Pain.* Ed. A. Soulairac, J. Cahn, & J. Charpentier. Academic Press, New York.

WOODFORDE, J.M. & MERSKEV H. (1972) Personality traits of patients with chronic pain. *J. Psychosom. Res.* **16**, 167.

Chapter 3
Anatomy and Physiology of Pain

Modern anatomical and physiological pain theory goes part of the way to explain how pain is appreciated and the pathways that are involved.

Before expanding on this it must be realised that in the human being the appreciation of pain is modified by the mental state of the patient and a purely anatomical explanation for pain cannot provide the whole story. Further, in pathological pain states, pain is experienced without any observable noxious stimuli and appears to be self-generating and perseverating. Finally, as physiological experiments have to control variables as much as possible and are therefore simplified with this in mind, the conclusions drawn from such experiments cannot be accepted uncritically. The information provided may be quite incorrect as the experiment may not correspond to conditions in the intact animal.

Thus the account of the anatomy and physiology of pain that follows has been kept deliberately fairly broad and too much fine detail has not been included. To state that a patient has skin, a spinal cord, a brain, and can appreciate pain would produce agreement in all anatomists and physiologists. Any further steps to explain the how and the why of pain perception would be controversial.

The traditional concept of the pain mechanism was that the pain was a process in which stimulation of peripheral nerve endings produced electrical excitation. This activity travelled along nerve fibres to the dorsal horn of the spinal cord. These fibres synapsed with second order neurons and the axon of those neurons crossed to the opposite side of the spinal cord anterior to the central canal. They ascended in the spinal cord as the spinothalamic tract in the antero-lateral quadrant. The spinothalamic tract had its input into the ventral postero-lateral thalamic nuclei and thence on to the somatosensory cortex. The sensation of pain was felt at thalamic level and higher.

In an attempt to explain those features which did not fit into the traditional theory above, usually called the 'specificity theory of pain', a new concept was invoked and given the title of 'pattern theory of pain'. The basic idea here was that the appreciation of pain was not due to stimulation

27

along specific pain pathways but occurred as a result of the interpretation of patterns of stimulation which reached the higher discriminating centres. These patterns were set up by noxious stimuli affecting non-specific receptors with an intense stimulation, and they travelled over non-specific pathways. In other words there was a spatio-temporal pattern of stimulation which was interpreted by the central nervous system as pain. This theory was also obviously incorrect but did add something new in suggesting that the central nervous system had a discriminating and interpreting function.

The gate control theory of Melzack and Wall is the basis of modern pain theory. It does not, however, provide a complete explanation of pain mechanisms but does provide a better explanation than previous theories. In the gate control theory it is postulated that large diameter A fibres (A-Beta fibres) and smaller diameter A fibres (A-delta fibres) and C fibres are activated during noxious stimulation of peripheral receptors. There is a difference of activity in the two sorts of fibres. It is suggested that at spinal cord level there is a 'gate' which allows pain stimulation to pass through it to higher levels. The small fibre stimulation tends to open the gate and that of the larger fibres tends to close it. The statement of the 'gate' opening and closing is merely descriptive, what is really meant is that activity of one or other type of fibre depresses or facilitates synaptic transmission at spinal cord level. This type of gate is not only to be found at the presynaptic level but was expected by Melzack and Wall to be found at post-synaptic level and also at other levels in the central nervous system.

In addition to the local effects, the gate was under the control of the higher centres by means of a central control mechanism. Thus cortical and subcortical supraspinal neurons modulate the gate and as this modulation must occur very rapidly, there must be a very rapid ascending and descending pathway. It is thought that stimulation of the central control neurons is via the large rapidly conducting fibres of the dorsal column system.

This basic theory can be expanded to take into account other known facts about pain mechanisms. Until recently it was believed that there were no specialised pain receptors but this is no longer accepted as there are known nociceptors which respond only to levels of stimulation which produce tissue damage. However, most noxious impulses arise in receptors which at lesser levels of stimulation transmit impulses representing innoxious irritation. Thus, stimulation of mechanoreceptors along small C fibres may at minimal levels be appreciated as, say, pin prick, at much more severe levels of stimulation it is appreciated as pain. This is due to the number of receptors stimulated and to an alteration of the frequency of stimulation which travels to the spinal cord. Thus, the sensation of pain is a spatio-temporal one and is transmitted in a code which can be translated by the central nervous system to give the position of the noxious stimulus in relation to the body image and also the type and intensity of the noxious stimulus. There is no single code which is used throughout the central nervous system but it has to be realised that the code is modulated at each central nervous system level. Chronic pain may be appreciated because of damage to one or other part of the system so that either the stimulus is coded incorrectly or a correct code is translated incorrectly. Nor must it be taken that this explanation has any validity as it is a method of trying to express in words what is suspected to be the physiologic mechanism of the appreciation of pain.

There are many facts known about different parts of the anatomical pain appreciating system but where these fit into the physiological appreciation of response to pain is not known with any real degree of accuracy though the way some sections of the mechanism behaves is known to some degree. Much of our understanding of pain mechanisms is based on pure speculation which hopefully fits the facts as they are appreciated at the time of speculation.

It is obvious there must be receptor organs, that some form of transmission must occur centrally and that this transmission probably and normally progresses from spinal cord to the brain. Further, at some level, there must be appreciation of pain and, but not necessarily at the same level, the appreciation of the intellectual connotations of the pain.

RECEPTOR ORGANS

There has been much study of the peripheral nerve endings and there are many of these. They act as transducers converting chemical, mechanical, or thermal stimulation into electrical activity. The molecular basis of transducer function in receptors has still to be elucidated. Nerve endings can be differentiated or undifferentiated. Throughout the skin and body are free nerve endings which are non-myelinated nerve fibres and form a widespread overlapping network. Some of these free nerve endings arise from small myelinated nerve fibres. Each group of free nerve endings arising from a particular nerve fibre remain separate, they do not connect with each other.

Encapsulated nerve endings exist such as Ruffini corpuscles, the Golgi tendon organ, Lanceolate terminals, Lamellated terminals, Merkel discs, and so on. Sometimes a number of different receptors are combined to form a specialised sensory structure such as a sinus hair which has the following receptors. A Merkel cell, neurite complex, straight lanceolate terminals, branched lanceolate terminals, branched circular terminals, Golgi–Mazzoni corpuscles, and unmyelinated endings. As each type of receptor responds to different types of stimulation (or perhaps different ranges of the same stimulation) it can be seen how such structures can transmit complex information and how the one system can distinguish different varieties of stimulation.

Since these receptors maintain their individual connections to their parent nerve fibre it can be seen how as, say, a given stimulation to the skin produces stimulation along certain nerve fibres and as this stimulation varies in intensity from being maximal at the centre of stimulation to being attenuated at the periphery of the stimulation, that a spatial representation of the stimulation can be transmitted. Provided of course there is somewhere in the central nervous system where appreciation of sensation is spatially arranged. At spinal cord segmental level there is reflex activity in response to stimulation, it is thought that appreciation of pain occurs at higher levels.

In a similar fashion the various nerve endings transmit information of the type and degree of stimulation. This is arranged in a temporal fashion with stronger stimuli to the receptors corresponding to increased frequency and a longer duration of activity. It must be remembered that once an action potential is initiated the size of the response and its rate of transmission is dependent on the size of the axon and not the strength of the stimulus. However, it can be seen that by the spatial arrangement of receptors in the skin and the varying response of different types of receptors the information the organism requires on position and type of stimulus can be transmitted.

Receptors can be divided into three types:

1   *Nociceptors* which until recently were not thought to exist in a pure form, in other words, it was thought some receptors responded to noxious stimuli at the upper range of their normal activity. A nociceptor is a receptor which only responds to levels of activity which are damaging to the organism.

2   *Thermoreceptors.* So far only cold receptors have been positively identified. Warm receptors have not been identified in mammals, though it is suggested that they lie at the junction of the cutis and subcutis and probably have unmyelinated axons.

3   *Mechanoreceptors.* There are two morphological types of these. In one the axon terminal is the transducer. In the other the axon terminal together with a Merkel cell forms the receptor complex. There are many types of mechanoreceptors and these are of two types in their response to stimuli. The one is a slowly adapting mechanoreceptor (such as a Ruffini corpuscle), the other is a rapidly adapting mechanoreceptor (such as the Lanceolate terminals).

SENSORY FIBRES

The receptor of whatever type is connected to a sensory fibre and these also are of various types. The earliest fibre classification of Gasser and Erlanger included A-beta and A-gamma fibres in addition to A-alpha and A-delta and applied to both motor and sensory fibres. After a single strong electrical stimulus the potentials recorded from a cutaneous nerve show peaks of three types, an initial one, an intermediate one, and a delayed one. The first peak is due to A-alpha myelinated fibres with a conduction velocity of 36–102 m/sec. The second peak is due to A-delta myelinated fibres with conduction velocities of 4–20 m/sec, and the third to C unmyelinated fibres with conduction velocities of 0·5–2·5 m/sec.

Lloyd devised the classification of types I, II, III, and IV for muscle afferents. Group I is divided into two types, Ia, primary spindle afferents and Ib, Golgi tendon organ afferents, with conduction velocities of 72–120 m/sec. Type II is from secondary spindles with velocities of 36–66 m/sec. Group III are small myelinated fibres with velocities of 4–20 m/sec, and Group IV are unmyelinated ones with conduction velocities of 0·5–2·5 m/sec. It will be seen that there is correlation between the two methods of classification.

Five groups of cutaneous afferents can be classified according to their response to stimuli. A receptor which discharges when the stimulus is stationary is defined as a position detector. A receptor sensitive to increases in the velocity of the stimulus is classified as a velocity detector when an increased rate of discharge results. If receptor activity increases at the on and off of a stimulus then it is classified as a transient detector. A nociceptor is a receptor which signals tissue damage and differentiates between noxious and innocuous events. And receptors, sensitive to heating or cooling, or both, or to the rate of heating or cooling are thermoreceptors. Receptors can respond to both thermal and mechanical stimulation.

Nociceptor afferents are grouped in the A-delta and C groups of cutaneous afferents. It is known that nociceptor afferents are slowly conducting and a correlation exists here between this fact and the known latency of pain sensation. Sharp objects have a shorter latency of pain, which is produced on certain skin positions. This fact seems to correlate with the mechano-nociceptors of the A-delta group. It has long been known that a sudden painful stimulus has a dual representation, there being a faster and a slower component. These facts may correspond to the way nociceptor afferents are grouped into the A-delta and C afferents. The C fibre group contain the polymodal nociceptors which are sensitive to several stimuli (such as heat, chemical, and mechanical stimulation) and the behaviour of these correlates with the threshold for the pain of heat (45–46 °C) in the human and the changes of this threshold with repeated stimuli.

It has already been mentioned how the gate control theory suggests that modulation occurs at spinal cord level but for the appreciation of pain there is much more than this. Painful stimuli are localised in time and space as previously stated but to be painful a stimulus must activate other mechanisms. These mechanisms produce actions leading to aversive behaviour, often with anatomic and emotional responses as well. As Melzack and Wall state in their original paper, a painful stimulus originates a series of reactions. First, the reflex removal of the affected part. The organism then turns towards the injury, the head and body swivel, the eyes move, and the damaged area and surrounding terrain is also observed. Judgement of cause and its effect are made and compared with previous happenings and so on. The response to damage from a knife and from a snake are completely different. There is a little information available to explain the mechanisms which allow these evaluations of, and response to, painful stimuli.

Afferent sensory fibres enter the spinal cord and make contact with cells in one or other part of the grey matter. This grey matter is not arranged in any simple fashion but is divided into ten laminae. This work was done by Rexed on the cat and in fact if a fairly thick section of the cat spinal cord is made these laminae can be seen by the naked eye. The basic concept is that each lamina may receive its own direct input but also has an input from the previous lamina if the activity in that lamina is high, and in turn if its own activity is high it will transmit to the succeeding lamina. Thus lamina 5 receives input from lamina 4 which also contains some input from 3, 2, and 1. Lamina 5 will then transmit to the higher centres by means of long axons, but also to lamina 6 and thence 7.

There is thus no single pathway for any sensory input to take but rather there are multiple pathways. Hence there can be no destruction of 'the' pain pathway and this may account for the pain relief, which follows destructive procedures at spinal and cord level, lasting for a finite time only.

Some laminae appear to be particularly involved in the transmission of pain sensation, lamina 5 being one of these. It is excited by small myelinated fibres (group III) which are activated by pin-prick and hot and cold receptors. It transmits through spinothalamic fibres. Lamina 1, 2, and 3 are the substantia gelatinosa; 4, 5, and 6 are the nucleus proprius. Lamina 7 and 8 correspond to the intermediate nucleus. Lamina 9 is the motor neurones of the ventral horn and lamina 10 is around the central canal.

Group IV unmyelinated fibres enter through the substantia gelatinosa. If there is a severe peripheral stimulation then both group III and group IV fibres will be activated. Lamina 5 may then be sufficiently stimulated, directly by group III and indirectly by group IV through the previous laminae, not only to activate spinothalamic fibres but also to stimulate laminae 7 and 8 which give off spinoreticular fibres. There are many more spinoreticular fibres than spinothalamic ones and in this way a much larger onward transmission of stimulation is possible.

The ventrolateral system of the spinal cord consists of a relatively small number of spinothalamic fibres, forming the spinothalamic tract and a relatively large number of spinoreticular fibres forming the majority of the anterolateral tracts. These spinoreticular fibres enter the brain stem reticular formation.

A cordotomy which sections the anterolateral portion of the spinal cord produces analgesia, i.e. freedom from pain, on the opposite side of the body below the level of the section. Cordotomy may be effective because of a reduction in total sensory input to the higher levels rather than section of specific pain fibres.

Before considering what happens to information transmitted to higher levels, some thought should be given to the information arriving at spinal cord level. Mention has been made of pain theories, receptor organs, and the arrangement of the laminae of the spinal cord, but it must be obvious that more information is arriving at the spinal cord level than can be conveniently handled. In other words how do the central nervous mechanisms eliminate the surplus information? Information in the central nervous system presents as nervous activity therefore the question being considered is how does the surplus activity get eliminated? As with so many mechanisms in the central nervous system they do not only occur at spinal cord level but at all stages in the processing of nervous activity in its movement to higher levels. This movement may ultimately produce an awareness of the original stimulus and various discriminating, cognitive, and effector actions result. However this may not be the case and the nervous activity is suppressed completely, or produces effects at the unconscious level only. The processes producing this effect are almost certainly similar to those in the spinal cord.

If it is accepted that for instance, in the cat the dorsal roots on one side of the spinal cord contain about half a million fibres, it is likely that there is a surplus of activity which must be controlled and eliminated. This elimination can occur at one of three sites (or all three).

(A)   At the receptor organ by modification of the sensitivity of the receptor. This is not a common method in the mammalian sensory system though it does occur in a few places such as the muscle spindles. Also at this level there is receptor fatigue, which may be the reason why after injury the first severe agony dies down.

(B)   Post synaptic inhibition can occur at the second order neuron. There are inhibitory interneurons which hyperpolarise the second order neurons acting directly on the soma and dendrites of these cells. Thus, the second order neuron requires a larger stimulation to activate it.

(C)   By means of presynaptic inhibition at the presynaptic terminals of the afferent fibres. While this process has been shown to occur at the axon terminals of most primary afferent fibres it has not been demonstrated in unmyelinated fibres (group IV).

Primary afferent depolarisation occurs through the third method mentioned above. It is suggested that it occurs by means of axo-axonal inhibitory synapses which are on the primary afferent terminal close to their end. Very small levels of depolarisation here can reduce the size of, or block, the action potentials to a marked degree. There is a reduction in the production of transmitter release at the terminals and the amount of activity transmitted is correspondingly reduced.

The simplest pathway postulated consists of two interneurons, the second of these forming the presynaptic terminal and being inhibitory. It is called the D-cell. Eccles (1962) suggested the D-cells were at the base of the dorsal horn, and Wall that the substantia gelatinosal cells act as D-cells and control the membrane potential of cutaneous afferents. It is not clear how many interneurons are involved in these pathways, but, in fact, both pathways do occur.

As far as pain is concerned, primary afferent depolarisation occurs in the cutaneous afferents and there is a negative feedback system.

Primary afferent hyperpolarisation (Disinhibition of primary afferents.) Primary afferent depolarisation can be transient or tonic. If the influence of a tonic primary afferent is removed (Jänig 1967), the removal is seen as a primary afferent hyperpolarisation. During the primary afferent hyperpolarisation transmission is improved. Mendell and Wall (1964) reported the presence of primary afferent hyperpolarisation following stimuli to high threshold cutaneous afferents during selective blocking of the larger fibres in the nerve. They suggested that 'if a pure group IV (C fibre) volley is fired into the cord an entirely positive dorsal root potential is generated'. This was one phenomenon which helped to produce the gate control theory of pain by suggesting that there was a link between disinhibition and the perception of noxious stimuli. However, despite many attempts these results have not been repeated by other workers.

The term 'hyperpolarisation' is a poor one as it suggests something quite out of the normal range. This is not the case. If a neuron has a certain basic excitability, this activity is reduced under primary afferent depolarisation and increased under primary afferent hyperpolarisation. The reduction or increase is within the normal range. At the same time the stimulus necessary to fire the cell is increased in primary afferent depolarisation and decreased with the primary afferent hyperpolarisation. This type of control lends itself to small gradations, and a very delicate control of activity is possible.

There are segmental and descending pathways which can induce and remove tonic presynaptic inhibition and it may be a mechanism of this type which produces long-term suppression and graded modulations of somato-sensory input, including pain, into the central nervous system.

CENTRAL PATHWAYS

The brain stem reticular formation neurons responding to noxious stimuli and A-delta fibre stimulation receive ventrolateral spinal input. It is further believed that the medial (intralaminar) nuclei in the thalamus receive the input from noxious stimuli. Damage to, or destruction of, these nuclei (e.g. centre-median) can relieve completely the response to painful stimuli without affecting movement or discriminative functions. Medial thalamic lesions can be surgically produced to relieve the pain of cancer; however, as these lesions only produce benefit for six weeks to three months if unilateral and for perhaps twice this time with bilateral lesions, the indications for this method of treatment are limited. Radiation of painful stimuli occurs at all levels below and above the thalamus and it would seem that this multi-registration of pain produces the poor results of thalamotomy.

The primary afferent fibres of the dorsal column terminate in the gracile and cuneate nuclei and impulses are relayed on in the medial lemniscus which carries them to the ventral postero-lateral nucleus of the thalamus of the opposite side. A final relay carries this information to the somato-sensory cortex of the post central gyrus. This whole system has been relatively recently evolved and its neurons tend to be long with concentrated restricted terminations. However, its apparent simplicity is deceptive as it is, in fact, an immensely sophisticated system with the possibility of subtle modifications of information at every synapse. Thus, not only is modulation present and possible at the laminae of the spinal cord, it is present and possible at brain stem and higher levels.

The ventral postero-lateral thalamic nucleus also receives fibres ascending in the antero-lateral spinal cord in the spinothalamic tract. This is the classic pain pathway. The ventral postero-lateral thalamic nucleus responds to well localised non-painful stimuli which travel via the spinothalamic tract. Lesions in this region of the thalamus do not relieve pain but produce deficits in discrimination. For instance, loss of touch but without loss of pain can occur.

However, many fibres ascending in the antero-lateral spinal cord synapse in the reticular formation of the brain stem forming a network of ascending and descending pathways with extensive connections. There is some projection to the medial thalamus and these intralaminar nuclei of the thalamus seem to be particularly related to the appreciation of pain. They contain some neurons which respond primarily to noxious somatic input and some which respond to non-somatic impulses. These are arranged to give broad spatio-temporal responses. As mentioned, lesions in this region of the thalamus have been used to relieve intractable pain without motor or sensory deficits.

Thus, there are two broad pathways to the thalamus; there is a phylogenetically older multi-synaptic spinothalamic pathway which connects with the medial reticular formation of the medulla, midbrain, and tectum, and thence to the thalamic nuclei. This probably serves as an alerting system. The other is a phylogenetically recent monosynaptic pathway ascending in the ventral spinothalamic tract which enters the ventral postero-lateral thalamic nuclei. Ventral postero-lateral thalamic neurons project to the somato-sensory cortex. Here then is an arrangement for rapidly transmitting impulses from the periphery to the ventral postero-lateral thalamus and on to the cerebral cortex which may provide a mechanism for localisation of somatic stimuli. Thus there may be one spinothalamic pathway subserving pain and another subserving discrimination. The latter providing the information on which a co-ordinated response is based. There may be other pathways concerned with the appreciation of pain just as there are a number of pathways which control sensory discrimination.

There are emotional and affective correlates of pain. The arousal system (the reticular formation) has connections with the hypothalamus which forms part of the limbic system and which is known to produce autonomic responses and aggressive and defensive behaviour. Parts of the temporal lobe are particularly concerned with this type of behaviour. This with the direct projections to the cerebral cortex through the intralaminar and other thalamic nuclei provides a slight understanding of some of the pathways concerned in the appreciation, discrimination, and motivational aspects of pain.

NEUROTRANSMITTER SUBSTANCES

It has been known for some time that there are neurotransmitter substances in the central nervous system (C.N.S.). This section of neurophysiology is advancing at such a rapid rate that it is impossible to make an entirely definitive statement and the reader requiring up-to-date information will have to consult current literature. Some things are known, or at least are highly likely, and a few of these are mentioned here. For example, the substance glycine appears to be the major inhibitory neurotransmitter in the spinal cord and brain stem and has been demonstrated to mediate post-synaptic inhibition (Curtis *et al.*, 1968), and that gamma-aminobutyric acid (GABA) is most likely to be the major inhibitory neurotransmitter substance in the brain (Krnjević and Schwartz, 1967). In addition, the degeneration of the nigrostriatal dopamine pathway is associated with the pathophysiology of Parkinson's disease, while blocking other dopaminergic receptors has a useful effect in the treatment of schizophrenia (Clement-Cormier *et al.*, 1974). As will be seen later, there is a descending serotonin-ergic pathway of great importance in the relief of pain (Oliveras *et al.*, 1975). Further, it is well known that cholinergic receptors and norepine-phrine alpha and beta receptors have been studied in the C.N.S.

It is obvious that receptor sites have no value unless there is a suitable agonist and possibly antagonist for that site. The following are some important facts in relation to the transmission of pain.

(1) Morphine in a dose of 15 mg has a profound effect on a man weighing about 75 kg, i.e. the weight to dose relationship is $5 \times 10^6 : 1$.

(2) A slight change in the morphine molecule, say by altering the methyl group to an allyl group, produces a profound effect on the potency of the resulting drug, in this case by the change from morphine to nalor-phine (Lethidrone) which is a narcotic with partial antagonist properties, i.e. an agonist/antagonist substance.

(3) A pure antagonist such as naloxone (Narcan) can reverse the effects of morphine in the very small dose of 0·4 mg.

(4) The laevo-rotatory optical isomers of opiates are physiologically active. The dextro-rotatory ones are usually inactive.

(5) Two models for assessing morphine agonist/antagonist activity are available, the guinea-pig ileum and the mouse vas deferens. An electrical current passed through a suitable preparation causes a contraction of muscle. The contraction is prevented by morphine and morphine-like

substances and this is counteracted in turn by naloxone (Kosterlitz
et al., 1973).

(6) These two preparations are sensitive to sodium ions with low concentrations favouring the agonist and higher concentrations enhancing the
antagonist effect.

These facts suggest that there is an endogenous opiate or opiates present
in the C.N.S. with a corresponding receptor site or sites with agonist/
antagonist phases. These receptor sites are related to the relief of pain and
there is a model for assessing the activity of the endogenous opiates. Recent
research has shown the presence of endogenous opiates and receptor sites
(Hughes *et al.*, 1975, Feldburg and Smyth, 1976, Pert and Snyder, 1973).
These discoveries take us a little way along the path elucidating the whole
problem.

Receptor sites. The receptor sites were demonstrated by making use of
the laevo-rotatory isomers, the method involving the stereospecific binding
of tritiated levorphanol (Dromoran; Pert and Snyder, 1973). The receptor
sites have since been mapped and are found near synapses. Some of the
densest concentrations of receptor sites occur in the marginal zone and
substantia gelatinosa of the spinal cord, the descending spinal trigeminal
nucleus, the brain stem raphe nuclei, the hypothalamus and medial thalamus,
the neostriatum, and the limbic lobe.

Enkephalin. Two pentapeptides, methianine-enkephalin (meten-
kephalin) and leucine-enkephalin were discovered to be naturally occurring morphine-like substances (Hughes *et al.*, 1975). These naturally
occurring enkephalins have similar activity to the narcotics with similar side
effects on bowel activity, mood, nausea, and addiction. They can be synthe-
sized and their duration of activity is short. They are antagonized by
naloxone. Immunofluorescent techniques were used to show enkephalinergic axons in the myenteric plexus of the gut, the substantia gelatinosa,
and in many regions of the brain including the globus pallidus, the amyg-
daloid nucleus, and the hypothalamus. Met-enkephalin forms part of the
amino acid chain of pituitary beta lipoprotein. There is a large fragment of
beta lipoprotein called the C-fragment, which like the enkephalins shows
agonist properties. It is known as beta-endorphin.

Substance P. There is strong evidence that this substance isolated from
gut and brain (von Euler and Gaddum, 1931) is a transmitter substance in
small primary afferents responding to painful stimuli. It has been suggested
(Jessel and Iversen, 1977) that the presynaptic gate (Melzack and Wall,
1965) may be the result of enkephalinergic neurones in the substantia

gelatinosa inhibiting noxious transmission presynaptically by blocking or modulating the activity of substance P in primary afferents to relay neurones.

Descending control. Stimulation of the periaqueductal grey matter (P.A.G.) produces analgesia in the rat (Liebeskind *et al.*, 1974), and this effect is also found in man (Richardson and Akil, 1977). The effect is reversed by naloxone. It is believed that neurones in the periventricular and periaqueductal region activate the medullary nucleus raphe magnus and this transmits down the fibres projecting to the spinal cord (Oliveras *et al.*, 1975) which appears to be the final common pathway for the suppression of pain. Destruction of the nucleus raphe magnus will block the analgesic effect of morphine. This pathway is serotoninergic.

It is probable that this descending pathway projects to the dorsal horn and has its inhibitory effect there. It does appear, under some circumstances, that serotonin activity is necessary for descending pain suppression and conversely that reduction in serotonin activity increases appreciation of pain.

Beta-endorphin. The role of beta-endorphin is not known. It has a much longer action than that of the transmitter enkephalin substances. It is possible that enkephalinergic mechanisms may release long-acting endorphins. It is probable that the endorphins do not only have a role in pain mechanisms but act as, or release, hormones affecting other systems.

Peripheral nerve stimulation. It may be that such practical techniques as transcutaneous stimulation as well as brain stimulation are mediated by an enkephalinergic mechanism. Acupuncture also is known to produce pain relief which is abolished by naloxone (Sjolund *et al.*, 1977 and Pomeranz, 1977).

REFERENCES

BEECHER H.K. (1946) Pain in men wounded in battle. *Ann. Surg.* **123**, 96.

BOWSHER D. (1957) Termination of the central pain pathway in man: The conscious appreciation of pain. *Brain*, **80**, 606.

BOWSHER D. (1962) The topographical projection of fibres from the anterolateral quadrant of the spinal cord to the subdiencephalic brain stem in man. *Psychiat. et Neurol.* (Basel), **143**, 75.

CHARPENTIER J. (1967) 'Pain'. Chapter in *Analysis and Measurement of Pain in Animals*, p. 171. Academic Press, New York.

CLEMENT-CORMIER Y.C., KEBABIAN J.W., PETZOLD G.L. & GREENGARD P. (1974) Dopamine-sensitive adenylate cyclase in mammalian brain; a possible site of action of antipsychotic drugs. *Proc. Nat. Acad. Sci. U.S.A.* **71**, 133.

CURTIS D.R., DUGGAN A.W. & JOHNSTON G.A.R. (1968) The hyperpolarisation of spinal motorneurons by glycine and related amino acids. *Exp. Brain res.* **5**, 235.

EULER V.S. VON & GADDUM J.H. (1931) An unidentified depressor substance in certain tissue extracts. *J. Physiol.* (Lond.), **72**, 74.

FELDBERG W. & SMYTH D.G. (1976) The C-fragment of lipotropin—a potent analgesic. *J. Physiol.* (Lond.), **260**, 30P.

HUGHES J., SMITH T.W., KOSTERLITZ H.W., FOTHERGILL L.A., MORGAN B.A. & MORRIS H.R. (1975) Identification of two related pentapeptides from the brain with potent opiate agonist activity. *Nature* (Lond.), **258**, 577.

JESSELL T.M. & IVERSEN L.L. (1977) Opiate analgesics inhibit substance P release from rat trigeminal nucleus. *Nature* (Lond.), **268**, 549.

KATZ B. (1952) *Different Forms of Signalling Employed by the Central Nervous System.* H.K. Lewis, London.

KEELE C.A. (1962) Sensation aroused by chemical stimulation of the skin. In *The Assessment of Pain in Man and Animals*, p. 28. Eds. C.A. Keele and R. Smith. Livingstone, Edinburgh.

KELLAREN J.H. (1939) On the distribution of pain arising from deep somatic structures with charts of segmental pain areas. *Clin. Sci.* **4**, 35.

KOSTERLITZ H.W., WATERFIELD A.A. & BERTHOOD V. (1973) Assessments of the agonist and antagonist properties of narcotic analgesic drugs by their actions on the morphine receptor in the guinea-pig ileum. In *Advances in Biochemical Psychopharmacology*: Vol. 8, *Narcotic Antagonists*, p. 319. Eds. M.C. Braude, L.S. Harris, E.L. May, T.P. Smith & J.E. Villareal. Raven Press, New York.

KRNJEVIĆ K. & SCHWARTZ S. (1967) The action of alpha aminobutyric acid on cortical neurons. *Exp. Brain Res.* **3**, 320.

LIEBESKIND J.C., MAYER D.J. & AKIL N. (1974) In *Advances in Neurology*: Vol. 4, p. 261.

LIM R.K.S. (1967) Pain mechanisms. *Anaesthesiology*, **28**, 106.

MELZACK R. & WALL P.D. (1965) Pain mechanisms; a new theory. *Science*, **150**, 971.

OLIVERAS J.L., REDJEMI F., GUILBAUD C. & BESSON J.M. (1975) Analgesia induced by electrical stimulation of the inferior centralis nucleus of the raphe in the cat. *Pain*, **1**, 139.

PERT C.B. & SNYDER S.H. (1973) Opiate receptor; demonstration in nervous tissue. *Science*, **179**, 1011.

POMERANZ B. (1977) Brain's opiates at work in acupuncture? *New Scientist*, **73**, 12.

REXED B. (1954) The cytoarchitectonic organisation of the spinal cord in the cat. *J. Comp. Neurol.* **23**, 259.

RICHARDSON D.E. & AKIL H. (1977) Pain reduction by electrical brain stimulation in man, part I: acute administration in periaqueductal and periventricular sites. *J. Neurosurg.* **47**, 178; part II: chronic self administration in the periventricular grey matter, ibid. 184.

SJOLUND B., TERENIUS L. & ERIKSSON M. (1977) Increased cerebrospinal fluid levels of endorphins after electro-acupuncture. *Acta. Physiol. Scand.* **100**, 382.

WEDDELL G., PALLIE W. & PALMER E. (1954) The morphology of peripheral nerve termination in the skin. *Quart. J. Micr. Sci.* **95**, 483.

FURTHER READING

BONICA J.J. (1974) *Advances in Neurology, Vol. 4.* Ed. J.J. Bonica. Raven Press, New York.

BRODAL A. (ed.) (1972) *Neurological Anatomy in Relation to Clinical Medicine*, 2nd edn. Saunders, Philadelphia.

FREDERICKSON R.C.A. (1977) Enkephalin pentapeptides—a review of current evidence for a physiologic role in vertebrate neurotransmission. *Life Sci.* **21**, 23.

NOORDENBOS W. (ed.) (1959) *Pain.* Elsevier, Amsterdam.

RUCH T.C., PATTON H.D., WOODBURY J.W. & TOWE A.L. (1961) *Neurophysiology*, 2nd edn. Saunders, Philadelphia.

Chapter 4
Pain in the Head

PAIN IN THE HEAD

This particular chapter is not meant to cover all the possible diseases that can cause pain in the head but it does cover the major ones. These can be divided into a relatively small number of conditions, which are:

(1) Primary or secondary malignancy.
(2) Migraine in its various forms.
(3) Headache and atypical facial pain.
(4) Trigeminal Neuralgia.
(5) A miscellaneous group which includes pain from the teeth, sinuses, cervical vertebrae, and some myofascial syndromes.

PRIMARY AND SECONDARY MALIGNANCY

It is rare for the first diagnosis to be made in the Centre for Pain Relief. These patients are sent already diagnosed, for advice on treatment and for this to be carried out. Nevertheless, it is absolutely imperative that a full examination of the patient, including the nervous system be performed. It is not sufficient to accept the findings of other clinicians without verification, if only because some of the physical signs in advanced cases can change over a very short period. Also it is important to note the state of the patient on being first presented so that a proper record of any neurological, muscular, or other deficits can be obtained. It is necessary to demonstrate to the patient and their relatives that these deficits exist and to record that this has been done on the case record sheets. It is not unknown for a patient to blame the pain centre physician for producing a deficit which was present before the treatment began. It is also important, of course, to be quite frank with the patient and their relatives as to the possible complications that may arise from the suggested treatment. If there is the possibility of a further or increased neurological deficit, or a risk, this must be very carefully and explicitly spelled out. In some countries patients accept that the physician is doing his best and will accept an unexpected complication philosophically. In others, there is the ever-present danger of litigation and heavy damages. In these countries the physician will protect himself not only by performing the most meticulous of examinations and treatments but also by careful explanation as suggested above. It is not unknown for patients or relatives to be asked to sign a statement that they understand the hazards involved and that they accept them.

If the tumour is intracranial, then sooner or later the increase in size will produce severe headache. While regression of the tumour may occur following treatment by radiotherapy or chemotherapy this takes time and a quicker method of relieving headache is necessary. A method which usually produces rapid relief is to give Dexamethazone. A loading dose of 10 mg is given with 4 mg six-hourly afterwards. Relief of the headache should occur within forty-eight hours. When intracranial tension is increased there is little likelihood of a response with doses lower than those suggested.

Primary malignancy of the head and neck is not usually a painful condition until the inoperable stage is reached with direct invasion, or spread to the near-by tissues and glands. In cases where the primary condition has been treated by surgery or radiotherapy and then recurred, a similar situation arises. While there is a prospect that eradication of the tumour is possible then treatment is directed to this end and further surgery, radiotherapy, chemotherapy, or regional perfusion carried out. Later when these measures have failed the most important feature will be to make the patient as comfortable as possible. Relief of pain may well be the most important of these, but not necessarily so. For instance, in patients who have had a laryngectomy for a carcinoma of the pharynx, the most important problem may be to keep a clear airway. However, in most cases the relief of pain will be the most useful single thing that can be done for the patient.

The difficulty in relieving pain in this region is due to the very rich and varied innervation of the tissues. Many sensory nerves are involved, such as the upper cervical spinal nerves, the trigeminal, glossopharyngeal, and vagus. Thus unless the distribution of the pain is confined to the distribution of one of these, no single nerve block will suffice to ablate painful sensation. Indeed as there appear to be anastomoses between various small branches of these nerves, occurring in the deeper structures of the face and neck, it may be impossible to block off all the nerves involved. Under these circumstances peripheral treatment of nerves is useless and the only active hope is to destroy nerve pathways more centrally, and this means at the cervico-medullary junction of the spinal cord, the medulla, or the thalamus. Alternatively the appreciation of pain can be altered by means of such procedures as leucotomy.

Sometimes it is possible to produce a marked relief of pain, even if it is not possible to produce a complete one, when the pain is in the field of two groups of sensory nerves. For instance, if the lower jaw is affected, pain will be travelling over both the trigeminal and the cervical nerves. A block of both of these will give satisfactory analgesia or anaesthesia over the whole of this area provided the deeper structures are not affected.

Another method which can be considered for cancer pain around the face is the instillation of hypertonic saline into the basal cistern. The instillation of the saline has to be performed under general anaesthesia as the side-effects are considerable and unpleasant. This method is not used at the Liverpool Centre.

If the pain is confined to the distribution of the cervical nerves then paravertebral blocks using absolute alcohol or 6 per cent phenol solutions may be effective. The use of an image intensifier X-ray machine will make this type of injection much easier to perform. An alternative method is to use intrathecal phenol in glycerine solution in 1 in 15 strength. In this case it may be necessary to anaesthetise the patient if it is too painful for them to lie on the affected side. The method of carrying out this technique is described in Chapter 7.

Finally, but by no means least, it should not be forgotten that there are neurosurgical techniques which can be applied for surgical section of the relevant nerves. For instance, if a posterior fossa approach is used not only can the trigeminal and other cranial sensory nerves be sectioned but by extending the operation to the upper cervical spines, these nerves can be sectioned producing anaesthesia of the superficial tissues of the neck and the 'cape' area, as well. This is a considerable and extensive operation and only patients in very reasonable condition would be able to survive for any length of time afterwards.

There are two groups of tumours which may give difficulty in diagnosis, the naso-pharyngeal carcinomas and tumours which arise around the neck of the first rib.

The naso-pharyngeal tumour produces pain by invasion of tissues in the deep structures. It is continuous without any remissions and can be any intensity up to the most severe boring pain. The pain is usually confined to the distribution of one trigeminal division but this is not invariable and in any case the pain will usually spread to more than one division at later stages. There may be a nasal obstruction or discharge which is often blood-stained. Gradually cranial nerves become involved producing the relevant palsy.

The presence of a malignancy in this particular position can be suspected but not diagnosed for certainty in the early stages. Radiographs of the skull especially the basal view may show the tumour if the X-rays are compared at monthly intervals. It is to be hoped that the introduction of computerised tomography will help in the diagnosis. When the position of the tumour is known it may be possible to biopsy it through one of the sinuses.

Treatment of this condition is by combined methods but the prognosis is not good. As far as the treatment of pain in these patients is concerned it may be possible to block it if the pain pathway is through one or two of the cranial nerves or on occasion the upper cervical nerves in addition. In most cases initial success may be obtained by these simple measures but the continued spread of active tumour widens the involvement and either intracranial and cervical nerve root sections are used or a thalamotomy is required. These procedures being used after the usual surgery, radiotherapy, and cytotoxic drugs have failed.

Tumours arising near the neck of the first rib produce diffuse pain and the problem here is to think of the possibility in the early stages when pain is not a feature but stimulation of the sympathetic nerves by involvement of the stellate ganglion may be a feature. The patient may present with excessive sweating of the hemi-face and arm. At a later stage when destruction produces depression of activity a Horner's syndrome will develop and at this stage will direct attention to the neck of the first rib. Treatment is as for a tumour at the upper pole of the lung and pain relief follows standard methods for that region.

In most cases the diagnosis is made on the history. Pain from malignancy in the head and neck has the same characteristics that pain from malignancy has in other parts of the body. It is continuous and over a period of a month or so becomes steadily worse. Unlike most non-malignant pains it responds to the analgesic drugs but when it is severe never entirely disappears. It is of an aching, deep-seated, boring nature which wakes the patient up at night after a few hours sleep. More analgesic tablets are taken and after an interval the patient gets off to sleep for a few more hours. This is a typical story and if there is any doubt about the diagnosis it can often be made on this history.

In similar fashion the diagnosis of migraine, trigeminal neuralgia, cluster headaches, tension headaches, and many others which are to be discussed shortly can in most cases be made on the history. Careful and painstaking history is an essential part of any investigation into a patient's pain. It is as well to bear in mind that a neurotic patient or one who has for many years been suffering from migraine, can develop other conditions and new pains from pathological processes which are completely or partially hidden by the old complaints. That is why the development of a new and constant pain, or an alteration in an old one, has to be treated with great respect.

MIGRAINE

The classical concept of migraine is of a periodic disturbance of function of the cerebral blood vessels associated with unilateral headache, nausea, and vomiting. 60 to 70 per cent of those affected are females and 5 to 10 per cent of the population have the condition at one time or another during their life. The peak incidence is reached in the child-bearing years of women and then falls as age increases.

In migraine patients more than 50 per cent have migraine attacks more often than once a month. About one-quarter of patients suffering from migraine have their first attack before the age of ten years, and it is uncommon for the condition to present after 45. If grandparents are included 55 per cent of patients have a positive family history (Selby & Lance 1960). Bickerstaff concluded that hereditary influences are the most important in the aetiology of migraine, and though not proven genetically was probably dominant, the transmitted factor being an abnormal response of some blood vessels to stimuli.

There does not appear to be a primary relationship between migraine and epilepsy or allergy, though there is no doubt that one of these conditions can trigger off another. For instance, the vasoconstrictive stage of migraine may trigger off an epileptiform attack.

FEATURES OF MIGRAINE

Headache

This is the most important single feature of the condition, and is the characteristic symptom. The classification of the various types of migraine will be given later and, as will be seen, although headache is usually a feature of an attack from the beginning this is not necessarily so. It may be the only manifestation of an attack or may follow other symptoms or signs.

In two-thirds of patients migraine headache is unilateral and is bilateral in the other third. It may vary the side from one attack to another but in about one-fifth of patients is always on the same side (Selby & Lance). It usually starts as a boring pain on one side of the head, in a small localised area. This is often in the temple and spreads until the whole side of the head is involved. The pain may extend over the whole of the head and down to the face as well. It sometimes radiates to the neck and shoulders, and conversely in some patients may start in the upper neck and the adjacent occipital region and radiate forward. The pain may remain limited in which case it is confined to the territory of one of the arteries, such as the temporal or occipital. The headache is present on the side opposite to that of the sensory phenomenon.

The dull headache gradually increases in intensity, becomes more severe, and acquires a throbbing character. This throbbing may be lost as the attack continues, but while present is intensified by all forms of exertion and by stooping.

The attack may start at any time of the day but more often the patient wakes up with the headache present. In about two-thirds of patients the headache lasts for less than one day but in others it may persist for days. Persisting headaches in patients with migraine who previously have not suffered from this variety must be thoroughly investigated to exclude newly developed or developing disease. It can be that other types of headache, such as tension headaches, are alternating with the patient's migraine attacks and these can be distinguished. Occasionally a patient develops 'status migrainosus' where headache is present every day for up to a week, the patient waking with migraine each day.

Other disturbances. Nausea is usually present during the headache stage to the extent of about 90 per cent of patients. Vomiting does not necessarily occur but the majority do vomit and in the milder forms of migraine, vomiting seems to relieve the headache.

In one-fifth of patients one or more loose stools are passed and this does not depend on the severity of the headache, being just as likely to occur in mild as in severe cases.

Vasomotor changes are often obvious. The face is pale and the extremities cold. There is often an increased pulsation and tenderness of the superficial temporal arteries and some patients notice that pressure over the affected vessel reduces the intensity of the headache. Congestion of the face, conjunctiva, and nasal mucosa occurs but more commonly the face is pale and sweating in an attack.

About three-quarters of patients with migraine suffer from photophobia during an attack and prefer a darkened room. Noise also is usually disliked and these symptoms may be a manifestation of hyperactivity of the special senses.

After an attack there is often a polyuria. About 65 per cent of patients complain of sensitivity of the scalp both during and after the attack. In many migrainous patients there is a persistently, mildly abnormal electro-encephalogram.

CLASSIFICATION OF MIGRAINE

A most useful classification of this condition was made by the Ad Hoc Committee of Classification of Headache (1962). They divided vascular headaches of migrainous type into the five main groups of Classic, Common, Cluster, Hemiplegic, and Lower half varieties of migraine.

The main consideration was the separation of the first two types. Classic migraine includes those patients with typical prodromata, consisting of sensory, motor, or visual disturbances. These patients tend to have unilateral headache. The second group is the common migraine type and this has vascular headache without the striking prodromata of the classical group, and these headaches are less often unilateral. It must be stated here that this is not a strict demarcation as there is a certain variation between these groups and a patient who normally has the common type may well occasionally have a classical attack, and vice versa. The features of the various types are now discussed.

Classical

Sensory symptoms are not consistent but are characteristic, visual disturbances being the commonest. These are symptoms of cortical origin and as far as vision is concerned have an homonymous distribution which involves corresponding halves of both visual fields. A gradually developing hemianopia occurs usually preceded by visual hallucinations. These scotomatas are common, occurring in about one-third of migraine sufferers. About 10 per cent of patients experience fortification spectra, so called because the zig-zag shape of the hallucination appears like the walls of a fortified town looked at from above. Another name for this phenomena is teichopsia. One-quarter of patients have photopsia, which is seeing unformed flashes of light either white or coloured.

Hemianopia can begin in the periphery and progress inwards or in the central region and move outwards. The onset may begin with a central bright spot which then expands to the periphery. The edge of the expanding area showing photopsia and teichopsia. Once the spreading edge has passed, an area of blindness is left behind, so that when the spread has been completed over the whole of the half-visual field the patient is left with an homonymous hemianopia. This phenomenon takes about twenty minutes or less for completion, and the blindness then fades away gradually in the corresponding order of its development in a further ten minutes or so.

The above is the usual picture but there are many types of visual disturbance which can occur, such as telescopic vision which is produced when the peripheral fields are affected in their entirety. There may be homonymous quadrantic anopia, and very occasionally, there is a bilateral hemianopia which produces temporary complete blindness.

All these symptoms originate in the occipital lobe and they are by far the most common. Other symptoms arise from other areas of the cortex or brain stem and the next most common to the visual ones are paraesthesiae and numbness of such parts of the person as the periphery of the limbs and the circumoral region. Paraesthesiae round the mouth and tongue and both hands can arise either from the cortex or the long tracts in the brain stem, and the upper limb is affected most, the lower limb rarely so. The usual picture is that tingling begins in the fingers, gradually spreads up the limb, the process taking about thirty minutes. The lips, face, and tongue are affected later either unilaterally or bilaterally. The face can be affected without the limbs and these paraesthesiae may occur after the onset of the visual hallucinations or may precede them.

In about 4 per cent of patients strictly unilateral paraesthesiae are associated with hemiparesis or dysphasia and are of cortical origin. In a similar fashion hallucinations of taste and hearing occur but are very rare.

Common

Common or non-classical migraine is not associated with sharply defined transient visual, and other sensory or motor prodromata or both. This is the usual type of migraine that presents. As mentioned previously there is no sharply defined border between these two types and they can shade one into the other and vary from one type to the other at different times in the course of the disease. It is not unusual for the condition to alter gradually throughout life, presenting as a different type at different decades. This is not unexpected as the process producing the symptoms and signs of the various types of migraine is the same but merely has its major effect in a different part of the brain stem or cortex.

Warning. Often a patient suffering from migraine will have a warning that an attack is imminent. There may be an unusual sense of well being and vigour, the patient may feel tense or excitable. There may be a feeling of weakness, fatigue, or unreality. The patient may have marked pallor or there can be an increased sensitivity to light or noise. Occasionally the preliminary symptom is an unusual degree of hunger. If symptoms or signs of this type develop they can be made use of in the treatment of the condition by immediately initiating active medication. In this way the attack can be aborted or at least minimised.

Precipitating factors are well known and many patients know that if they carry out certain types of activity an attack will almost certainly follow. Anxiety, excitement, or depression may be such causes in susceptible people. A change of routine such as over-exertion can do it, as can loud persistent noises, or bright lights. Thus a visit to the cinema is always followed by an attack in some patients—often the young ones. In similar fashion watching television may do the same thing. Alterations of diet such as when dieting may precipitate an attack. The weather is said to affect some people and many women have more frequent attacks during their periods.

Certain foods can precipitate migraine attacks and people susceptible to this form of sensitivity know that they have to avoid certain kinds of food. Chocolate, milk, or cheese are well known in this respect but it can be fried foods or certain kinds of fruit.

It is commonly believed that migraine patients are more anxious, tense, and intelligent than the average. It is probably true to say that they are more anxious and tense but there is no evidence that they are more intelligent. Nor is it true that migraine is brought on by stressful conditions, though there is no doubt that this does occur in a small number. More frequently it occurs in the period of relaxation after stress has been present, and for this reason may occur at the weekends.

There is some relationship of migraine with hormonal changes, as evidenced by the fact already mentioned that in a large proportion of women there is a relation between the menses and the development of the headache. Again a large percentage of women who suffer with migraine get relief during pregnancy, while others may develop the condition for the first time. Somerville studied the plasma levels of oestradiol and progesterone and his work suggested that it is a withdrawal of oestrogen which is the precipitating cause when migraine is linked to the menstrual cycle or to pregnancy. Oral contraceptives exacerbate migraine but not enough is known of the underlying mechanisms, as yet, for alteration of hormonal balance to be of much use.

As with cluster headache, alcohol and other vasodilators can precipitate an attack of the condition and the standard treatment involves the use of vasoconstrictive drugs.

Origin of the migraine headache is believed to be in the vascular system and in particular the extracranial arteries. In those patients who develop visual hallucinations there is little pulsation in the superficial temporal artery in the earlier stage, while there is obvious pulsation during the stage of the headache. As the headache develops in intensity the pulsation tends to increase. Thus it appears that the arteries of the scalp dilate and cause the headache although the patient's face is usually pale reflecting a vaso-constriction of the smaller vessels.

The control of the extracranial blood vessels is faulty in migraine and there may be a corresponding fault in the intracranial ones. As previously mentioned neurological symptoms occur in many patients (65 per cent) about half of these having a visual disturbance. It appears that there is a phase of cerebral vasoconstriction followed by a vasodilatation but that the large cerebral vessels do not take part in this. Evidence of this has accumulated from cerebral angiography, cerebral blood flow investigations, electroencephalography, and observation of the retinal vessels. There does not seem to be any abnormality in the nervous control over the intra- and extra-cranial vessels, and for instance, operation on the stellate ganglion or cervical sympathectomy is not effective in relieving the condition. Similarly more complicated procedures such as section of the greater super-ficial petrosal nerve have little value.

There is no doubt that the focal symptoms of migraine are preceded by a vasoconstriction and the spread and progress of these is due to a wave of inhibition which slowly spreads over the cerebral cortex and which prevents normal activity. For instance, changes in the electroencephalogram can be recorded on the opposite occipital cortex during the stage of visual hallucina-tions and while it must be acknowledged that the focal symptoms and electro-encephalographic changes are produced by the wave of inhibition, it is not known for certain whether this is initiated by the vasoconstriction or some other mechanism is involved. Sometimes the vasoconstriction persists and partial or complete blindness has resulted from thrombosis of a branch of the central retinal artery or of the central artery itself. Similarly permanent defects have resulted from thrombosis of vessels in the cerebral cortex or brain stem.

Although the theory given above is commonly accepted for migraine headache, it is not the only possibility. Recently Blau (1978) suggested that 'the headache is due to stimulation of nociceptive nerve endings in the walls of meningeal vessels' and further postulated that 'the aura arises from calibre changes in meningeal vessels that penetrate the outer cortex, resulting in localised inhibition or excitation'. Further work is required before this can be accepted.

Serotonin is a naturally occurring vasoconstrictor which seems to have a key role in the development of migraine. The principal breakdown product of serotonin is 5-hydroxyindoleacetic acid (5-HIAA) and this substance is excreted in excessive amounts in some patients during a migraine headache. At the onset of a migraine attack there is a slight rise in the plasma level of serotonin but the level falls with the onset of the headache (Anthony 1968). This phenomenon is quite specific for migraine and does not occur in cluster headaches or headache from other causes. If serotonin levels are lowered artificially by reserpine an attack of migraine can be precipitated in susceptible people. The same patients can benefit by an injection of serotonin.

Other humeral agents. Apart from serotonin there is no substance with a certain relationship to the migraine attack. Acetylcholine, histamine, and noradrenaline do not appear to be the cause of migraine attacks, or in fact, to have any relation to them. Bradykinin does not reproduce the migraine headache and prostaglandins as yet have not been proved to have any definite role. It may well be that there is no single precipitating factor and that a migraine attack is initiated by a number of interacting humoral factors.

Unilaterality, whatever the mechanism of migraine production there is no knowledge at the present time as to why the migraine headache is usually unilateral.

Treatment

Treatment is designed to prevent, abort, or diminish the attack. Thus, in those patients who have a known idiosyncrasy to a particular food it must be avoided; similarly, if the attack is brought on by bright lights or a visit to the cinema these situations must also be avoided. Any known allergy is treated and any psychological or personal problems which, by causing stress, might initiate or increase the tendency to attacks, are dealt with. Migraine in susceptible patients is common at the menses and may be more severe in those patients taking the contraceptive pill and it may be worthwhile considering a trial of hormonal therapy in severe cases. However, the results from this type of therapy are not very certain. A common feature in migraine and pregnancy is that water retention occurs before both, and it is worth trying a reduction in salt intake combined with a diuretic during the premenstrual period.

Drug therapy is the standard method and there is a large pharmacopoeia to choose from but the drugs preferred are the ergot derivatives or the serotonin antagonists, the rationale being that these drugs constrict the extracranial arteries. One of the problems in using the ergot derivatives is that they themselves can produce nausea and vomiting but as ergotamine tartrate relieves about half the cases of their headache completely and in half of the remainder cuts the period of the attack down to a shorter period these disadvantages are acceptable. An antiemetic such as prochlorperazine (Stemetil) 5–25 mg can be given beforehand in those patients known to be nauseated or who vomit, or during the severe phase if the attack is not aborted. Diazepam (Valium) 10 mg intravenous or intramuscularly is a useful sedative with antiemetic properties.

Ergot. The usual treatment advocated for the average migraine sufferer is that they should take 1–3 mg of ergotamine tartrate orally at the first indication of an impending attack. The same drug can be given by intramuscular injection in dose of 0·25–0·5 mg. If necessary these can be repeated in half an hour but there is no point in repeating further if there is no effective result. When a very rapid action is required there are sublingual tablets which are said to be absorbed more quickly, or an aerosol form such as the medihaler-ergotamine can be used. The instructions in the latter method must be carefully carried out so that the measured dose is inhaled deep into the lungs. Each dose is 0·36 mg and can be repeated twice if necessary at five-minute intervals, but the maximum is six in any twenty-four hours and the makers recommend no more than fifteen in any week.

One of the problems with ergotamine therapy is that if daily medication is used the patient may develop a rebound headache when the tablets are omitted. If it becomes necessary to take the patient off these tablets they need to be weaned off them gradually.

There are a number of compound tablets combining ergotamine tartrate with other drugs which can be used, some of these contain an antiemetic, e.g. Migril (containing Cyclizine). There are also suppositories which are valuable in those patients who are particularly nauseated during the attack.

Serotonin antagonists can be divided into two types, one of these, e.g. methysergide (Deseril) 2–6 mg per day, will suppress migraine in about 20 per cent of patients and relieve it in about another 40 per cent. However, it has side-effects the most important of which are connected with peripheral vasoconstriction as it produces its effect by potentiating constrictor responses by noradrenaline and by serotonin. It is, at times, only a weak serotonin antagonist and seems to have a similar action to serotonin as far as vasoconstriction of the scalp vessels is concerned.

Methysergide is contra-indicated in peripheral vascular disease, hypertension, coronary disease, and peptic ulcer (as acid secretion is increased). However, if the patient with one of these contra-indicated diseases has migraine of severe degree which does not respond to other drugs, and a trial of methysergide proves of great value, then the patient may have to continue on it using an expectant regime.

In the doses suggested there is very little danger of the main complication which can occur with methysergide which is fibrosis, which occurs retroperitoneally, in the pleura or on the heart valves. If this fibrotic condition occurs it usually resolves when the drug is withdrawn and it is reasonable to stop this medication for one month in every six. When on medication these patients should be seen regularly.

The second type of serotonin antagonist has an antihistamine and antiserotonin effect and does not potentiate the vasoconstrictor effect of serotonin. Such a drug is cyproheptadine (Periactin) 2–4 mg q.d.s. and drowsiness is the commonest complication. The drug is normally used to stimulate appetite and produce weight gain and as far as migraine is concerned these are unwanted effects.

Beta-blockers. These are drugs which block the beta adrenergic receptors and thus reduce vasodilator responses. A commonly used drug of this type is propanalol (Inderal) 10 mg t.d.s. or q.d.s. The theory behind the use of this drug is that the dilatation of the peripheral arteries is believed to be caused by the adrenaline being taken up by beta-receptors in the arterial walls, and therefore beta-blockade should prevent this happening. There are conflicting reports as to how effective this method is, but it is worth a trial after other more commonly useful drugs have been tried and failed. This drug is useful occasionally in other forms of facial pain.

Central reflex blockers. There are a number of drugs which depress both vasomotor and vasoconstrictor reflexes of peripheral arteries. They are neither alpha- nor beta-blockers nor ganglion blockers. Such a drug is Clonidine (Catapres) 0·1 mg t.d.s. It can also be used if standard methods fail.

Monomine oxidase inhibitors. Sicuteri (1974) has shown that there is an alteration in monoamine oxidase activity in migraine sufferers and this represents indirect evidence of monoamine involvement. Theoretically, a drug such as phenelzine (Nardil) should benefit the patient by allowing serotonin and amines such as noradrenaline to accumulate. This is to some extent how methysergide has its effect but the problems of controlling the patient's diet while on phenelzine to keep it free of amines make this a hazardous drug to use.

Miscellaneous

There are a number of drugs which are sometimes used in the treatment of migraine, unfortunately they are not very, or often, effective. The drug carbamazepine (Tegretol), usually used to control trigeminal neuralgia, for which it is a specific, is said to be effective in migraine. This is not our experience and there is an incidence of side-effects.

Methdilazine (Dilosyn) 8 mg b.d., has antihistaminic and antibradykinin activity combined with weak antiserotonin effects. It is not a very effective drug, but there is some rationale involved in trying it in patients who do not respond to any other regime.

Many other drugs have been used in the treatment of resistant forms of migraine. They are usually ineffective having benefit at the same level as placebo drugs, and there does not seem to be any reason why they should be mentioned here.

Practical treatment will depend on the type of migraine the patient suffers from. The occasional migraine attack is dealt with in the manner already mentioned, by immediate medication when the first prodromal sensations occur. If the patient is one of those who can forecast when the attack is due then medication commences at the relevant time. For those patients whose attacks are frequent, unexpected, and severe a trial of continuous (interval) treatment should be carried out. If ergot is used in this way regularly the danger of its vasoconstrictor effects must be kept in mind, a dose of ergotamine tartrate up to 1 mg daily should not produce untoward effects in the normal patient. A general sedative drug such as phenobarbitone can also be given but should be abandoned if its addition makes no improvement.

The aim of the treatment is to prevent all attacks if possible, and in those cases where this cannot be done then to decrease the length, severity, and number of the attacks. If the ergotamine drugs are ineffective then one or other of those listed above is used. The author would suggest that the most useful drug after ergot is methysergide, and it is important to realise that the patient can still use ergot in the acute stage while on methysergide daily treatment.

MISCELLANEOUS MIGRAINE

CLUSTER HEADACHE

This condition is also known as periodic migrainous neuralgia. It is a severe, often an exceedingly severe, unilateral head or face pain which lasts for minutes or hours. Commonly lacrimation of the ipsilateral eye occurs once or more per day for a period of weeks or even months. The name cluster headache refers to the pain tending to present in bouts, the intervening period being completely free of pain.

There are many different names given to this condition reflecting the problem of its aetiology, such as vidian neuralgia, histamine cephalgia, greater superficial petrosal neuralgia, and many others.

Clinical features

The clinical features are quite different to those of either classical or common migraine. First, the sex incidence is different, in that most series give a preponderance of males to females of about four to one. In most patients suffering from this condition the illness begins in the second and third decades.

Pain

The site of pain almost always affects the same side of the head in each bout, but in a few patients the pain can vary from side to side in different bouts. About 60 per cent of patients feel the pain deeply in the tissues in and around the eye. Radiation of the pain usually occurs to the surrounding areas of the face and may involve the whole side of the head. Commonly it is not confined to the circum-orbital region but radiates to the supra-orbital area, temple, maxilla, upper gums, and on occasion the lower jaw, gums, and chin. The ear and neck can also be involved. The nostril on the affected side aches and burns, and this type of sensation is sometimes described in the palate.

The pain is described as severe with a most unpleasant quality to it tearing or boring and there is often some element of heat mentioned, such as burning. The pain is constant, but is sometimes throbbing in type. Usually between each attack the pain clears up but this is by no means always the case and some patients describe a dull pain persisting somewhere in the distribution of the acute pain, in between the attacks. Occasionally a dull ache precedes the attack for hours or days, and sometimes there are a few sudden jabs of pain in the face or head during a bout.

The bout commonly lasts from 4 to 8 weeks and the number of daily attacks is from one to three, they often appear at the same time of each day the pain lasting from a few minutes to a few hours. They can end quite suddenly or may slowly fade away. Although these headaches are called 'cluster headaches' because they cluster together in bouts, some patients, although undoubtedly suffering from them, do not have them in regular daily episodes. These are called 'non-cluster' headaches and about one-fifth of patients fall into this category.

Associated features are numerous. Ipsilateral lacrimation is the most common symptom and is occasionally bilateral. Injection of the conjunctiva on the affected side usually occurs and a Horner's syndrome (drooping of the ipsilateral eyelid and miosis) is present in about one-third of attacks and sometimes persists. Excessive bilateral sweating can occur and may be present in a patient with a Horner's syndrome. Apart from lacrimation which will produce a running nose, a blocked and secreting nostril does occur as a separate feature.

Hyperalgesia of the face and scalp occur and in severe cases the patient cannot touch these parts. About half the patients feel nauseated and may vomit but this type of symptom is less common than in migraine. Similarly, focal neurological symptoms or signs are unusual though occasionally they do occur. Facial flushing is present more commonly than pallor as contrasted to migraine, and the veins may dilate. The superficial temporal artery on the affected side may become more prominent, tender, and pulsatile.

Alcohol. During the period of a bout many patients suffering from this condition find that an attack of pain can be precipitated by an alcoholic drink. In most cases pain is initiated only if the patient is having a period of activity in the cluster headache disease, but sometimes this can occur in between attacks. Some vasodilator substances can precipitate an attack, such as histamine or nitroglycerine as can such things as stressful conditions, changes in the weather, hay fever, and others.

Origin. The origin of cluster headaches is not certain but there are a number of common features between this condition and migraine. The principal one is that there is a dilatation of the extracranial arteries which is almost always unilateral in cluster headaches and may be bilateral in migraine. As in migraine some patients find relief from their pain by pressing on the superficial temporal artery.

The internal carotid artery is also involved in most of these patients as shown by the retro-orbital pain and paralysis of the ocular sympathetic. It is believed that this is due to compression of the sympathetic plexus in the carotid canal by the wall of the internal carotid artery which is distended. Facial sweating may or may not be present with or without a Horner's syndrome, and this helps to localise the site of the sympathetic lesion as facial sweating occurs through the sympathetic pathway along extracranial vessels.

In migraine it has been shown that serotonin plasma levels fall during an attack. There is no significant alteration in this substance in cluster headaches. However, the blood level of histamine increases during cluster headache (Anthony & Lance, 1971). Antihistamine drugs have not been of value in the treatment of cluster headaches but histamine is believed to play a role in the genesis of this condition. There thus appears to be a definite distinction between migraine and cluster headache on biochemical grounds.

Treatment. The treatment of cluster headaches is not straightforward. Originally when it was thought that histamine was the complete answer to its development the system known as histamine desensitisation was advocated. This is now in disrepute as rarely is the condition improved by this technique. As the disease has normal remissions, it is very difficult to decide whether a particular treatment is effective or whether it merely coincides with a remission. Lance mentions that the substance Pizotifen (Sanomigran), which is a potent antihistamine and antiserotonin agent, may prevent further attacks of pain. The suggested dose is 0·5 mg tablet t.d.s. during the bout.

The normal treatment for cluster headache is to give the same agents as are used in migraine to relieve the extracranial dilatation. The rationale is to relieve that part of the syndrome which is known to cause pain. Initially ergotamine medication is used regularly by mouth two to three times per day. If the attacks come mainly at night the drug can be given as a suppository before settling down for the night. If necessary ergotamine tartrate can be given by injection and if all these methods of presenting ergot compounds fail, then methysergide orally in dose of 2 mg t.d.s. can be tried. The dose can be increased if necessary. There are side-effects of methysergide which are mentioned under the treatment of migraine.

The pain in cluster headaches is usually severe but sometimes, and by no means rarely, the pain can be of such an intensity that the patient will just sit rocking back and forth till the bout passes, or will literally knock their head against a wall—'anything just to do something' as one patient put it. Large doses of analgesic drugs can be, and are, taken, if necessary these should be given by injection. In those patients who get some warning of an impending attack, the use of an ergotamine inhaler will provide a rapid method of absorbing that medication if the patient gets any relief from the drug. Taken in this way, the drug is absorbed into the blood stream within a minute or so.

Blocking the stellate ganglion does not provoke an attack of cluster headache, thus the suggestion that a deficiency, or relative deficiency, of sympathetic activity is the precipitating cause does not seem to hold good.

Various neurosurgical operations have been done on one or other part of the parasympathetic system without much effect. For instance, White and

Sweet stimulated the greater superficial petrosal nerve during craniotomy. This was done under local anaesthetic and therefore the parasympathetic fibres travelling to the sphenopalatine ganglion were stimulated. These are fibres which control lacrimation and rhinorrhea, but during White and Sweet's stimulation nine out of fourteen patients had pain localised to the ear, eye, and adjacent parts of the face and head. In six patients having cluster headaches this nerve was divided and initially had an encouraging degree of clinical relief, but they mentioned that their data was too fragmentary to permit any final decision on the value of neurectomy. This is the general feeling about active surgical treatment for cluster headaches.

If all else fails then peripheral nerve diagnostic blocks in the distribution of the pain can be tried. If these relieve the pain during an attack then similar blocks using semi-permanent blocking agents such as phenol or alcohol can be carried out. In severe and intractable cases a gasserian ganglion block may be necessary. It cannot be emphasised enough that before a semi-permanent block is used in these cases a diagnostic block should be tried first. Before the block is carried out the patient should be warned of the side-effects of this type of treatment, namely that an anaesthetic portion of the face will result.

On a few occasions the author has found that injection with simple local anaesthetic solutions in the region of the pterygo-palatine fossa has had a long-acting beneficial effect on the frequency and severity of attacks. The method can be repeated and is performed on the purely empirical grounds that it occasionally works. Presumably the beneficial effect of this block (when it occurs) is related to the near presence of the maxillary nerve, branches of the maxillary artery as it passes through the pterygo-maxillary fissure, and many branches to and from the sphenopalatine ganglion. All these are structures which are implicated in some unknown fashion in the production of the pain of cluster headache.

HEMIPLEGIC

This type of migraine tends to run in families, and is sometimes called familial hemiplegic migraine. Migraine attacks occur and during them there is a consistent neurological deficit involving sensation and motor power on one side of the body. Symptoms and signs start in one place, say the hand, which begins to feel numb and weak, and this gradually progresses up the arm to shoulder and body or face. It may progress to the whole of one side of the body. Often if the face is affected there is loss or slurring of speech, and in severe attacks there may be vomiting, confusion, or stupor. After the onset of the paretic attacks severe headache usually develops in about one hour.

There are other types of paretic migraine such as that called ophthalmo-plegic migraine, where there are recurrent attacks of headache associated with paresis of one or more oculomotor nerves. Ptosis and dilatation of the pupil may occur before or during an attack, and is followed by an ocular palsy. This palsy may become permanent or may last some hours or days after the initial onset. The third nerve is the most commonly affected, thus lateral gaze is preserved.

There is no doubt that this type of ophthalmoplegic migraine does occur, but any ocular palsy which lasts more than a few hours should be treated with great suspicion until evidence of intracranial aneurysm, neoplasm, or other slow-growing space occupying lesion is excluded.

Neurological consultant help is indicated in this and for that matter in any patient in whom the diagnosis is in doubt, and apart from a complete neurological examination, including auscultation for intracranial bruits, specialist investigations such as carotid angiogram, electroencephalogram, and scans may be indicated.

Facial palsy associated with migraine is rare on its own but can be present. Retinal migraine is also rare and is due to vascular constriction during the migraine attack, and if this persists after the attack, or for long periods during a prolonged attack, then thrombosis of one or other branch of the retinal artery can result. In this way complete blindness of one eye occurs if the central retinal artery is affected, or partial blindness depend-ing on which branch of this artery is thrombosed. If recurrent retinal constriction occurs there may be eventual optic atrophy, and other com-plications are retinal and vitreous haemorrhages.

Bickerstaff described vertebro-basilar migraine where the symptoms include vertigo, loss of vision, and signs of brain stem involvement, such as ataxia, dysarthria, and paraesthesias. Usually these symptoms are followed by a throbbing occipital headache and by vomiting and there is a tendency to faint during the migraine attack. This variety of migraine is due to the migrainous process being limited to the brain stem but any part of the central nervous system seems capable of being affected and thus there are varieties of migraine which are consistent in some patients but which do not have the classical or common features. These are known as migraine equivalents.

Migraine equivalents are a variety of periodic illness which occurs in the migraine patient where headache is not a feature and the mechanism is believed to be the same as in other forms of migraine. The varieties are many and pleomorphic, for instance, there is a type known as abdominal migraine where nausea, vomiting, and diarrhoea are the main features: in the same way, psychic disturbances can present such as confusion and alterations of mood and behaviour. Sleep rhythm can be altered, or there can be pain in the chest or pelvis. Bizarre forms of this kind will need thorough investigation before being accepted as due only to the migrainous condition.

Lower half headache

This variety, also known as facial migraine, is an episodic facial pain and its features are similar on the one hand to migraine and on the other to cluster headaches. The pain in this condition is invariably unilateral and usually starts in the second division of the trigeminal nerve, the angle of the nose or the palate being common sites. The pain spreads to the rest of the face or neck and there may be visual hallucinations of a minor degree and nausea and photophobia may be present. Often the affected side of the face becomes slightly swollen and the ipsilateral eye waters. If the pain is mainly in the distribution of the orbit and surrounding tissues there will be considerable difficulty in distinguishing the condition from that of cluster headache, particularly as both these types of vascular headaches can be brought on by vasodilators such as alcohol.

Some separation can be made as the lower half migraine headache tends to last longer than the usual cluster headache (for hours instead of minutes), and there are usually symptoms or signs of common or classical migraine features. The fact that cluster headaches tend to occur in bouts and then at frequent intervals during a bout is another distinguishing factor.

All these varieties of migraine are managed in the same way as mentioned previously for migraine.

HEADACHE AND ATYPICAL FACIAL PAIN

PSYCHOGENIC HEADACHE

There are a number of types of facial pain and headache which come into this category. Before elaborating on these it is as well to remember that many, if not most, patients who suffer from intractable pain from whatever cause develop some degree of depression or anxiety. This does not mean that these patients are mentally ill but treatment of their depression or anxiety may well improve their underlying painful condition. In general terms the longer a painful condition has been present, especially if unrelieved, the more likely it is that psychological factors become prominent and can be relieved by appropriate medication. The more important of the varieties of head and neck pain, which are of particular relevance to pain centre work, are now mentioned. Some are mentioned merely in relation to the specialist or consultant they should be referred to.

Psychiatric

A psychogenic headache is one where the headache is combined with obvious psychiatric abnormalities, commonly acute depression, hysteria, or schizophrenia. There is no method of treating such patients except by psychiatric means and they have to be treated by the specialists in this type of medicine as soon as possible. Their pains may be systematised into the delusional pattern of the patient and will fluctuate with the degree of abnormality present in the thought processes at that time. It is always difficult for those not trained in the abnormal mental field to decide whether a particular patient has a painful condition with psychological overtones or has an abnormality of the thought processes with pain as an abnormality of these. In any case of doubt psychiatric advice must be obtained.

Atypical facial pain

This is a condition which gives great difficulty in treatment. The history is quite typical and so often the description of its genesis from one patient to another is so much a carbon copy that one must accept a common aetiology. However, such a common aetiology has not so far been placed on a scientific basis, nor has any method of treatment proved of much avail.

Pain in this condition is usually unilateral and is present deep in the cheek or angle of the nose. Invariably there is a history of trauma to this region, or a tooth may have been extracted before the pain occurs. This latter statement is open to some doubt as many patients suffering with this condition put their pain down to a dental cause and one by one have some or eventually all their teeth extracted in the affected jaw. This process may continue until the patient is edentulous with the pain spreading to other parts of the head, neck, or jaws in severe attacks. In similar fashion if the pain is put down to an infected sinus the patient may have a series of ear, nose, and throat operations without any subsequent benefit. The doubt arises as to whether the pain was present before the operation or was precipitated by the early trauma, but there are some cases where there is no doubt that a relatively minor knock on the face was the precipitating factor.

The type of pain described by the patient is of a constant and boring quality which is ever present. Although most patients mention that the pain is always there, they will admit that it 'goes away' at times. If this point is pursued they will say they mean that the severe pain they suffer from has eased and merely left a residual minor constant pain. The patients may be woken up from their sleep by the pain and will then take medication for it, or if for any other reason they wake at night the pain is always present.

Treatment of this condition is extremely difficult and at the present time it is regarded as a depression. Treatment is therefore by means of Imipramine (Tofranil) 25 mg t.d.s. initially, or Amitriptyline (Tryptizol) 25 mg initially. Monoamine oxidase inhibitors may be used but these are best given under psychiatric supervision. Electroconvulsive therapy has been used in these patients and has proved of value only in the early period after the convulsive therapy. It appears to be of particular benefit at the stage where the patients memory is deficient and this does not appear to be a particularly satisfactory way of producing benefit. Unfortunately the same remark can be made of most of the treatments used in this type of pain.

It is reasonable to make sure there is no obvious cause of the pain such as an infected tooth, or a sinus with a fluid level in it, or other evidence of sepsis round the head and neck. It is reasonable that if there are obvious abnormalities demonstrated that they should be corrected, and having said that the author would remark that correction of abnormalities in this condition bears little relation to relief of the pain and is certainly unreliable. Nevertheless if there is overt disease present it should be corrected.

If the pain is in the distribution of one or other branch of the trigeminal nerve, say the infra-orbital or maxillary, it is worthwhile performing a diagnostic block to see if this relatively simple measure will relieve the pain. The simpler of these blocks is performed first and if it fails those covering a wider area are used. If all fail, then there is no point in proceeding further with this method, but if a block is successful it should be repeated at least twice at intervals of two to four weeks. Only if benefit is obtained on all these occasions should a long-acting block with alcohol, for instance, be performed. There is a great tendency for these patients to respond to any new method on the first occasion.

If all other methods fail then, as previously mentioned in regard to cluster headaches, it is worthwhile injecting in the region of the pterygo-palatine fossa with a simple local anaesthetic agent such as 1 per cent lignocaine combined with a long-acting corticosteroid such as methyl-prednisolone acetate (Depomedrone) 40–80 mg. This is done on a purely empirical basis and seems to provide some of these patients with a period of freedom from pain or a period of diminished pain.

It is very easy with pain of this type to label all the patients suffering with it as having abnormalities of their mental processes. There is no doubt that some are of this kind, but most specialists in the field of pain have seen patients with atypical facial pain whose pain arose in the manner described above, become worse and intractable, and which did not respond to any treatment, and yet all tests and psychiatric opinions were regarded as normal. These are patients where there is no doubt about their mental normality and this suggests that there is an as yet unknown cause for some atypical facial pain.

Post-traumatic headache

Headache following head injury is common and to some slight extent depends on the original degree of injury, for instance, it tends to disappear quickly (when it occurs) in patients who did not have post-traumatic amnesia, and there is a higher incidence in patients who had a laceration of the scalp. Nevertheless, there does not appear to be a great deal of correlation between the severity of the injury, shown by coma, fracture, or disorientation and the severity and length of headache. The great problem in those patients who develop brain damage is that it is difficult to separate mental and physical features, and in addition, there is the prolonged time-scale during which recovery can take place. As Jennett (1978) states 'the combination of mental and physical handicap not only complicates assessment but also tends to make the total disability greater than the sum of its parts'. For patients who do not have a gross degree of brain damage and can be classified into those groups who have made a good recovery or have only a moderate disability, there will be a proportion who have headache, and this may or may not coincide with a post-traumatic psychosis. There is also the question of compensation or litigation for the accident causing the head injury, and it is commonly accepted that in most cases the speediest way of resolving any disability under these circumstances is to settle the litigation. Even then there will be a proportion of patients who seek to justify any residual mental disability in physical terms by persistent headache. This may well be initiated by the sympathy and help it produces, and if persisted in for any length of time will become permanent, as the patient obtains too many benefits in a society where they may be at a disadvantage, at least for a period after the injury.

The above can be said to be suffering from compensation neurosis, a pain habit or frank malingering. There are appropriate treatments for each of these but the outcome is not very satisfactory.

The headache following trauma is due either to alteration in response of the intracranial vessels, or occurs in the distribution of extracranial arteries. In the former case, following concussion the intracranial vessels dilate and the patient develops a throbbing headache increased by movement of the head or by straining. Neurological signs may be absent and there may be other symptoms present. This type of headache can persist for many months.

The latter type of headache is often present when there has been damage to the scalp over or near a large vessel and the pain is often periodic producing a condition which has some features of migraine and is treated in the same way.

There is a third type of pain which may develop after head injury due to damage to the upper cervical spine. This is described later under whip-lash injuries which produce pain in the occipital region and on occasion around the orbit and side of the head. The simplest and most useful active method of treating this condition is to inject near the relevant C.2 nerve root with a local anaesthetic solution which can usefully be combined with a long-acting corticosteroid.

Muscle contraction headache

This is another of the headaches which can be classified in the group of psychogenic pain, and it is, of course, commonly present after head injury also. There are numerous names given to it such as tension headache, nervous headache, or rheumatic headache. The condition is not difficult to diagnose and is very different from migraine, though in some patients there is an alternation between migraine headache and tension headache. There is no point in treating a tension headache as though it were migraine.

Most people at some time in their lives suffer from a tension headache, but this is usually an isolated experience and can be recognised for what it is—a response to eye strain or muscular tension.

The incidence of the condition is widespread being similar to that of migraine. It can begin early in life and last throughout life with some patients suffering daily headaches for years. A most constant feature of the condition is a sustained contraction of the neck muscles which can be seen on physical examination. It can also be seen on the electromyograph. The tension in the patients' muscles is not confined to the occipital ones and it is obvious that these patients find difficulty in relaxing any of their muscle groups this being seen in the arm or jaw as easily as in the neck.

The headache of tension headache is usually bilateral and has none of the prodromata of migraine. It is dull and persistent and may vary during the day though it tends to get worse as the day wears on, and usually occurs in the back of the neck and in the occipital region, but it can occur in the frontal region, side of the head, or can be round the head like a cap or band. Some patients who tend to clench their teeth place strain on to the temporo-mandibular joint and the pain is present in front of the ear, radiating to the temple. Similarly those patients who tend to frown or have their brows constantly wrinkled have frontal headaches. About three-quarters of patients who suffer from this condition are females. The pain is often described not so much as a pain as a feeling of pressure or tightness or weight on the head. It can feel like a tight band round the forehead squeezing the head as though in a vice and in severe cases or during exacerbations it is present all over the head.

Many of these patients are of the anxious highly strung type and many authorities believe that a large proportion of them suffer either with an anxiety state or depression of greater or lesser degree. As Lance says, many patients with tension headache are 'born two drinks down on life', they are never really relaxed and are rarely elated.

There are many conditions which produce muscle contraction headache where the process producing the tension is obvious. One which has already been mentioned is due to pressure on the tempero-mandibular joint, which can develop from mal-occlusion of the jaw and an abnormal bite. It can result from infection of the neck muscles, a cervical disc, cervical spondylosis or other bony abnormalities of the cervical vertebrae. Treatment of these conditions will be the specific for that condition when it can be applied. As far as muscle contraction headache itself is concerned, treatment is symptomatic, and a simple analgesic of the aspirin type is given combined with a tranquilliser, preferably with a muscle relaxant action as well. Of these latter drugs diazepam (Valium) 5 mg four-hourly is excellent. In addition the usual methods for relieving tension can be used. Physiotherapy, heat or short wave diathermy to the tense muscles is indicated, and this can be combined with psychotherapy but in most cases psychotherapy is too time-consuming to be practicable. However, often there are simple suggestions for altering the patient's way of life which helps to remove some of the strain and tension out of it. Formal relaxation exercises are well worthwhile but training the patient to do these may require patience after a lifetime of tension, in fact, some of these patients refuse to believe that they are tense and the first line of treatment will be to demonstrate the patient's inability to relax their own muscles.

If relief from the condition does not occur in about 1–2 months after treatment is initiated it is worth trying the effect of the antidepressant drugs such as meprobamate (Miltown) 400 mg t.d.s. or amitriptyline (Tryptizol) 25 mg t.d.s. The patient should be informed that these drugs produce side-effects of drowsiness, tremor, and dryness of the mouth.

TRIGEMINAL NEURALGIA

Trigeminal neuralgia is also known as Tic Douloureux because during a severe paroxysm of pain the face is contorted by agony. Classical trigeminal neuralgia is such a well-defined entity that there is little difficulty in arriving at a diagnosis. Certain features are commonly present, the most important of these being as follows. It is a disease of age, being uncommon in youth, and two-thirds of patients are over the age of 50. It is more frequent in woman than man, the incidence varying with the authority but is of the order of two to one. The pain occurs in bouts which are self-limiting and during a bout the pain is confined to one or other part of the trigeminal nerve distribution. Each bout can persist for many months and as the disease progresses there is a tendency for the remissions to become shorter and the bouts to become longer.

The type of pain and its frequency is typical of the condition, it being described as a superficial, severe, electric-shock like pain, intense and brief. During the attack of pain the patient may be unable to move and sits clutching the affected part of the face. The attacks are always brief, lasting one or two minutes, and the patient is completely free of pain in between. However, attack may succeed attack, one after the other with only a short interval between, and in severe cases these occur at a few second intervals so that the patient is hardly free of pain; in fact the patient may describe it as continuous and careful questioning will be needed to bring out this point. Between attacks some patients have a persistent dull ache or discomfort present but in the classically described disease no pain is present except during the attack.

TRIGGER POINTS

In the acute stage of the condition and during it the patient may stop eating, shaving, or washing as often one or other of these activities initiates the pain. This occurs by touching certain special areas called trigger zones which are characteristic of the disease, and which are usually found within the painful region but not always. Common places for trigger zones are the side of the nose, the upper or lower lip, and the mucous membrane of the upper or lower jaw, or the tongue. Some patients never have trigger points. As might be expected, if touching a particular trigger point initiates pain, the patient will not touch, shave, or wash that particular part of the face, and the diagnosis may sometimes be made as the patient walks into the consulting room with, for instance, an unshaven upper lip on one side, or with a clean face except for one portion which has obviously not been washed for some time. If the pain is precipitated from the tongue then talking and eating will be avoided; the patient can lose considerable weight and become quite dehydrated because of this. If the patient is seen in an attack the posture adopted is quite typical as mentioned above, they stop whatever they are doing—in mid-sentence perhaps—clutch the face and remain immobile until the attack is over.

Alterations of sensation of the face occur in patients who have no pain between attacks. Hypersensitivity is the commonest but hyposensitivity when it does occur must be regarded as a symptom of some significance until it is proved otherwise, as the presence of analgesia or frank anaesthesia is to be regarded as evidence of intracranial pressure on the fifth nerve and investigated accordingly. For this reason during the physical examination of the patient it is essential to examine both sides of the face to pin prick and touch. A small area of unexplained analgesia or hypoalgesia must be investigated.

PAIN DISTRIBUTION

The trigeminal nerve is divided into three sensory divisions, and a small motor one, and during an attack of trigeminal neuralgia pain is limited to one or more divisions of this nerve. A pain starting in the cheek which shoots towards the upper jaw, lip, and under the eye is common and denotes second division pain, while third division pain starts in front of the ear and shoots down to the chin and tongue, or it may start in chin or tongue and shoot towards the ear. First division pain is rare on its own but it is sometimes difficult to decide whether a pain in the forehead is first division pain or not. A good working basis is that if the patient describes the pain as being in the eyebrow and shooting laterally along the brow towards the zygoma it is probably second division pain, while if it is described as starting in the brow or forehead and shooting upwards along the distribution of the supra-orbital nerve it is first division pain.

It is not uncommon for the second and third divisions to be the site of trigeminal pain on their own, the frequency with which this happens being roughly equal. In about 30 per cent of cases the second and third divisions are involved together, and it is a common feature that when pain is confined to one division it will spread to a neighbouring one after a longer or shorter time, sometimes after many years. Pain in the first division on its own occurs in less than 3 per cent but in combination with the other divisions in about 30 per cent of cases. Most of these are combinations of the second and first divisions as third and first combinations are present in less than 1 per cent. Bilateral trigeminal neuralgia is rare, being of the order of 3 per cent and its treatment is important as under some circumstances severe complications can be produced. The important point is that if bilateral damage occurs to the motor root then movement of the jaw becomes affected. It hangs open and the patient cannot chew, this being more likely to occur if the condition is treated by means of an alcohol injection. It is safer to use either an alcohol injection on one side and a surgical root section on the other, or bilateral root section rather than a bilateral injection into the gasserian ganglion. Of course, if the condition can be treated by peripheral nerve blocks, such as infraorbital or mandibular nerve blocks, then the danger mentioned will not apply.

It might be thought that the incidence of trigeminal pain would be the same on the two sides of the face but such is not the case. The right side of the face is affected more frequently than the left in the ratio of about two to one. There is no certain reason why this is so but it may be due to the anatomy of the petrous part of the temporal bone which tends to be different on the two sides of the body. It is said that when trigeminal neuralgia occurs it is more often on the side where the apex of the petrous temporal bone is highest and this tends to be the right side.

CAUSE OF PAIN

Many reasons have been suggested for the increased incidence of trigeminal neuralgia in old age, such as it being part of the atherosclerosis which occurs in the older age groups, or to the narrowing of the foramina that occurs with increased age, to the loss of myelin sheaths, or the displacement of the brain stem with increasing age. In women there is the post-menopausal osteoporosis which may occur.

The paroxysmal nature of trigeminal neuralgia has been compared to the paroxysmal discharge of the epileptiform attack and it has been postulated that a discharge of this type producing the pain of trigeminal neuralgia would be due to centrally located trigeminal neurones. This is a theory which has gained considerable acceptance and has been interpreted as evidence in favour of a central aetiology for the disease (King, 1967). However, this is not accepted without dispute that the aetiology is a peripheral one (Kerr, 1967). The problem has not been resolved and the argument still continues. Fortunately the treatment of the condition does not depend on the theory of its production.

TREATMENT

Treatment can be demarcated into a number of well-defined groups: (1) Drug therapy, (2) Peripheral nerve blocks, (3) Avulsion of nerves, (4) Gasserian ganglion injection, (5) Other needle methods, (6) Trigeminal rhizotomy, (7) Other operations on the gasserian ganglion, (8) Medullary tractotomy.

(1) *Drug therapy*

The most useful drug available in this respect is carbamazepine (Tegretol) which has been found to have a specific effect in trigeminal neuralgia. It is an anticonvulsant and in trigeminal neuralgia a starting dose of 100 mg t.d.s. is used and this can be increased to 200 mg q.d.s. if the pain is not controlled on the lower dose. There are a number of problems which may prevent its use in any particular patient. The first is that it has toxic effects such as dizziness, depression, and skin rashes but sometimes the cerebellar symptoms settle down in a few days if the drug is persisted with. If skin rashes appear then the patient must abandon the drug. Serious though these complications are they are not as dangerous as the pancytopenia which can develop. For this reason a weekly white cell count should be performed for the initial four weeks after the patient first goes on to this drug, and after that these should be done at monthly intervals. It is emphasised that this frequency is the least that should be carried out. A patient who has active trigeminal neuralgia controlled by Tegretol and who develops a reduction in white cells or in platelets will have to be withdrawn from the drug. The painful paroxysms will then appear in their full severity and the patient and their medical advisor will be in some difficulty as both surgical and injection therapy will have hazards. Probably the most reasonable method of treatment under these circumstances is to replace any missing coagulation factors and carry out an alcohol block of the gasserian ganglion. A lesser peripheral block should be performed if it will relieve the pain and can be carried out dexterously and speedily.

The second problem with the use of Tegretol is that its effect tends to diminish with time and that therefore the pain may begin to break through again and will require injection or surgical treatment.

Tegretol suppresses the pain in about 70 per cent of cases and a similar drug that can be used is phenytoin (Epanutin) 100–200 mg t.d.s. This drug is not as successful as Tegretol but it also has an anticonvulsant effect which lends support to the theory that trigeminal neuralgia is a form of peripheral epilepsy in the sensory neurones of the trigeminal pathways. Epanutin has complications which include allergic phenomena and haematological disorders such as leucopenia. Sometimes when one of these drugs does not have a satisfactory effect in controlling the pain of trigeminal neuralgia the combination of both of them does but it is not advisable to keep patients on this regime for any great length of time. In any case, from time to time, it is reasonable to stop or reduce these drugs to see if the patient has entered a period of remission.

(2) *Peripheral nerve blocks*

If the pain of the trigeminal neuralgia is confined to one or other peripheral nerve distributions then blocking that nerve will relieve the pain for the period of the block. This means two things: firstly, that this method can be used diagnostically to determine whether a particular nerve block is effective and if positive continue with a long-acting neurolytic agent such as alcohol. Secondly, it will be axiomatic, as peripheral nerves regenerate, that the anaesthesia in the distribution of the block will wear off in time and therefore as sensation returns there is a likelihood of recurrence of the trigeminal pain. There is one proviso in this in that if normal sensation returns in a period of remission pain will not reappear. The value of peripheral nerve blocks is that they tide the patient over a period when they are perhaps not prepared or not fit for surgery, and in addition it gives the surgeon the opportunity to demonstrate to the patient the 'feel' of a numb face or tongue.

Apart from these considerations there is a great advantage where the pain is in the distribution of a limited peripheral nerve distribution such as the infraorbital, maxillary, or mandibular, and anaesthesia of the skin can be kept to the minimum possible by blocking a branch and not the whole nerve. The technique of performing peripheral fifth nerve blocks is described elsewhere (see Chapter 14).

(3) *Avulsion of peripheral nerves*

This method is designed to produce the effect of long-acting injections on peripheral nerves more certainly and for a longer period of time. Portions of the nerve have been excised but the logical extension of this is to exterpate the nerve branch completely. The simplest method of carrying this out is to make an incision near the nerve at a convenient place, expose it, clamp it, and avulse it. Certain branches lend themselves more than others to this technique which is not used very much nowadays, but of those used the supraorbital nerve is the most common. Here the surgeon tries to do the minimum which will permanently relieve the pain and still leave the patient with a normally sensitive cornea. The other nerve sometimes dealt with in this way is the infraorbital nerve. The method has fallen into disuse nowadays, principally because it is not successful. Although nerve tissue is removed it is not always possible to remove the whole of the nerve so the avulsion is incomplete. Sometimes an accessory nerve or additional branch is present. Further, regrowth tends to occur in about six to twelve months depending on how large a piece of nerve is removed and how proximal the gap is. A cut peripheral branch of the trigeminal nerve grows at a rate of 0·2 mm approximately per day. The nerve can be avulsed or cut repeatedly but as the regrown nerve may be present in scar tissue in thin stringy bundles the technique becomes progressively more difficult.

(4) *Gasserian ganglion injection*

Just as there are various approaches to blocking the maxillary and mandibular nerves so there are a number of different approaches to the gasserian ganglion. In particular the names of Harris and Härtel will always be associated with these methods which were designed to insert a needle through the foramen ovale into either the gasserian ganglion or the rootlets as they enter this ganglion. The so-called anterior approach to the foramen ovale would appear to be the simplest and most straightforward approach to it, and the method is described later (see Chapter 14). It can be used also as an approach to the mandibular division of the trigeminal nerve merely by placing the needle tip in the centre of the foramen as seen in the base view of an X-ray film and, after a small injection of a local anaesthetic to demonstrate the extent of blocking the nerve in that area, 1·0 ml or less of absolute alcohol is injected in divided doses. Sweet has advocated then rotating the bevel of the needle upwards and injecting further amounts of alcohol of 1 to 3 cc. This increases the length of nerve destroyed and may spread far enough to reach the ganglion, and there may be temporary sensory loss in the other divisions.

Anatomy of the gasserian ganglion is crucial in understanding the finer points of the various techniques for destroying the ganglion or the rootlets entering it. A brief account is given here although it is also mentioned in Chapter 14.

This ganglion is situated in the trigeminal impression near the apex of the petrous part of the temporal bone on its superior surface. It is semilunar in shape being convex in front and concave behind, and in thickness is only about 3 mm. Its length from front to back is about 12 mm and the sensory root of the trigeminal nerve enters the posterior aspect of the ganglion where it is expanded, forming a number of separate strands. The divisions of the ganglion arise from the convex portion, being three in number, the ophthalmic, maxillary, and mandibular. The ophthalmic is the smallest proceeding forwards in the outer wall of the cavernous sinus, lying below the fourth nerve. It divides into smaller branches on approaching the superior orbital fissure. The maxillary nerve lies in the lower part of the outer wall of the cavernous sinus, passing forward horizontally through the foramen rotundum to the pterygo-palatine fossa. The third division is the mandibular nerve, the largest of the three, it passes downwards into the foramen ovale and leaves the cranium by entering the infratemporal fossa. The motor root of the trigeminal nerve joins the mandibular nerve in the foramen ovale.

The posterior part of the ganglion lies in a recess of the dura mater called the Cavum Trigeminale or Meckel's cave, but it is very important to realise that the front part of the ganglion does not lie in this recess but is closely covered with dura. Thus a surgical approach to the ganglion from the anterior aspect can be performed without opening into the subarachnoid space.

On the antero-medial side the ganglion is closely related to the posterior part of the cavernous sinus and medially and inferiorly to the carotid artery in the foramen lacerum. Sympathetic fibres are received from the internal carotid sympathetic plexus. The greater superficial petrosal nerve lies beneath the ganglion as does the small motor root. Laterally lie the structures of the middle fossa.

In the outer wall of the cavernous sinus lie a number of cranial nerves which are, from above downward, the oculo-motor, the trochlear, the ophthalmic division and the maxillary division, while in the cavity of the sinus is the cavernous portion of the internal carotid artery and the abducens nerve.

Henderson in his monograph on the anatomy of the gasserian ganglion and its relations to injections and operations pointed out that there was a sinus which extended from the cavernous sinus deep to the origins of the first two divisions at the ganglion and to some extent surrounding them.

Injection of alcohol into this could account for the persistence of first and second division anaesthesia, while that of the third division wore off. He also showed that the distances of the various portions of the trigeminal pathways was variable. Important measurements being that the distance from the internal foramen ovale to the trigeminal ganglion (i.e. the mandibular division) varied from zero to 10 mm. The length of ganglion between this anterior point and the posterior edge of the ganglion averaged 5 mm, while the rootlets from the posterior edge of the ganglion to the trigeminal pore (or porus) varied from 5 to 15 mm and corresponded inversely with the anterior distances. Thus a short mandibular division coincided with long roots, and a long mandibular division with short roots. The distance between the anterior edge of the foramen ovale and the posterior superior edge of the petrous bone at the porus trigeminae (this is where the root crosses the apex of the petrous part of the temporal bone, lies under the superior petrosal sinus and pierces the dura at that point, immediately under the tentorium) is approximately 15 to 25 mm.

It should be noticed that using the anterior approach to the foramen ovale (Härtel's approach) an insertion of the needle fairly close to the corner of the mouth tends to place the tip of the needle somewhat lateral to the ganglion as the needle enters the foramen laterally, while a more lateral insertion of the needle further away from the mouth combined with a more medial insertion through the foramen tends to place the needle tip more medially in the ganglion. Thus the former approach is to be preferred if the third division is to be blocked, and the second if the second and first are required. The technique is not quite as simple as is implied by this as a definite effort has to be made to direct the needle along the correct line. Traditionally the target is the pupil of the eye and this tends to place the needle tip laterally, while if a medial placement is required it should be directed to the inner corner of the eye as recommended by Sweet and Wepsic (1974).

DESTRUCTION OF GASSERIAN GANGLION AND ROOTS

As might be expected, many different methods have been advocated and abandoned over the years. Those methods which are not of much value will be mentioned only.

(*a*) The lateral approach of Harris is the same as that used for a mandibular block from the lateral approach except that the needle is inserted as far below the zygoma as possible and above the coronoid notch. The foramen ovale is directed downwards and outwards and thus in many cases it is possible to enter the skull from the approach suggested. However, the anterior approach is much more straightforward, provides a better 'line' to the ganglion, and lends itself to various types of destruction of the ganglion. It is the commonest used nowadays.

(*b*) The anterior approach of Härtel has been described elsewhere (see Chapter 14), and some of the finer points have been mentioned above. There are a number of others; for instance, the needle tip can be placed in the ganglion itself, though this is not easy owing to the narrow thickness of the ganglion. However a deliberate attempt can be made to do this by making sure the needle enters the centre of the foramen and also, if possible, lies parallel to the slope of the petrous ridge. The needle enters the cranium from anterio-laterally alongside or through the mandibular nerve. In the former case insertion is painless, in the latter there will be referred pain in the mandibular distribution. This can be exceedingly painful at times and a slow insertion with small increments of local anaesthetic solution injected ahead of the needle tip will prevent this. Alternatively a small quantity of a short-acting general anaesthetic can be given at this stage, but this means that there will be a delay after each movement of the needle while the patient regains consciousness. As mentioned previously the anatomical relations between the foramen, the ganglion, and the roots are not constant as far as distances are concerned, and this means that on any particular insertion one cannot be sure where the tip of the needle is lying.

Henderson performed post-mortem studies and found that using an injection site lateral to the corner of the mouth and aiming at the pupil, about one-third of the insertions entered the rootlets; the remainder were either in front of the ganglion, or went through the lateral portion of the ganglion. Sweet's suggestion of aiming the needle more medially than the pupil seems a better line which places it either inside the ganglion or in the rootlet area. Jefferson also performed post-mortem studies and showed that when the needle was inserted deep enough for the tip to lie at the junction of middle and posterior fossae, it was 5 to 10 mm posterior to the profile of the clivus. He made his injections with the needle tip 5 mm posterior to the clivus when it was amongst the rootlets. In this situation cerebro-spinal fluid could often be obtained.

Sweet discusses the anatomical placement of the needle in some detail and summarising this and the above it would appear that if the needle tip is to be placed amongst the rootlets it should on X-ray films be 10 to 15 mm deep to the foramen, and lie about 5 mm or a little more posterior to the clivus, in the lateral view. In the basal X-ray view the tip should lie 1 to 5 mm medial to the antero-medial edge of the foramen ovale for the third division and 5 to 10 mm medially for the second. This unfortunately leaves considerable variation and fractional methods of injecting local anaesthetic or destructive agents should be used to monitor the development of trigeminal anaesthesia. In a similar fashion fractional methods of using a radio frequency heat lesion technique are used.

When the needle has been inserted according to the above and by the anterior approach described later, it should be advanced not more than 5 mm beyond the foramen ovale and a small quantity of local anaesthetic agent injected, of the order of 0·25 ml to 0·5 ml. There are differences to be found in the results from this small amount of local due to the variable diffusability of different anaesthetic agents. Thus lignocaine will tend to spread further than procaine, in addition it tends to last longer for equivalent concentrations. A long-lasting local such as marcaine (Bupivacaine) should only be used when the purpose of the block is to show the patient what the 'feel' of an anaesthetic portion of the face is like before making a decision as to a permanent effect. Under normal circumstances procaine 0·5 per cent is quite sufficient. There are two effects which are to be observed, the first is what analgesia develops and in what areas, the second is whether any alteration in the pupil or ocular muscles occurs.

Analgesia

In the first case it is important that if analgesia is required in the third division and develops first in the second that a further increment of local is injected to see whether the next division to be affected is the third or the first, alternatively the needle may be withdrawn a little before the increment is injected. Some operators, after the initial injection of local has shown that the needle is more or less in the correct place, will go ahead with the injection of pure alcohol if that is the agent to be used. It must be remembered that in this case the increments of alcohol used should be small, of the order of 0·05 ml and is best injected by means of a 1 ml syringe. Ample time should be allowed for the analgesia or anaesthesia to develop in between injections. As long as anaesthesia of the trigeminal nerve is proceeding in a progressive fashion, increment after increment is injected until the required spread of analgesia has developed. Some operators do not even inject a small amount of local but inject small amounts of pure alcohol from the beginning. This is painful for the patient but has the merit that there is no doubt how much of the anaesthesia is due to local and how much due to alcohol. If the amounts of alcohol injected are small any untoward effect that develops will clear up in hours or days provided no further alcohol is injected.

Ocular palsy

The second effect to be observed is whether or not the nerves controlling
the eye are affected. Often if the needle hits the ganglion in its insertion
there is an immediate dilatation of the pupil which passes off in a few
minutes. However, if paresis of any of the ocular muscles develops then it
is unwise to proceed with the injection of alcohol at that site or the paresis
and resulting double vision may well be permanent, or at least, last a very
long time. Repositioning of the needle will be necessary taking into account
the X-ray views and no further injections will be made until the original
local anaesthetic effect has worn off.

In addition to ocular palsy the sensitivity of the cornea must be monitored.
It is most unusual for loss of the corneal reflex to occur when the third
division is the one where anaesthesia is developing during injection, but
if analgesia has progressed to the second division or started in the second
division then testing must be carried out after every incremental injection.
Usually there will be anaesthesia or analgesia of the first division at the same
time as corneal anaesthesia develops but this is not necessarily so. It should
also be remembered that if the needle tip lies inside the ganglion then a very
small quantity of alcohol, of the order of 0·15 to 0·3 ml, can produce complete
anaesthesia of all three divisions of the trigeminal nerve, including the
corneal reflex. This happens exceptionally, but when it does occur, happens
with great swiftness.

The fifth nerve motor root lies very close to the ganglion and as one might
expect, in many cases there is a palsy of this branch with consequent loss
of action of the muscles of mastication. Activity often returns but by no
means as a matter of course. Most patients find that the loss of this activity
on one side is no great handicap but if a bilateral trigeminal nerve neuralgia
should develop then it is most important that bilateral fifth nerve motor
palsy should be avoided at all costs as the jaw will hang open and normal
chewing movements will not take place. Bilateral open operation or,
unilateral operation with a unilateral injection, or other combinations of the
various methods available should be used instead.

Corneal anaesthesia has grave penalties under certain circumstances.
Absence of the corneal reflex means that foreign bodies in the eye will not
be appreciated and infection, corneal ulceration, perforation of the globe,
and eventual loss of the eye is not uncommon. The patient with an absent
corneal reflex must be instructed in ocular hygiene and informed to seek
medical help if conjunctival injection or obvious infection of the eye appears.
If necessary a tarsorraphy should be performed. Neuropathic keratitis is

a very real complication and when the first division is not affected it is well worth the time and effort trying to preserve the sensation in this division. Corneal clouding also occurs and of the various complications that can occur after medical or surgical treatment of trigeminal neuralgia, those concerning the eye are the most urgent.

Anaesthesia dolorosa

From the patient's point of view this is the worst possible complication following trigeminal neuralgia treatment that can occur. There are, however, a grading of patients from those who complain of some paraesthesias of a minor nature in the anaesthetic area; to others where the paraesthesiae are more constant and present in all the waking hours; to the florid condition where there is constant severe burning, or aching pain combined with such descriptions as the 'pain crawling under the skin', or 'as though there was ground glass under the skin'. There are many descriptions for this condition, and all unpleasant.

It is generally agreed that some of those patients who are at risk in developing this condition can be picked out by performing a long-acting peripheral nerve blocking procedure before the destructive procedure at the gasserian ganglion or roots. They develop lesser or greater sensations of paraesthesiae and should be avoided for the more permanent techniques. The condition of anaesthesia dolorosa may develop soon after the injection but may take months or years to appear. Treatment of this condition is very difficult and it seems that nothing short of leucotomy or a stereotactic lesion in the thalamus or midbrain will help. Further surgery to the gasserian ganglion does not seem to offer much hope.

Trophic lesions

These do not occur very often but when they do they can be devastating to the patient's appearance. It is due to the patient constantly rubbing or even picking at one area on the anaesthetic skin. A common site is the corner of the nose either through constant blowing and rubbing with a handkerchief, or to scratching or picking at the ala. An ulcer results and loss of tissue occurs. This process continues and extends and eventually the whole side of the nose may disappear. The process can take place without trauma, owing to trophic changes in the anaesthetic skin but this is rare. The patient may deny damaging the tissue and believe this to be true, while observation will show that they have developed an automatic habit and are in fact 'working' on the area.

Herpes

After most operations and after some ganglion injections an herpetic lesion
will develop on the lip and mucous membranes in the anaesthetic area. The
causal virus is the herpes simplex and occurs so frequently after operation
as hardly to be classified as a complication.

Percentage complications

These vary depending on the authority quoted. Marguth summarised some
of the data from the international literature comprising about 20,000 cases.
There were 3,500 cases of peripheral surgery and injections, with 50–80 per
cent relapses and 5 per cent complications. Alcohol injections and electro-
coagulations totalled 9,000 but were not separated. Relapses were 25–40
per cent with 10–15 per cent complications. 10,000 sections of the retro-
ganglion root produced 5–10 per cent of relapses and a similar complication
rate. Dandy's operation showed 670 cases with 15 per cent relapses and
5–10 per cent complications.

White and Sweet reviewed some 6,000 cases of surgical rhizotomy which
showed mortalities varying from 0·4 per cent to 4·5 per cent with complications having an equally wide spread. As mortality must vary with the age
and general physical status of the patient, and as these patients are usually
in the later decades, this mortality is not unreasonable. White and Sweet's
mortality in 305 cases being a most acceptable 1·3 per cent.

As far as the percentage complications of injection of the gasserian
ganglion is concerned the complication rate using alcohol seems very high,
for instance, Härtel had more than 10 per cent incidence of keratitis, and
changed his technique. Harris treated a tremendous number of patients
running into many thousands and about two-thirds of his patients were still
pain free three years later. In general terms the earlier workers in this field
tended to use larger amounts of alcohol in their injections and produced
longer periods of anaesthesia with more complications. It is true to say
that with modern techniques using X-ray control and minimal amounts of
alcohol the results are no better, but perhaps produced with less complications. As a result they also do not last as long.

There is little difference between the operation and gasserian ganglion
injection as far as the complication of anaesthesia dolorosa is concerned. It
appears that many patients who have these procedures, perhaps as many
as 40 per cent, develop some form of paraesthesias. However, if one
is considering only the most severe of these as qualifying for the name

anaesthesia dolorosa then the incidence is of the order of 2 per cent. There are no simple methods of treatment.

Other injection techniques

These involve the injection of alcohol with the patient placed in different positions; or the use of different injection materials; or the abandonment of injection methods in favour of electrical ones (see (5) later). Previously discussed are injection techniques where the position of the needle is varied.

Patient position

Penman (1953) used a radiographic technique, after penetration through the foramen ovale to position the needle tip among the trigeminal rootlets. He obtained considerable success with this method which was designed to obtain complete anaesthesia, but at the expense of a considerable complication rate. Ecker and Perl (1958) modified this method; in particular they placed the patient's head so that the hypobaric alcohol would float into Meckel's cave. They positioned the patient supine with the head extended, the needle lying perpendicular to the operating table. The third division fibres are the highest in this position and thus the injected alcohol rises towards them. They are affected first and to some extent the corneal sensation is preserved. The alcohol is injected in small increments of 0·05 ml and the total dose used is 0·3 ml. In a further paper in 1965 they obtained relief in more than 95 per cent, but even with this technique there was a 10 per cent incidence of corneal anaesthesia.

If the substance used for injection into the gasserian ganglion or the roots is heavier than cerebro-spinal fluid then the position is different from the one described above. For instance, if phenol in glycerine is used then the patient is placed in the sitting position with the head flexed forward on the chest, the needle pointing vertically upwards. Injection of hyperbaric solutions cause these solutions to fill Meckel's cave initially and then overflowing additional solution falls into the spinal canal.

Other injection materials

These are many but those which have had reasonable results have been boiling water; various strengths of phenol, normally in myodil or glycerine with wax; and the combination of alcohol and local anaesthetic solutions in 50 per cent mixtures has also been used. The use of these different materials has been part of the effort to produce acceptable relief of pain with a low incidence of complications. In particular they form part of the search to avoid unwanted corneal anaesthesia. The method of Jefferson (1963) using 5 per cent phenol in glycerine seems to be the best of these techniques.

Jefferson technique

The injection needle is inserted through the foramen ovale in its central or medial third and advanced until it is approximately 5 mm anterior to the clivus. In this position the needle tip is normally amongst the trigeminal rootlets and cerebro-spinal fluid can be obtained from the needle. The patient is placed in the position described above, namely sitting up with the head flexed on the chest and the needle pointing vertically upwards. The volume of Meckel's cave varies (up to 0·2 ml) and Jefferson's average injection was 0·45 ml in increments of about 0·1 ml. The benefit of this technique is that in most cases it relieves the pain of trigeminal neuralgia without producing a completely anaesthetic face. Although corneal anaesthesia developed in one-quarter of his patients, no patients developed corneal ulcers or anaesthesia dolorosa. The penalty for this satisfactory state of affairs is that the pain tends to recur at shorter intervals than when using alcohol and only 5 out of 50 were pain free at the end of eighteen months. However, the method is easily repeated and a similar result to that of the first occasion can be obtained on the second.

(5) *Other needle methods*

These consist of the electrocoagulation methods, the first of these being that of Kirschner. He used a diathermy apparatus, a needle insulated except for the terminal 1 cm which was placed through the foramen ovale into the gasserian ganglion. A stereotactic apparatus combined with radiographic control placed the needle in the correct place. This apparatus incidentally has been the basis for many instruments capable of placing a needle in the ganglion. The speed and simplicity of this method led to its widespread use on the continent of Europe where many thousands of cases have been treated in this fashion, and in fact, continue to be treated so today in some units. The complications with this method were severe and many were reviewed by White and Sweet in their recent book (1969). White and Wepsic have advocated a modern method of heat coagulation of the gasserian ganglion by means of a controlled thermocoagulation. Their method is very different indeed from the blunderbuss technique of Kirschner. The heat is provided by a radiofrequency electric current (i.e. a diathermy current).

RADIOFREQUENCY COAGULATION METHOD

This method is based on the hypothesis that it is the less myelinated fibres that carry sensations of pain and that these might be selectively destroyed by heat. The patient is sedated with a neurolept anaesthetic and during the period of coagulation the patient is given a short period of methohexitol

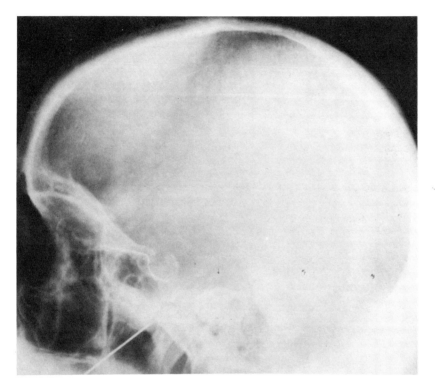

FIGURE 6. Needle held up on edge of foramen ovale. Lateral view.

(Brietal) sleep. A period must then elapse until the patient recovers enough to understand questions. Thus the method takes time, in fact, is rather tedious, but the end results are worthwhile.

The cannula electrode is inserted through the foramen ovale by the anterior approach. If the second or first divisions are required the electrode penetrates the skin further lateral to the corner of the mouth than if only the third division is required. Also if only one division is to be affected then the terminal 0·5 mm of the electrode is bare whereas 10 mm are bare if more than one is required. No stereotactic frame is used. In the Liverpool Pain Relief

Centre o·5 cm has been adequate for one, two, or three divisions, and the
1·0 cm electrode is rarely used.

During insertion the needle electrode is directed 3·5 cm to 4·0 cm
anterior to the anterior wall of the external auditory canal in the sagittal
plane at the lower border of the zygoma. In the coronal plane it is directed
to the lateral border of the lachrymal caruncle. Using these directions the
needle electrode tends to pass through the foramen ovale at its middle or
medial portion. This ensures that as the electrode penetrates deeper it takes
up a position medially and lies within either the ganglion or the rootlets.

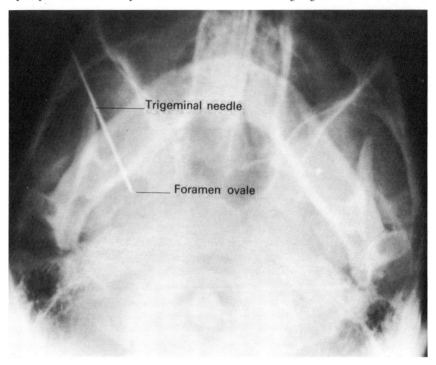

FIGURE 7. Needle held up on edge of foramen ovale. Submento-vertical.

The position of the electrode is confirmed by X-ray films (Figs. 6–9). The
electrode enters the foramen at about 7 cm depth, and the most satisfactory
length of electrode is 10 cm. When the electrode is positioned correctly
a measurement from hub to skin is made where it emerges from the skin to
provide some indication of the required depth and whether it moves
subsequently.

The needle electrode is inserted to a sufficient depth to obtain cerebro-
spinal fluid as this means the tip must lie behind the ganglion and most of

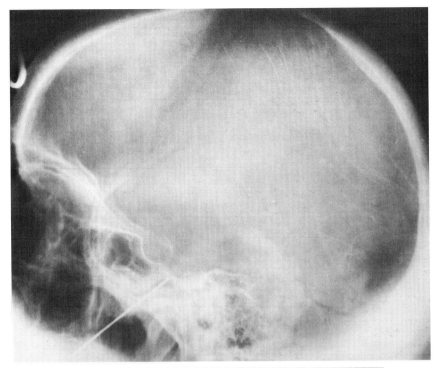

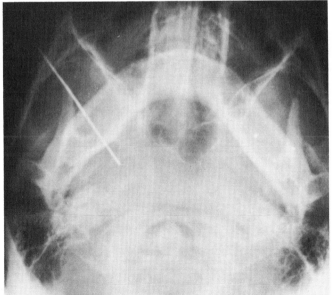

FIGURES 8–9. Varying positions of needle during insertion.

the lesion will be in the rootlets, ganglion, or both. The radiographic position varies markedly as would be expected from the work of Henderson and Jefferson. One constant feature is that the more the tip of the electrode is medial and posterior to the clival profile, the more likely is first division sensory loss. Under these circumstances the heating process must be very carefully and slowly carried out to avoid unwanted corneal reflex loss.

Electrical stimulation corroborates the position of the needle tip, a square wave pulse being used. The threshold is usually low being about 0·2 volt at 50 hertz. At the threshold value the sensation felt by the patient is not painful and can be described quite calmly as a touch, tingling, buzzing, or other similar sensation on or under the skin. The paraesthesiae obtained at stimulation are an accurate guide to the division or divisions which later become analgesic (see Figs. 10 and 11).

As an added precaution the sensation the patient feels when the electrode is allowed to heat up gradually can be used to distinguish the division in which analgesia will develop when a full heat lesion is made. This starts at about a temperature of 50 °C and is a sharply localised burning pain usually in the same division. When it is not in the same division it may be referred to either or both of two divisions and if one of these is the first division it is reasonable to withdraw the electrode a few millimetres until stimulation does not occur in that division.

The lesion is made after the stylette is withdrawn from the needle electrode and replaced with a thermister. This monitors the tip temperature of the needle electrode and this is kept down to a level which it is believed will selectively destroy the smaller pain fibres and leave a proportion of the larger myelinated fibres carrying other sensation. The initial lesion is made at 50 °C for 1 minute or 60 °C for 0·5 minute, and then 60 °C for 1 minute. The temperature is then gradually increased by 5–10 °C monitoring the degree of sensory loss after each increment. The final electrode temperature is not above 90 °C for 90 seconds.

Anaesthesia is used during each lesion so that the patient does not appreciate the severe pain that would be felt when the electrode is heating up rapidly. A minimal amount of a short-acting intravenous anaesthetic is used so that recovery occurs as rapidly as possible. While the lesion is being made autonomic nervous system signs may appear in one of the divisions and this indicates the spread of the lesion into that division. Thus if these appear in the forehead and first division analgesia is not required the current is switched off. If a very slow rate of heating the electrode is used it is said that anaesthesia is not necessary as destruction of the nerve and development of analgesia keeps ahead of pain sensation. The analgesia can be

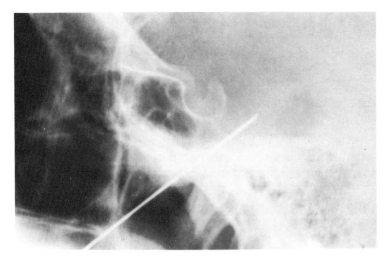

FIGURE 10. Needle has been inserted too far.

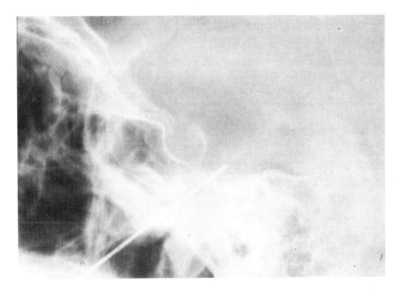

FIGURE 11. Needle has been withdrawn a little.

monitored very accurately and by control of the heat lesion it is possible to preserve some touch sensation in the face.

When the procedure nears its end it is wise to proceed with smaller increments either of time or electric current strength as there may be a sudden development of complete anaesthesia with a minimal final lesion.

Sweet and Wepsic point out two interesting facts. First, that they could carry on with the lesion to the stage of full analgesia to pin prick without producing anaesthesia to touch sensation, and secondly, the less there was of sensory loss to pin prick the greater was the incidence of recurrence of pain.

Results are very satisfactory and at least comparable to any other method. In the well-documented series described by Sweet and Wepsic long-term follow-up was available in 125 patients of from $2\frac{1}{2}$ years to 6 years, and the recurrence rate in this group was 22 per cent. There was a tendency for the recurrence rate to increase with the passage of time.

Comment

Although this method of treating trigeminal neuralgia tends to take longer than the traditional method of alcohol injection it appears to have much merit. It provides a better control over lesion development, a reduction in morbidity, and most of the patients have been free of major paraesthesiae. This latter benefit applies only to the true trigeminal neuralgias. The author has no doubt that this is the method of choice in the non-operative techniques of treating trigeminal neuralgia and is so used at the Centre for Pain Relief.

(6) Trigeminal rhizotomy

It is not proposed in a book of this type to go into the surgery of trigeminal neuralgia in any great detail but some indication of the various surgical methods in lesser detail is required. The basis for the methods that are to be mentioned is that the most certain method of curing the pain of trigeminal neuralgia is by section of the posterior rootlets in the middle fossa. There is a penalty to pay for this and one must be certain the patient understands that the affected part from thenceforth will be permanently anaesthetic. It is most important that the patient understands this most clearly, and in particular that if the third division is sectioned, the tongue and mucous membrane of the lower jaw will be affected, and that if the section involves second and third divisions then the whole of the internal surface of the mouth on one side will be numb, as well as the outer surface of the face. It is perhaps as well before this procedure is performed on the more vacillating patients to perform a gasserian ganglion block on them using a simple local anaesthetic. In this way they can appreciate the feeling that will be present in the future.

One of the benefits of this method is that it is possible to spare the motor root which is not always possible with the injection. Although not an absolute ability the operations do provide the possibility of differential section of the trigeminal rootlets so that the lesion can be confined to the third division only, or second and third division as required. In this way corneal sensation can be spared and the dangers of keratitis and corneal ulceration obviated.

There are two methods of approach to the trigeminal rootlets in the middle fossa, the temporal extradural route, and the temporal intradural route. The benefit is said to be that the latter method avoids the middle meningeal artery and veins round the foramen ovale, but principally that damage to the facial and greater superficial petrosal nerves can be avoided. As ever there are pros and cons for each approach and individual surgeons make their own choice.

There is a third approach to the trigeminal rootlets, through the posterior fossa. This is the operation known as Dandy's, which did not gain much of a following as the operative mortality was much higher than the temporal routes. One of the features of this operation was Dandy's belief in accessory rootlets at the pons which were not cut in total sections and which fact was supposed to explain the absence of loss of skin sensation after these operations. More recently it has been postulated by some surgeons that small arteries near the pons may produce damage in nearby fibres of the trigeminal roots as they enter the pons and the release of these is all that is necessary to relieve the pain of trigeminal neuralgia.

There is some doubt as to whether the approach via the posterior fossa will ever become as popular as that into the middle fossa. The posterior fossa approach is technically more difficult and there is a higher morbidity if not mortality.

(7) *Other operations on the gasserian ganglion*

These consist of a series of operations where it can be said quite truthfully that nobody is sure what the surgeon is doing and yet the results in terms of relief of pain and lack of complications are good. At various times surgeons have approached the gasserian ganglion or the trigeminal rootlets with different operative techniques and for one reason or another have got near enough to the ganglion or the roots to touch or explore them, and yet have been unable to complete the operation which has been abandoned. In many cases these patients have become free of their trigeminal neuralgia for periods that on average have been longer than a normal remission. Further the relief of pain starts immediately or very soon after the operation. It has been postulated that there has been 'damage' to the sensory pathways of the trigeminal nerve and that there may be false synapses between the nerve fibres. Thus, if these can be separated mechanically, freedom from pain should result. An alternative theory and one which is diametrically opposed to that above, is that it is trauma to the pain pathways which produces the effect of trigeminal neuralgia. If this is so then one would expect that decompression rather than further trauma would be beneficial. Whatever the mechanism involved it appears that trauma in one form or another is the treatment which gives relief from the neuralgic pains.

There are two methods, therefore, in relieving the pain of trigeminal neuralgia by these non-destructive operations. In the one the nerve is decompressed, for instance, by incising the dura to relieve tension, in the other mild trauma or compression is applied to the nerve, ganglion, or rootlets. Some surgeons have gone so far as not to operate at all but inject 3-6 ml saline rapidly into the gasserian ganglion after blocking it with local anaesthetic. Most of them operate, expose the intracranial portion of the trigeminal pathways, and apply trauma in various ways, such as rubbing the ganglion with a pledget of wool, or with a blunt instrument, sometimes in addition, the ganglion is painted with phenol.

It is impossible to decide whether there are artificial synapses between the fibres of the trigeminal nerve pathways, and that disturbing these fibres destroys the false pathways, or whether the benefit is merely due to direct injury to these pain pathways. The weight of evidence lends itself to the latter conclusion mainly because it appears that the more trauma applied to the ganglion and the more deficit of sensation produced in the face from this, the more likely does it appear that there is a longer period of relief from pain than would be expected from either a remission or from an alcohol block.

The only thing that can be said for certain about this method is that it works in a high percentage of patients for quite long periods of time. Sweet suggests that this operation may be of particular benefit in that group of patients whose behaviour or complaints of continuous facial sensations make surgeons wary of rhizotomy. The operation would also appear to be of value in those patients with bilateral trigeminal neuralgia, and those with pain in the first division.

(8) *Medullary tractotomy*

The spinal or descending tract of the trigeminal nerve has a long course. It stretches from the point of entry of the roots into the upper pons, down through the medulla oblongata, and into the upper cervical cord. If incisions are made above or below the level of the obex in this tract, relief of trigeminal pain can occur and there is a well-marked anaesthesia in the trigeminal nerve distribution in the face. Incisions made above the obex have certain disadvantages as the restiform body covers the descending trigeminal tract at this level and disturbances of gait and movements of the hand can occur. Incisions below the obex do not have this disadvantage and this is where the operation is performed, when it is used today. There is some controversy as to which level is the best but somewhere in the region of 3 to 5 mm below the obex seems commonly accepted.

The operation appears to have a limited role to play in the treatment of trigeminal neuralgia.

REFERENCES

ANTHONY M. & LANCE J.W. (1971) Histamine and Serotonin in cluster headache. *Arch. Neurol.* **26**, 225.

CHAWLA J.C. & FALCONER M.A. (1967) Glossopharyngeal and vagal neuralgia. *Brit. Med. J.* **2**, 529.

CLASSIFICATION OF HEADACHE. (1962) The Ad Hoc Committee on Classification of Headache. *Arch. Neurol.* (Chicago), **6**, 173.

COSTEN J.B. (1934) A syndrome of ear and sinus symptoms dependent upon disturbed function of the temporomandibular joint. *Ann. Otol. Rhinol. Lar.* **43**, 1.

ECKER A. & PERL T. (1958) Alcoholic gasserian injection for relief of tic douloureux. Preliminary report of a modification of Penman's method. *Neurology* (Minn.), **8**, 461.

HENDERSON W.R. (1965) The anatomy of the gasserian ganglion and the distribution of pain in relation to injections and operations for trigeminal neuralgia. *Ann. roy. Coll. Surg. Eng.* **37**, 346.

HORTON B.J. (1941) Histamine cephalgia. *J. Am. med. Ass.* **116**, 377.

JEFFERSON A. (1963) Trigeminal root and ganglion injections using phenol in glycerine for the relief of trigeminal neuralgia. *J. Neurol. Neurosurg. Psychiat.* **26**, 345.

JENNETT B. (1978) Sherrington Lecture, Liverpool University Medical School.

KERR F.W. (1967) Evidence for a peripheral etiology of trigeminal neuralgia. *J. Neurosurg.* **26**, 168.

KING R.B. (1967) Evidence for a central etiology of Tic Douloureux. *J. Neurosurg.* **26**, 175.

MEADOWS S.P. (1966) Temporal or giant cell arteritis. *Proc. R. Soc. Med.* **59**, 329.

PENMAN J. (1953) Some developments in the technique of trigeminal injection. *Lancet*, **1**, 760.

SELBY G. & LANCE J.W. (1960) Observations on 500 cases of migraine and allied vascular headache. *J. Neurol. Neurosurg. Psychiat.* **23**, 23.

SWEET W.H. & WEPSIC J.G. (1974) Controlled thermocoagulation of the trigeminal ganglion and rootlets for differential destruction of pain fibres. *J. Neurosurg.* **40**, 143.

WHITE J.C. & SWEET W.H. (eds.) (1969) *Pain and the Neurosurgeon*. Charles C. Thomas, Springfield (Illinois).

ADDITIONAL READING

BLAU J.N. (1978) Migraine: A vasomotor instability of the meningeal circulation. *Lancet*, 2, 1136-9.
LANCE J.W. (1973) *The Mechanism and Management of Headache*, 2nd edn. Butterworths, London.
WILKINSON M. (1971) *Cervical Spondylosis*. Heinemann, London.
WOLFF H.G. (1963) *Headache and other Head Pain*. Oxford University Press, London.

Chapter 5
Pain in the Neck and Upper Limb

It is useful to have a classification of disorders of the cervical spine and neck which produce pain. Also included are conditions which refer pain to the arm and hand, and general conditions which refer pain to the upper quadrant of the body.

1. Deformity
    (a) congenital; e.g. the Klippel–Feil syndrome.
    (b) acquired; e.g. a fractured vertebra.

2. Infections
    (a) in bone—tuberculous and pyogenic infections of the cervical spine.
    (b) surrounding tissues—fibrositis, cervical glands.

3. Arthritis
    (a) ankylosing spondylitis.
    (b) osteoarthritis of the cervical spine.

4. Referred pain
    (a) chronic infection around the shoulder joint.
    (b) from the cervical plexus.
    (c) from the brachial plexus.
    (d) the costoclavicular syndrome.
    (e) median or ulnar nerve compressions.
    (f) myocardial disease.

5. Mechanical
    (a) prolapsed intervertebral disc.
    (b) costoclavicular syndrome (again).
    (c) cervical spondylolisthesis.

6. Tumours
    (a) benign.
    (b) malignant.

7. Miscellaneous
    (a) fractures.
    (b) other direct injury.
    (c) cervical fibrositis.

This list is not meant to be exhaustive but it contains the more important conditions. Some of these are now discussed and are grouped for convenience.

1. DEFORMITY

Cervical spondylolisthesis
In this condition the dens or odontoid process is not firmly fixed to its vertebra and therefore tends to move with the atlas. The reason for this is due to a congenital failure to fuse, to an inflammatory softening of the transverse ligament of the atlas, or there may be instability due to a previous injury. In all of these the upper spinal segment is displaced forwards in relation to the lower ones and thus the spinal canal becomes progressively narrowed with a high risk of compression of the spinal cord developing.

When this condition is present there is always pain. If the condition is congenital, or due to trauma, there is discomfort and stiffness and a flexion deformity will be seen. If the condition is due to inflammation then the head is usually held rigid owing to spasm of the cervical muscles.

Treatment is by immobilisation or surgery but the most important diagnostic feature is merely to consider the possibility that this condition may be present.

The Klippel–Feil syndrome
This is not of itself important and the owner of such a condition may go through life without symptoms. In this condition there is a fusion of one or more vertebrae in the cervical region and this reduces the mobility of the cervical spine. The joints above and below the affected vertebra tend to have a compensatory larger range of movement and for this reason and because of an increased wear and tear, osteoarthritic conditions tend to develop at these levels. Movement becomes limited and painful both above and below the fused vertebra and osteophytes can encroach on the foramina.

Fractured cervical vertebrae
The results of this condition depend on whether the fractured vertebrae

heal in good position or not. This, of course, apart from any damage to the cervical cord or nerve roots themselves at the time of the fracture. If the healing of the vertebra takes place in good position then there is no particular reason for osteoarthritis of the cervical spine to develop at a later date. However, if alignment is not good, then this condition will result and if there is a 'step' in the cervical canal produced by one body not being aligned correctly with that above or below, there may be marked narrowing of the antero-posterior diameter of the cervical spine with resulting myelopathy.

2. INFECTION

Tuberculosis

Tuberculosis is infrequent in Western countries compared to its incidence only 25 years ago, but it must not be forgotten that tuberculosis of the cervical spine, or for that matter of any part of the spine, is a possibility. The pain produced by this condition is persistent and unremitting and can be mistaken for a malignant condition. The bacilli reach the spine by the blood stream from a focus elsewhere in the body. The infection usually begins in the anterior portion of the vertebral body or in the intervertebral disc. Destruction of bone and disc ultimately leads to an anterior collapse with cervical kyphosis. Destruction of this degree would occur in a long-standing case but nowadays this degree of infection would be unusual. In a severe infection the formation of pus would lead to abscess formation and the spinal cord could be damaged by direct pressure of the abscess or from a secondary thrombosis of the blood vessels.

The disease occurs in children and young adults and when the cervical vertebrae are affected there will be pain in the neck and the occipital region aggravated by movement. There may be difficulty in swallowing and possibly an abscess or sinus may appear at the side or back of the neck. Neurological symptoms may be present, the upper limbs being affected first.

When examined, the head is held rigid and the cervical muscles are in spasm. If cervical kyphosis is present, one or more of the spinus processes is more prominent than the others. All movements of the head and neck are restricted and cause pain and there may be tuberculous lesions elsewhere. The radiographs are typical and the E.S.R. is raised.

Pyogenic infection of the cervical spine

This is rare, and as in tuberculous spondylitis there is destruction of bone and the intervertebral disc with or without abscess formation. Again, the spinal cord may be damaged by direct pressure or by thrombosis.

Pyrexia and an acute or sub-acute onset is normal, with the clinical features being very much like those of tuberculous spondylitis but the course of the disease is much more rapid. An infective process somewhere else in the body is usually present. X-rays are typical, showing a local osteoporosis or erosion of bone with reduction of the disc space and possibly new bone formation. The E.S.R. is raised and a polymorphonuclear leucocytosis is usually present.

The treatment of both tubercular spondylitis and pyogenic spondylitis are similar in that the appropriate antibiotic treatment is indicated. The problem may well be that pain and spasm are present in the early stages without there being any indication of an infective process. Possibly the main problem is that which occurs when a tuberculous spondylitis needs distinguishing from a secondary malignant tumour which presents in bone in a very similar fashion.

Cervical fibrositis

This is sometimes known as muscular rheumatism. It is an inclusive term commonly used for a fairly clear-cut clinical condition, characterised by pain and tenderness with associated muscle spasm and stiffness of the muscles at the base of the neck. No other objective sign is present unless the painful syndromes due to a trigger mechanism are included in this term. There seems to be two types of the condition, as when a muscle, its fascia, or its tendon are affected in a diffuse fashion; and secondly, where pain and muscle spasm are due to a trigger mechanism with one small portion of the muscle acting as the trigger point. At the trigger point a nodule is usually found, a so-called rheumatoid nodule which varies from pea size to larger more easily palpated structures.

In the diffuse muscular condition there may be no demonstrable pathology at all or merely a mild inflammation. When hard nodules do develop there may be a demonstrable fibroblastic proliferation producing them. In the cervical region these nodules are often found in the posterior muscles at the base of the neck, the trapezius muscle being notorious in this way. As the trapezius takes its insertion from the nuchal line down to the dorsal vertebral spines and out towards the spine of the scapula, nodules in the cervical trapezius arise over a wide area down from the occipital region to the supra-scapular area.

The outstanding feature in these conditions is that there is pain at the base of the neck posteriorly with radiation towards the shoulder usually on one side but it may occur bilaterally. The pain is inconstant, and may be knife-like or may gradually develop becoming dull and aching. This condition is not of course confined to the cervical region but can occur in any part of the body musculature, however, it is particularly noticeable around the upper and lower limbs girdles.

In muscular rheumatism there is no physical sign to be found except that the muscles are tender on pressure and the treatment is by physiotherapy, local heat, deep massage, and analgesic and anti-inflammatory drugs.

When nodules are found sharp lancinating pain can usually be produced by squeezing or pressing them and the treatment is to inject a local anaesthetic solution combined with a long-acting steroid. Insertion of the needle into the nodule and subsequent injection should produce the typical pain of which the patient complains.

These conditions which are of more or less severe degree can be classified into a general group known as the myofacial pain syndromes. They usually have trigger areas and the pain that is produced by stimulation of the trigger area may bear no relation to its situation. There is usually some muscle spasm when the trigger point is stimulated. Again treatment is by injection of the trigger point, local heat, physiotherapy, and so on.

These rheumatic conditions have to be distinguished from the pain and stiffness in the shoulder that is the early symptom of the frozen shoulder. In addition referred pain down the arm and in the shoulder occurs from irritation in the acromio-clavicular joints and in the supra-spinatous and other tendons. Appropriate treatment needs to be given for these.

Cervical glands
When present these can produce diffuse pain in a similar fashion to trigger nodules, presumably from a chronic non-suppurative infection, developing around the glands and affecting local structures. These painful structures can be treated by injection into and around them as for the trigger nodules provided of course that a diagnosis has been made, or rather that all other conditions have been excluded.

Osteoarthritis of the cervical spine
Also known as cervical spondylosis, but more accurately should be called spondylosis deformans. This is the term invented by Schmorl for the reactive changes in the spine which are the responses to degeneration of the intervertebral discs. The underlying pathology is due to alteration of the bone close to the disc with over-growth of bone around its margins. These overgrowths are known as osteophytes. Some authorities use the term spondylosis deformans to describe the clinical syndrome or

rather syndromes which result from the bony abnormalities. These abnormalities of the intervertebral discs are discussed elsewhere.

3. ARTHRITIS

Rheumatoid arthritis
There are a large number of inflammatory arthropathies of which the most commonly known is rheumatoid arthritis. This is a chronic non-bacterial inflammation of the joints associated with constitutional symptoms. There are other conditions in this group such as Stills disease which is confined to children and in which the spleen and lymphatic glands are enlarged; and Reiter's syndrome which has the combination of urethritis, arthritis, conjunctivitis, and hyperkeratotic eruptions of the skin; lupus erythematosus with its scaly erythema of the face or other parts of the body; and psoriasis. There are many others totalling over 150 different varieties but rheumatoid arthritis is the most common and in this disease the patient develops pain at some stage of the condition.

The disease lasts for a variable period and usually burns itself out in time but this time can be very long indeed and sometimes activity lasts throughout life. In this condition the synovial membrane of the joint is thickened by chronic inflammatory changes and the articular cartilage is softened and eroded. Eventually the joint is permanently damaged with small erosions of the bone end. Inflammatory nodules can form in the soft tissues and, in the hands tendons may become softened and may rupture and in this way deformity of the fingers is increased.

The patients are young or middle-aged and any joint can be affected though the peripheral joints in the hands, wrists, and feet are more usually affected than the spine or shoulders. The onset of the disease is gradual with initial pain and swelling of one joint but other joints are similarly affected in time. One of the particular features of this disease is that pain and stiffness are worse after inactivity and the patients are much worse on waking up in the morning and often dread the first hour of the day.

Some features of this disease can be grouped separately. Pain is present in joints and the surrounding tissues due to the inflamed tissues and there is also local pain on movement due to the articular tissues being altered and eventually disorganised. There is a systemic illness, the features of which are more or less obvious depending on the stage of activity of the disease but fever, tachycardia, loss of appetite and weight, and anaemia are not uncommon. Another feature is the anxiety and depression which is often present and is a result of the condition probably being due to its prolonged and chronic nature and the ineffectiveness of treatment. There are extra-articular rheumatic changes such as the subcutaneous nodules already mentioned; and an arteritis which is common and usually symptomless but occasionally affects the digital vessels producing gangrene in the fingers and nail beds. A peripheral neuropathy can develop, while episcleritis, ititis, and uveitis occur in some cases. Pleurisy with or without effusion and pericarditis are also seen. Valvular incompetence of the heart due to an endocarditis may be present, and renal involvement can develop.

The disease is mainly one of temperate climates and women are affected three times as frequently as men, the usual age of onset being between 25 and 55. There is usually a disorder of immunity in rheumatoid arthritis patients in that in the serum of most of them is the rheumatoid factor. This is an Igm globulin which reacts with human Igg antigen provided that the antigen is aggregated or fixed to particles such as latex balls, or red cells. It is believed that the rheumatoid factor does not cause rheumatoid arthritis but actually develops because of the disease. Rheumatoid arthritis is probably caused by circulating immune complexes but the reason for their development is unknown. The treatment of rheumatoid arthritis as might be expected from the multiplicity of signs and symptoms are both general and specific. Rest, sleep, and diet are important and the anaemia should be corrected. In the acute phase immobilisation of the affected joint is best but it is important that immobilisation does not mean fixation and passive movements of the affected joints must be carried out regularly. Wasting of muscles should be prevented but cannot be avoided in many cases because of the stiffness and pain in the joints. As soon as possible, active movements are carried out and these movements may be helped by local injections of steroids.

Sometimes operative treatment is useful, for instance, synovectomy is sometimes recommended at a fairly early stage of the disease. Radical operations can be used where superimposed osteoarthritic changes are present and for instance, arthroplasty may give satisfactory results. Often arthrodesis is the operation of choice and there are various operations used on the hand for correction of finger deformities or for tendon repair. Usually, the patient with rheumatoid arthritis appears at the Pain Clinic at a late stage in the disease, often in an old and rather decrepit female. Usually, pain arises from deformities of the hips and knees (particularly in the hips), and their mobility is seriously impaired by pain and contractions. There is not very much that can be done at this stage but if it is pain in the hip which is causing the problem then the block around the hip joint mentioned elsewhere can be tried. Sometimes and exceptionally, when only one hip is affected in an old patient who otherwise would be fairly mobile a percutaneous cervical cordotomy can be used if no orthopaedic measure is available. The danger of a cordotomy under these circumstances is that the patient may live beyond the time at which the cordotomy begins to wear off, or that the patient uses their new-found freedom from pain for greatly increased activity which may disorganise the already damaged joint. In this way, it is possible to produce a Charcot type of joint.

Specific treatment in these patients consists initially in the use of the salicylates which are analgesic drugs and in large doses are also anti-inflammatory. One of the problems with this type of drug is that irritation of the gastric mucosa occurs and nausea, vomiting, and haemorrhage is possible. Sometimes the drug Benorylate can be used. When this is absorbed it splits up in the blood stream into its constituent parts of salicylate and paracetamol. With most analgesic drugs there is a personal idiosyncrasy to some of them and it is worth trying different ones to find the best for that particular patient.

Other anti-inflammatory analgesics are Indomethacin but sometimes this causes headaches, peptic ulceration, and mental disturbance. The dose is 25 mg daily, increasing to 25 mg three times daily or it can be given as 100 mgm suppository at night.

Phenylbutazone 100 mg t.d.s. can produce gastric bleeding, blood dyscrasias, and rashes.

The steroid hormones are very effective in relieving these symptoms but when withdrawn relapse may occur and in prolonged use may have many side effects.

Gold, Chloroquine, and Penicillamine have all been used, sometimes in combination with those already mentioned.

Ankylosing spondylitis
The incidence of this disease is ten times as frequent in men as in women, usually beginning between 15 and 35 years. There seems to be a familial tendency not only with this disease but there may be mixtures with different members of one family having ankylosing spondylitis; non-specific urethritis; and for instance, Behcet's syndrome. The diagnosis of ankylosing spondylitis depends upon the X-ray appearance of lesions in the sacro-iliac joints.

The earliest changes are widening of the joints with blurring of the joint margins. Sclerosis of the sacrum and ilium follows and eventually destruction of joint spaces occur. The spine is affected and eventually all the vertebrae are joined by bone forming the so-called 'bamboo' spine (see Figs. 12 and 13).

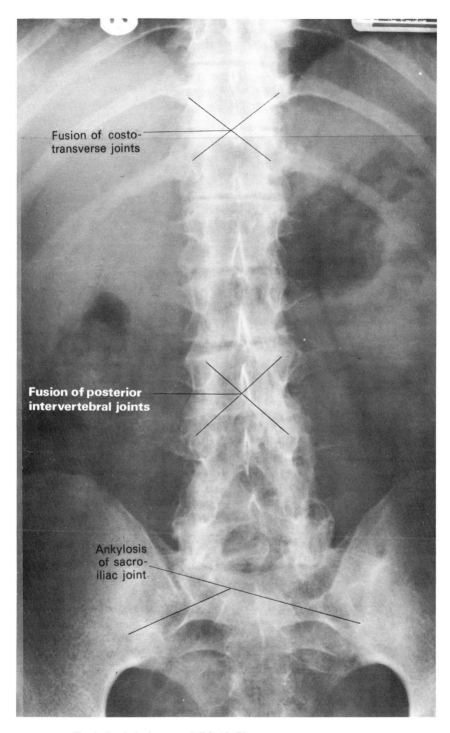

Fusion of costo-
transverse joints

Fusion of posterior
intervertebral joints

Ankylosis
of sacro-
iliac joint

FIGURE 12. Typical ankylosing spondylitis (A–P).

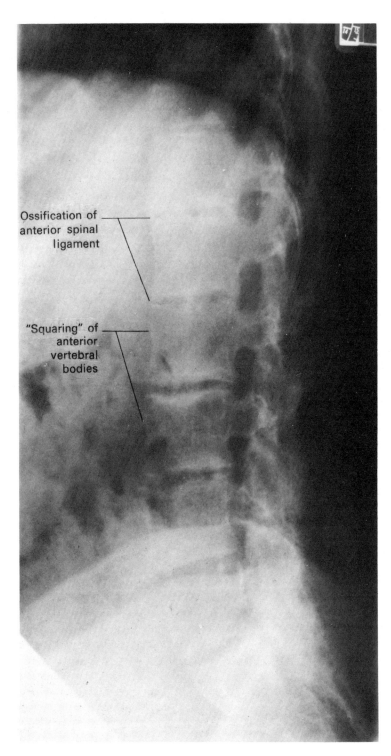

Ossification of anterior spinal ligament

"Squaring" of anterior vertebral bodies

FIGURE 13. Lateral view of Fig. 12.

The initial complaint is usually of low back pain. The patient is usually woken from their sleep in the morning and the condition is associated with a general stiffness of the spine. Iritis is common in about 20 per cent of patients and non-specific urethritis is frequent. Apart from loss of mobility of the lumbar spine, a common feature is that the respiratory excursion is poor, the patient having less than two inches of expansion. The heart can be involved and if so, aortic regurgitation is the commonest feature, the aortic valve being the one most commonly affected. As in rheumatoid arthritis, the E.S.R. is very high in the active stage of the disease and there is an anaemia.

At one time radiotherapy to the affected joints was used as this arrests or retards the condition but it is used much less nowadays because of the recognition that this increases the incidence of leukaemia. The cortico-steroids will give good relief but tend to be kept for the acute exacerbations only. Physiotherapy is important to reduce ankylosis and deformity and to maintain posture, and drug therapy is used to give relief of pain. The drugs of value are the same as those used for rheumatoid arthritis but there is one important difference between these two conditions in that exercise is useful and is in fact mandatory for the ankylosing spondylitis patient. Often it is the damage to their hips which produces the most difficult problem for these patients as they are often young male patients. Hip replacements have much to offer them.

Osteoarthritis

Osteoarthritis is due to wear and tear occurring in joints that have been damaged in one way or another. It is a degenerative process and the joints have usually been affected by a congenital defect, or by age, or by a deficient blood supply, or from a previous injury or disease. It is the commonest variety of arthritis.

The term arthrosis is also applied to this condition (osteoarthrosis) but this word strictly means an osteoarthritis where the changes in the joint cause actual symptoms such as pain or stiffness, a restricted range of move-ment or some other disability.

Usually, osteoarthritis is a condition produced during ageing by normal or abnormal use of the joint. This produces wear and tear on the cartilage which shows increasing evidence of degeneration from about twenty years of age onwards.

Obviously, the more highly stressed a joint is the more likely it is that its cartilage will degenerate. This means that the rather lightly stressed joints in the upper limbs are in general terms less prone to osteoarthritis and arthrosis than the more heavily stressed joints of the lower limb. Often the degenerative process has a predisposing cause which increases the damage produced from wear and tear.

The disease presents in the older patient, most of them being beyond middle age. When it occurs in the younger patient there is usually some reason such as a previous injury or disease of the joint. It develops slowly with pain increasing gradually over months and years. Movements become more and more restricted and deformation of some joints commonly occurs in the later stages. When affected joints are examined and moved, there is usually palpable or audible coarse crepitation. A fixed deformity may occur in any affected joint but is most often noticed in the hip joint.

Osteoarthritis can be classified into two types, the first of which is polyarticular degenerative arthritis of unknown aetiology. This is active in several joints at the same time and rarely occurs in early adult life. Secondly is a monarticular arthritis which is usually due to an injury producing mechanical derangement or abnormality of the joint. A congenital anomaly or a pyogenic infection in the joint will also produce this type.

The predisposing causes which increase the wear and tear on the joint cartilage are:

(1) An abnormal congenital development which places the joint surfaces at a mechanical disadvantage.
(2) Old age due to a reduced capacity for cartilage repair.
(3) An irregular joint surface from previous injury such as a fracture.
(4) Internal derangements such as a torn meniscus in the knee.
(5) Disease of the joint which leaves a damaged articular surface.
(6) A misalignment of the joint.
(7) Obesity which increases the mechanical stress on the joint due to the increased weight carried. This applying particularly to the weight-bearing joints.

The pathology in osteoarthritis is straightforward. Articular cartilage is slowly worn away and eventually underlying bone becomes exposed. This bone becomes hard and glossy from use as joint surface, the process being known as eburnation. At the same time, bone at the margin of the joint hypertrophies and forms a rim of projecting spurs known as osteophytes. There is a slight thickening and fibrosis of the capsule and synovial membrane of the affected joint but this is not a primary change being due to the continuous strains to which such a joint is exposed.

The course of the disease is very slow and in many cases does not require any treatment at all. In most patients the increasing pain, stiffness, and deformity is of an order which is best treated by conservative measures. But where these are severe, operative treatment is indicated. In general, treatment should start first with the simpler methods which means analgesics and anti-inflammatory agents should be used. These can then be combined with rest, perhaps with splinting and supports. Rest should be limited as otherwise movement will become progressively reduced. Therefore exercises with active and passive movements are required. Local treatment by heat and ice, and injections are useful adjuvants and when indicated should be tried. The use of sedatives and anxiolytic agents also has a place and as a final treatment surgery can be considered. At present, a most useful surgical technique in severe chronic osteoarthritis affecting the hip is the Charnley hip replacement.

The particular problems of osteoarthritis in the cervical and lumbar regions will be discussed separately.

4. REFERRED PAIN

Cervical rib

Sometimes there is a congenital over-development of the costal process of the seventh cervical vertebra. This over-development can be either bony or fibrous and when it is bony it is seen on X-ray as an extra or cervical rib. It may be present without causing any symptoms whatsoever, but it can cause both neurological and vascular problems in the upper limbs. This condition, because it is congenital, must be present from early life but it may not produce symptoms until there is drooping of the shoulder girdle which occurs in later adult life.

Cervical ribs can be unilateral or bilateral and can be quite small or of large dimensions. Their importance is that the subclavian artery and the lowest trunk of the brachial plexus arch over this extra rib and in some cases the nerve trunk is damaged at the point of pressure against it. The vascular changes are probably caused in a similar fashion by local damage to the subclavian artery. The flow of blood within this artery may be reduced in its peripheral portion, and it can thrombose, or emboli may be produced down the damaged portion.

It is certainly true that the lowest trunk of the brachial plexus and the subclavian artery will arch over a cervical rib if it is large enough but sometimes when the rib is not complete, there is a fibrous band occupying the position it would have occupied and symptoms are produced by this.

Thus there are neurological manifestations of which the main symptoms are pain and paraesthesiae in the forearm and hand. These are most severe towards the ulnar side of the hand and may be relieved temporarily by altering the position of the hand and arm. Motor symptoms will also be present and an increasing weakness of the hand develops. The distribution of the neurological deficit bears a relation to the lower trunk of the brachial plexus but does not follow the distribution of the peripheral nerves.

Usually the vascular features are not marked but can be severe at times, the radial pulse being weak or absent.

As mentioned previously, the presence of a cervical rib does not necessarily produce symptoms so it must not be assumed that symptoms in the upper limb are due to a cervical rib when one is demonstrated radiologically. Other causes of pain and paraesthesiae, of muscle wasting in the hand, and of other reasons for peripheral vascular changes, have to be considered. The differential diagnosis is very wide and amongst other conditions will be included tumours of the spinal cord and its roots, cervical spondylolisthesis, cervical spondylosis and prolapsed cervical disc, neuritis of the brachial plexus, ulnar neuritis, and median nerve carpal tunnel syndrome. Injuries round the shoulder joint and such conditions as subacromial bursitis will also need consideration, while the circulatory signs need to be distinguished from Raynaud's disease.

Treatment will depend on the severity of the symptoms but it is unlikely that developed neurological signs will disappear unless pressure on the brachial plexus is relieved. This is usually done by releasing the scalenus anticus muscle and the abnormal rib. Its fibrous extension are often removed as well.

Conservative treatment can be tried first and is designed to relieve any spasm of the scalenus anticus which is present. It can be injected regularly with local anaesthetics and at the same time, the usual treatments of physiotherapy, diathermy, massage, and exercises to strengthen the shoulder girdle are adopted.

Scalenus syndrome
Sometimes without radiological evidence of a cervical rib being present, the characteristic neuralgia and other neurological signs of a cervical rib syndrome are produced. The brachial plexus and the subclavian artery occupy the base of a triangle between the scalenus anticus muscle anteriorly and the middle scalenus muscle behind it with the upper surface of the first rib as the base. If for any reason the scalenus anticus goes into spasm or becomes hypertrophied, the space between the two muscles is reduced and

the scalenus syndrome is produced. This is the reason for trying local anaesthetic injections into the muscle.

Another mechanism is if the middle scalene muscle is pushed anteriorly, then again the space is narrowed. Sometimes a tough, fibrous band has been demonstrated in this muscle which causes kinking of the lower trunk of the brachial plexus.

The symptoms of a prolapsed cervical disc particularly at the C7-T1 level and the cervical rib or scalenus syndrome are very similar but can often be distinguished by the fact that wry neck and loss of sensation involving the thumb and index finger does not occur in the scalene syndrome.

Treatment is as for cervical rib and if conservative measures do not help the tendon of the scalenus anticus muscle is divided.

5. COSTO-CLAVICULAR SYNDROMES

Complete tear of the rotator cuff
The term rotator cuff refers to the rotator cuff of the shoulder joint. This is a tendinous cuff which comprises the supraspinatus tendon together with adjoining flat tendons which blend with it. These additional tendons are the infraspinatous posteriorly and the sub-scapularis anteriorly and they form a structure above the shoulder joint that is sometimes called the rotator cuff.

This tendinous cuff can give way under a sudden strain and often there is a pre-disposing degeneration of the tendon, usually due to age, also present. The tear tends to be mainly in the supraspinatus tendon but it can extend into the adjacent anterior and posterior tendons of sub-scapularis and infraspinatous. The tear is close to the insertion of these tendons and usually involve the capsule of the joint with which the tendons blend. The edges of this tear retract, leaving a hole which communicates between the shoulder joint and the sub-acromial bursa.

The patient is often a man over 60 and the history is that after falling, he complains of pain at the tip of the shoulder and down the upper arm and is unable to raise the arm. On examination, there is tenderness below the acromion and when the patient attempts to abduct the arm, no movement occurs at the gleno-humeral joint, but 40-60° of abduction is achieved by scapular movement. There is a full range of passive movement and if the arm is abducted beyond 90°, the patient can continue the abduction by the action of the deltoid.

The characteristic feature in cases of torn supraspinatus tendon is thus an inability to initiate the gleno-humeral abduction.

In young patients operation is usually undertaken to suture the tear, but in the older patient, operation is often avoided.

There are a number of injuries which occur in this area of the body of varying severity. They tend to form a series with one condition merging into the next. There are, however, some well defined entities amongst them and these are described now.

The supraspinatus syndrome

This is a clinical syndrome, sometimes called the painful arc syndrome in which there is pain in the shoulder and upper arm through the mid range of gleno-humeral abduction. There is freedom from pain at the beginning of the abduction and beyond 90°. It is a syndrome which occurs in a number of distinct shoulder lesions and in some respects is similar to the complete tear of the rotator cuff.

The pain is produced when a tender structure is nipped between the tuberosity of the humerus and the acromion process or possibly the coraco-acromial ligament. Normally, there is a small distance between the upper end of the humerus and the acromion process when the arm is abducted and this is particularly so in the range of abduction between about 45° and 160°. If a swollen structure is present beneath the acromion during this abduction, it may become nipped and this produces pain. With the arm in a neutral position or in full abduction the pain is either absent or reduced as there is increased clearance between the joint tissues. There are four principal conditions which give rise to this syndrome and these are:

(1) An injury to the greater tuberosity which may produce either a contusion or a fracture.

(2) There may be a minor tear of a supraspinatus tendon with the tearing of a few tendon fibres producing an inflammatory action with local swelling. However, impairment of the muscle action is unaltered as the tear in the tendinous cuff is incomplete.

(3) Supraspinatus tendinitis is the condition where there is an inflammatory reaction and sometimes a calcified deposit is present in the supra-spinatus tendon which can be seen on X-ray. This causes an inflammatory reaction in that part of the tendon where the deposit forms.

(4) Finally, there is a sub-acromial bursitis where the walls of the bursa are inflamed and thickened from mechanical irritation.

All these conditions have the same features which vary only in degree.

When the arm is against the body, pain is absent and during abduction pain begins at about 45° and persists throughout the whole arc of movement up to about 160°. After that the pain decreases or disappears. As the arm is lowered again, pain is felt in this middle range once more. The patient often develops trick movements which enable them to get the arm above their head and down to their side again without pain or without too much pain. The pain, however, can be so acute that the patient is unwilling to lift their arm under any circumstances.

Treatment of mild cases is not necessary as they are self-limiting. Mild activity and mobilising exercises combined with short-wave diathermy are beneficial for most of them, but if the condition is due to a calcified deposit the pain is intense and it may be necessary to incise the tendon or possibly aspirate the deposit. Various operations are used for the chronic case, the simplest method being to excise the acromion process up to the acromio-clavicular joint which prevents any nipping of inflamed tissues.

It is always worthwhile to inject a mixture of a local anaesthetic and a long-acting steroid into the sub-acromial bursa and the rotator cuff. This can be repeated at intervals in the milder chronic case, or can be used to accelerate recovery in the milder acute cases.

Rupture of the long tendon of biceps
Like the supraspinatus tendon, the long tendon of the biceps is prone to rupture without any violent stress or injury to it. This tendon does not rupture under ordinary stresses unless it has already been weakened. Degeneration due to age is the predisposing factor but this is probably increased by constant friction at the point where the tendon enters the bicipical groove of the humerus.

As in rupture of the supraspinatus, the patient is usually a man of about 60 or more and during active lifting or pulling he feels 'something giving way' in the front of the shoulder. A bulge of muscle is noted in front of the arm when the biceps muscle is contracted. Repair of the tendon is not usually necessary but can be carried out to help in flexing the forearm. The disability produced is surprisingly little and treatment is not necessary.

Biceps tendinitis
This condition corresponds to the supraspinatus tendinitis but does not produce such a severe disability as that condition does. The patient has pain in the front of the shoulder which is worse when the arm is used, and examination shows tenderness to pressure over the course of the long tendon of the biceps and particularly where it lies in the bicipical groove.

Short wave diathermy, a sling and avoidance of movement allows the condition to settle down. In addition or alternatively, injection of a local anaesthetic combined with a long-acting steroid made into the tender area in the bicipical groove often helps.

Frozen shoulder

This is sometimes called adhesive capsulitis or peri-arthritis of the gleno-humeral joint. There is pain and limitation of all the movements of the shoulder joint and although there is a tendency for spontaneous recovery to occur, this is slow and some patients who develop this condition never recover a full range of movement afterwards.

The cause of the condition is unknown but there seems to be a diffuse, inflammatory process involving the soft tissues around the gleno-humeral joint. Any condition which restricts the activity of the joint can produce a frozen shoulder and thus it may follow injury from a fall or fracture, or follow a tendinitis or bursitis or there may be no obvious injury present at all. It sometimes occurs after such conditions as a coronary thrombosis or cervical spondylosis which produce a restriction of shoulder movement through pain. There are many other causes, but they all seem to have some element of passivity of the patient in addition. In the early stages the shoulder is placed at rest with the arm in a sling, but passive movements must be carried out regularly to avoid adhesions and subsequent stiffness. When movement of the joint has been reduced for long periods, it may be necessary to manipulate it before active exercises can be used.

However, in the early stages, regular sympathetic block of the stellate ganglion or blocks of the suprascapular nerve or injections into the sub-acromial bursal may be effective when combined with physiotherapy.

The carpal tunnel syndrome

The carpal tunnel syndrome produces a compression of the median nerve within the carpal tunnel. It occurs five times more frequently in women than in men. Any condition which reduces the carpal tunnel capacity can produce the symptoms. Thus the condition is common when trauma or infection to or near the carpal tunnel produces oedema. Further any tumour occupying this space, such as a ganglion or lipoma, will also produce the syndrome. Conditions producing water retention such as obesity, diabetes, and pregnancy can all develop the condition. The most frequent symptom is paraesthesiae in the distribution of the median nerve and there is usually atrophy of the thenar muscles.

In mild cases symptomatic treatment can be used and a short period of immobilisation combined with injections of hydrocortisone into the carpal tunnel often gives relief. When signs and symptoms persist and are progressive the deep transverse carpal ligament is opened up by surgery. In most patients this will relieve the condition but there are some cases which are refractory.

Ulnar tunnel syndrome
Just as there may be pressure on the median nerve in the carpal tunnel syndrome, so there is an equivalent ulnar tunnel syndrome which results from compression of the ulnar nerve in a fibro-osseus tunnel at the wrist.

Tennis elbow
The condition called tennis elbow is probably not a single entity but a number of conditions, all of which produce pain and tenderness on the lateral side of the elbow. They often arise after an injury on the lateral side of the elbow, the patient reporting that they carried out a particular action and felt pain in their elbow immediately. It can also occur over a longer period presumably due to successive small traumas. Exactly what damage the injury produces is still under discussion but it is simplest to believe that it is due to one or more tears within the common tendon of origin of the extensor muscles. The alternative is to believe that it is a peri-osteitis produced by repeated sprains. In either of these cases injection of a local anaesthetic with or without a long-acting steroid into the painful region should relieve the pain. Unfortunately, this does not occur in all cases.

Other explanations of the cause of the tennis elbow are that there is an inflammation of an adventitous bursa, that there are calcified deposits within the common extendor tendon near the epicondyle, or that the annular ligament is responsible for the pain.

There are two other possibilities in that there can be hypertrophy of the synovium between the head of the radius and the capitulum and, secondly, that the pain may arise from the radial nerve which is anterior to the neck of the radius. There are other possibilities for pain in this region such as the musculo-skeletal syndromes at the shoulder joint.

The majority of patients with a tennis elbow obtain relief from simple measures such as rest and local therapy. Injections of local anaesthetics with long-acting steroids, when made into the point of maximum tenderness near the epicondyle help many patients but not all. It is certainly worthwhile repeating these injections when partial relief only is obtained.

The movements causing pain are those when supination and then pronation are performed with the wrist extended. This is a movement which is particularly valuable to tennis players but is an action which is used as much in work as in play.

If local treatment does not help then there are surgical procedures which can be tried if the pain and disability is severe.

6. MECHANICAL

Cervical intervertebral discs and the various ways in which they can produce pain are fully discussed in the chapter on the intervertebral disc (see Chapter 6). This material is not repeated here.

Some of the subjects of sections 6 and 7 of the classification have been mentioned. It is not proposed to expand them further.

REFERENCES

British Medical Journal. Editorial (1977) Pathogenesis of osteoarthrosis. *B.M.J.* 2, 979–980.
British Medical Journal. Editorial (1977) Painful shoulder and painful arcs. *B.M.J.* 2, 913–914.
DePalma A.F. (1957) The painful shoulder. *Postgrad. Med.* 21, 368.
Friedlander H.L., Reid R.L. & Cape R.F. (1967.) Tennis elbow. In *Clinical orthopaedics and related research*. Vol. 51. (Ed.) Urist, M.R. Philadelphia, J.B. Lippincott.
Moseley H.F. (1951). Ruptures of the rotator cuff. *Br. J. Surg.* 38, 340.
Wilson C.L. (1943) Lesions of the supraspinatus tendon; degeneration, rupture and calcification. *Arch. Surg.* 46, 307.
Young H.H., Ward L.E. & Henderson E.D. (1954) The use of hydrocortisone acetate (compound F) and the treatment of some common orthopaedic conditions. *J. Bone Joint Surgery*, 36-A, 602.

FURTHER REFERENCES

Hart F. Dudley (1975) Inflammatory disease and its control in rheumatic disorders. *B.M.J.* 4, 191–194. (32 useful references).

Chapter 6
The Intervertebral Disc

ANATOMY OF THE DISC

A normal disc can be divided into three parts, these being the cartilage plates, the nucleus pulposus, and the annulus fibrosus. The cartilaginous plates are connected to both the vertebral body and to the disc, and consist of hyaline cartilage. They merge on one side with the cancellous bone and on the other side with the nucleus pulposus. Towards the periphery they merge with the annulus.

The nucleus pulposus is the centre of the disc and consists of soft resilient fibro-cartilage. In the cervical and dorsal region the centre of the disc and the centre of the nucleus pulposus coincide, but in the lumbar region the centre of the nucleus pulposus is a little posterior to the centre of the disc.

The nucleus pulposus is incompressible but is readily deformable. It contains a loose network of fine fibrous strands between which are connective tissue and cartilage cells. The lower cervical discs have a volume of about 1 to 1·4 cm³ with a nucleus pulposus of about 0·2 cm³. A lumbar disc has a volume of about 10 cm³ and its nucleus has a volume of about 1·4 cm³.

The annulus fibrosus is the outer portion of the disc and gives it its shape and size. It is the strongest portion of the disc and serves to transmit tension throughout the spine. The attachments of the annulus fibrosus are extremely strong. Its deeper layers merge into the marginal lip of the vertebral body, while the superficial layers fuse with the periosteum of the outer surface of the vertebral body, actually fusing to the periosteum. Anteriorly and laterally the outer layers of the annulus fibrosus are indistinguishable from those of the anterior longitudinal ligament. Thus the anterior ligament and the disc provide a strong flexible connection between adjacent vertebrae. This is so strong that, in health, bone is much more likely to fracture than the ligament and annulus are likely to tear.

Posteriorly the annulus structure is not as strong as anteriorly and correspondingly the annulus fibrosus is weaker posteriorly. The posterior longitudinal ligament is less well developed than the anterior longitudinal ligament. It is much narrower and more open in its structure.

In health there are no blood vessels in the intervertebral disc, its nourishment occurs largely by diffusion from the adjacent cancellous bone of the centre of the vertebral body. A healthy nucleus pulposus has a high proportion of water which decreases as the years pass. From infancy to old age the percentage varies from about 90 per cent to about 70 per cent. It is this high proportion of water that makes the nucleus pulposus incompressible.

Inside the nucleus pulposus the pressure is usually high and this arises in two ways. Partly from the annulus fibrosus but also by such activities as the erect posture, muscular contraction, and by flexion of the spine.

The intervertebral discs render the spine flexible and resilient and allow movement to take place. Different parts of the disc have different functions. The annulus has strength with limited mobility whilst the nucleus pulposus separates the vertebrae and provides a frictionless mechanism acting somewhat as a ball-bearing. It absorbs shocks and its incompressibility transmits applied forces through the axis of the spine.

An important feature in the function of the disc is its degree of hydration. Normal hydration is necessary for normal width and normal function and where nutrition fails through destruction of vascular tissue near the cartilaginous plate the intervertebral disc space narrows.

The intervertebral discs also alter with age and again this is related to reduction in water content. However, this process can occur at a much earlier age, occasionally while the patients are in their teens. When this happens dehydration alters the normal functions of the nucleus pulposus which changes so that it is no longer incompressible. The nucleus pulposus is the first portion of the disc to deteriorate. Loss of nucleus pulposus material leads to inability to absorb shocks, to a narrowing of the intervertebral space, and eventually to degeneration of the annulus. The nucleus pulposus shrinks and becomes degenerated and thus the intervertebral space narrows so that the annulus fibres become loose. This causes slight bulging of the annulus beyond the edges of the vertebral bodies and reactive changes in the bone of the adjacent vertebrae.

There is a tendency for adjacent vertebrae to slide upon the loose tissue of the degenerating disc and sometimes this can be seen radiologically in the cervical region.

THE CERVICAL DISC

The degenerative disc bulges in all directions even vertically through the cartilaginous plate into the bone-forming Schmorl's node. Bulges in the anterior and lateral directions do not matter, but if local bulging occurs posteriorly it can encroach upon the intervertebral foramina or the spinal canal. This prolapse or herniation of the disc may press on nerve roots or spinal cord and these prolapses are produced by what is called the soft disc.

There is considerable controversy with the ethiology of the second type of disc lesion which is called the hard disc. Other names used for this particular type are osteophytes, hypertrophic bars or spurs, and cervical spondylosis. It is possible that this hard type of disc lesion is a later stage of the soft type.

When the intervertebral disc becomes degenerated the bone is no longer cushioned against the usual stresses and the vertebral body tends to expand and mushrooms out. The transverse surface of the vertebral body becomes irregular and a reactive sclerosis develops which can be seen in radiographs, as a dense margin to the intervertebral disc space. The edge of the intervertebral surface develops outgrowths of bone and transverse osteoarthritic bars or ridges in the mid-line posteriorly can arise and impinge to varying degrees upon the spinal cord. Laterally there may be osteophytes which compress the nerve roots.

Osteophytes are more common on the lateral margins rather than anteriorly or posteriorly. This probably being due to the effect of the two longitudinal ligaments. In the cervical region development of osteophytes is common within the spinal canal after middle age and these osteophytes may well interfere with spinal cord function and press upon nerve roots. In the cervical region osteophytes commonly encroach upon the intervertebral foramina compressing the nerves and the radicular arteries and by protruding between the transverse processes may even interfere with the vertebral artery.

It should be noted that at the edges the bodies of the cervical vertebrae articulate with the discs, the joint being known as the neurocentral or Luschka's joint. These joints are frequently the seat of degenerative changes and osteophytes developing here lie immediately anterior to the cervical nerve root and medial to the vertebral artery.

Spondylosis deformans produces alterations in the curvatures of the spine, usually accentuating the normal curves. The cervical spine is hyperextended to a greater or lesser degree and in severe cases the neck is shortened. This is in part due to the loss of intervertebral disc substance as the discs provide about $\frac{1}{5}$ to $\frac{1}{4}$ of the total length of the spine, and partly owing to the lordosis. This results in the laminae overriding each other and in addition the ligamentum flavum bulges into the posterior part of the spinal cord diminishing its capacity further. The relationships between the nerve roots, the nerve sheaths, and the intervertebral foramina are altered and it is possibly this alteration which accounts for some of the symptoms.

As previously mentioned spondylosis deformans produces transverse osteoarthritic bars in the mid-line which posteriorly press upon the anterior spinal cord and nerve roots. If there are laterally placed osteophytes present as well the nerve roots may also be compressed.

Post-mortem measurements of normal and spondylotic spines show differences in the cervical region. The normal spine has an antero-posterior diameter of approximately 14·3 mm, on average, while spondylotic spines with myelopathy are about 3·0 mm less than this. A radiological examination of the cervical subarachnoid space using Myodil (Iophendylate B.P.) will show whether narrowing is present, whether there is free flow of the Myodil, or whether spondylotic ridges are pressing upon the spinal cord. The measurements given above were taken at the narrowest antero-posterior diameter of the cervical spine and were measurements made at post-mortem. However, estimations of the antero-posterior diameter of the cervical spinal canal can be made by X-ray examination and under these conditions the diameter in normal adults can vary by as much as 7 mm.

It will be seen that in the so-called soft disc, which is a rupture of the annulus fibrosus with extrusion of portions of the nucleus pulposus, the rupture can be located in the mid-line, para-centrally, or laterally. When in the mid-line cord compression can be produced, when para-centrally both cord compression or nerve root compression or both can occur and if it protrudes laterally it produces nerve root compression. The level in the cervical spine at which the protrusion occurs decides the type of symptoms the patient develops. These patients all complain of pain down the arm which is due to compression of the nerve root itself. Thus in ruptures of the fifth and sixth cervical discs the pain is down the lateral aspect of the upper arm and dorsum of the forearm. If the protrusion lies between C5 and C6 vertebrae with compression of the cervical sixth nerve root then there is pain in the neck, shoulder, the medial border of the scapula, the lateral aspect of the arm, and dorsum of the forearm. In addition there may be numbness of the thumb and index finger and a mild weakness of the biceps muscle. There will be a decreased or absent biceps jerk.

If the rupture occurs between C6 and C7 with compression of the seventh nerve root the pain produced is essentially the same as in the cervical sixth nerve root, but numbness will be in the index and middle fingers, while there will be marked weakness of the triceps muscle and the triceps jerk will be reduced or absent. The frequency of ruptures of a cervical inter-vertebral disc, compared to the lumbar ones is about 1 to 25. Lesions of the cervical discs between C6 and C7 are about three times as common as those between C5 and C6. Rupture between C4 and C5 involving the fifth nerve root and those between C7 and T1 involving the eighth nerve root are much less frequent but do occur. The lesion between C7 and T1 gives pain in the neck, the medial border of the scapula, the anterior chest, the medial aspect of the upper arm, and forearm. There is numbness of the little and ring fingers and sometimes the middle finger and there may be marked to extreme weakness of the wrist and hand.

Treatment depends on whether there have been irreversible changes due to myelopathy, whether there is pressure on nerve roots which can be relieved, or whether it can prevent further deterioration. Conservative measures are aimed at immobilising the cervical spine. This prevents flexion and extension movements which produce indentation and deforma-tion of the spinal cord and prevents the intermittent ischaemia that this produces. Oedema of soft tissues may disperse and the spondylosis may not progress further. The latter is rather doubtful as there are very few figures available in the literature as to the effects of conservative treatment.

Two to four weeks traction with skull calipers may be used in those patients who have myelopathy with severe neck pain and brachial neuralgia. A period of traction should normally be followed by immobilisation in a collar. For the patient who does not need traction, the use of a collar is valuable and physiotherapy, heat, and mobilisation all help. Manipulation to overcome stiffness is used when necessary.

Active surgical treatment involves removal of the ruptured disc when it is the soft type of lesion producing the symptoms, but if the condition is due to bony spondylosis and myelopathy then other operations are necessary. Fusion of the intervertebral joint can be carried out by either an anterior or posterior approach with benefit. The Cloward operative approach allows transverse bars to be removed and the foramen to be cleared out. However, if a number of disc spaces require to be treated the posterior approach may be used.

It is possible that the Cloward operation may be used in the most severely affected disc spaces while a laminectomy provides a decompression posteriorly as well.

THE THORACIC DISC

Radiological signs of degeneration in thoracic discs are quite common but there is no great incidence of disease from this cause. The scarcity of these lesions is probably due to the fact that the thoracic spine is less flexible than either the cervical or lumbar spine and is therefore, less likely to be subjected to strain.

Thoracic disc prolapses can produce signs similar to that of cervical disc lesions and, for example, herniation between T1 and T2 will compress the first thoracic nerve root. This produces pain down the medial side of the arm with some numbness and weakness of the intrinsic muscles of the hand. However, the usual symptoms and signs of a thoracic intervertebral disc prolapse are from cord compression. Because of this fact, a definite diagnosis is dependent upon myelography.

Prolapsed thoracic discs can be loosely divided into three groups according to their clinical signs. First, the compression syndrome where symptoms and signs develop is due to this cord compression. These are in no way different from cord compressions due to any other condition such as an intraspinal neoplasm. There is a progressive paraparesis with impairment of all types of sensibility and there is disturbance of the sphincters. Nerve root pain is present and it is possible for a Brown–Sequard syndrome to develop. In addition to the root pain, spinal pain can occur and this as with other disc lesions, is aggravated by movement and is of a deep and boring type.

The second type is a progressive paraparesis and this is usually painful.

Third is the radicular type which has girdle and intercostal pain. The most likely cause of these signs and symptoms is a laterally placed protrusion and this type of disc lesions usually settles with rest and immobilisation.

Treatment of these discs is treatment for the compression syndrome and involves surgery.

THE LUMBAR DISC

This lesion is the most common cause of low back pain and sciatica and occurs more commonly than all the other causes of low back pain put together. In 95 per cent of cases the fourth or fifth lumbar disc, or both, are involved and in most of the rest, it is the third. As the fourth lumbar disc affects the fifth lumbar nerve, and the fifth lumbar disc affects the first sacral nerve, the pain produced is in the distribution of the sciatic nerve. However, these patients also have pain in the back and the precise origin of this pain remains unknown. There is no nerve supply to the interior of the disc while the posterior longitudinal ligament, the other ligaments, the periosteum and capsules of the joints are sensitive. Narrowing of the intervertebral space introduces abnormal stresses to the zygapophyseal joints. An affected root may cause pain in the back through the recurrent branches to the intra-spinal structures and articulations. The posterior primary divisions of the nerve supplies both the muscles and superficial tissues and presumably pain can be referred along this distribution.

Sometimes severe spasm of the erector spinae muscles is produced and when marked can be seen quite easily on observation. The muscles are tender to pressure, resist all movements, and these attempts at movement increase the pain. The mechanical effect of the prolapse upon the nerve root is fairly straightforward. The usual prolapse is in the lateral part of the posterior portion of the annulus fibrosis and is thus near to the intervertebral foramen. It does not, however, press upon the nerve which passes through that particular foramen, but on the next one down. The trapped root crosses the disc and descends under the next lamina leaving the spinal cord below that pedicle and lamina. Normally, an S1 root is affected by an L5/S1 disc prolapse and an L5 root is affected by the L4/5 disc prolapse. In large disc prolapses the prolapse presses upwards on to the foramen and thus will affect that nerve root but this is uncommon, except perhaps in the L5/S1 large disc prolapse, where a large lateral disc may spread upwards toward the foramen containing the L5 nerve root, and this may be affected as well as the S1 root.

Normally, when a nerve root is pressed upon by a prolapse, it can either lie to one side or other of the bulge of the prolapse, or on its apex. The nerve itself is tethered to some extent by the thecal sheath where it leaves the spinal theca. This is known as the axilla of the sheath and if the prolapse presses on the nerve at this point the nerve is completely tethered and cannot move out of the way. Relief of pain can be obtained when the nerve root slips from the apex of the bulge to one side of the bulge and this is probably how relief of pain by mobilisation and manipulation is obtained. The danger, of course, is that the prolapse may increase in size and even become a detached sequestrum by this manoeuvre.

A very large retropulsion of a lumbar prolapsed disc can press upon the cauda equina and will produce weakness of the sphincters. In addition there will be pain in the mid-line of the back and down the posterior thighs and legs, with numbness in the perineum, back of both thighs and legs, and the soles of the feet. There will be paralysis of the feet and weakness or paralysis of the sphincters and there will be absent ankle jerks. Massive mid-line lumbar disc extrusions of this kind usually occur at L4 or L5 (see Figs. 14 and 15). There is often a history of injury immediately or shortly before the

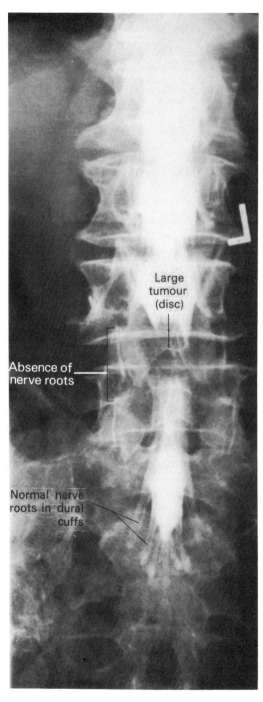

FIGURE 14. Large prolapsed disc in a 77-year-old man who had lifted a 30-foot long tree. (A–P radiculogram).

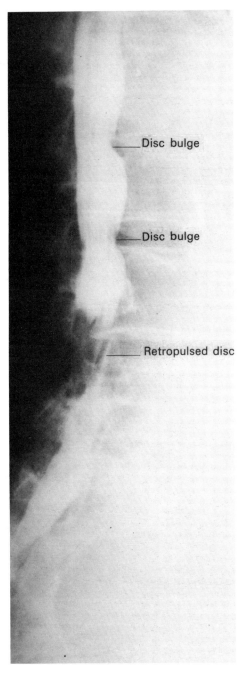

FIGURE 15. The same patient as Fig. 14 (Lateral).

onset of these gross symptoms. This, in fact, holds true for many of the disc prolapses which are often associated with vigorous muscular efforts such as lifting a heavy weight when the spine is flexed. The discs at each level have certain features in common but they also have variations which distinguish between them.

Thus a prolapse between L3 and L4 produces pressure on the fourth nerve root and gives pain in the sacro-iliac joint and the hip, the postero-lateral aspect of the thigh, and the anterior aspect of the leg. There is numbness on the antero-medial portion of the leg with weak extension of the knees. The reflexes are altered, the knee jerk being decreased or absent.

A disc between L4 and L5 compresses the fifth nerve root which produces pain in the sacro-iliac joint and hip, and the postero-lateral aspect of the thigh and the leg. There is numbness on the lateral aspect of the leg or the dorsum of the foot, and this includes the big toe. Weakness involves dorsiflexion of the big toe and sometimes of the foot. There is usually no change in the reflexes.

A ruptured disc between L5 and S1 compresses the first sacral nerve root and this produces pain over the sacro-iliac joint and the hip and the postero-lateral aspect of the thigh, the leg, and the heel. There is numbness on the lateral aspect of the leg and foot which includes the lateral three toes. Weakness is not common in this type of prolapse but if it is present then plantar flexion of the foot and the great toe is reduced. The ankle jerk is reduced or absent.

Treatment of retropulsed discs should be carried out by neurosurgeons or orthopaedic surgeons. Conservative treatment for any patient in severe pain involves total rest on a firm, flat bed and large doses of analgesics will be necessary. The minimum period of bed rest is about three weeks and the patient should not be allowed up to go to toilet. Milder symptoms may respond to simpler measures and in all cases exercises to strengthen the erector spinae muscles should be carried out when the pain has been relieved completely. Lifting weights, particularly with the trunk flexed should be prohibited for at least three months.

Injections are sometimes used, either into muscles which are in spasm, or extradurally to give total relief of pain for a time, and they can be made into the disc itself with Chymopapain (Discase) which digests the disc substance so that it absorbs more easily.

If complete rest fails to relieve the pain or when pain prevents a return to a normal life, operation is indicated. Other indications are when a number of severe prolapses have occurred and expectant treatment has not helped. In particular, any sudden development of neurological signs, paralysis, or disturbance of sphincter control should be regarded as an urgent indication for surgery as it suggests cauda equina compression.

LUMBAR SPONDYLOLISTHESIS

When the term spondylolisthesis is used on its own it always means lumbar spondylolisthesis. It is the name used to describe the spontaneous displacement of one of the lumbar vertebral bodies upon the segment below it. The displacement usually occurs anteriorly but can develop posteriorly.

Normally a lumbar vertebra is held rigidly in place by the anterior and posterior longitudinal ligaments and by the inferior articular processes of an upper vertebra resting on the superior articular processes of the vertebra below. In the main, forward displacement of a vertebral body is prevented by the inferior articular processes impinging on the ones below. If in the development of a lumbar vertebra there is a loss of bony continuity between the superior and inferior articular processes by a defect in ossification, the deficiency is bridged by fibrous tissue. When this stretches and gives way the common variety of spondylolisthesis occurs. The defect occurs in the neural arch of the vertebra and allows separation of the vertebra into two portions. The body with the pedicles and the superior articular processes, and of course the spinal column above it, slides forwards leaving behind the laminae and the inferior articular processes.

The fifth lumbar vertebra is the one usually affected but the fourth has this defect on occasion. Usually although a major displacement can occur there is a relatively minor irritation to the nerves. This produces a sciatica.

There are two other types of spondylolisthesis which may develop and in one of these types the posterior intervertebral joints are osteoarthritic and become unstable due to degeneration of the articular cartilage. This type can occur at any level in the lumbar spine but again is most common in the lower lumbar vertebrae, particularly between the fourth and fifth lumbar vertebrae. This type of spondylolisthesis may displace backwards instead of forwards. Neurological disturbance is quite unusual in this type, the displacement is not marked.

The least common type is where the posterior intervertebral joints are congenitally unstable because of malformation of the articular processes which are rudimentary. This variety occurs most frequently at the lumbosacral joint and the whole spinal column may move forward on the sacrum. The neural arch remains with the lumbar vertebra and thus the cauda equina can be trapped producing a cauda equina syndrome.

As mentioned, the common variety is due to a defect of the pars interarticularis of the fifth lumbar vertebra and the cause of the defect is unknown. The defect can be unilateral or bilateral and when it is unilateral the displacement is small. In bilateral defects displacement of the vertebrae may not occur and this is known as spondylolisthesis.

Spondylolisthesis is graded in four grades depending on the position of the anterior displacement of the fifth lumbar vertebra on the sacrum. A grade 1 displacement occurs when the anterior displacement is 25 per cent or less of the antero-posterior diameter of the first sacral segment. In grade 2 the displacement is between 25 and 50 per cent of the antero-posterior diameter of the first sacral segment. In grade 3 it is between 50 and 75 per cent and in grade 4 it is greater than 75 per cent.

In spondylolisthesis symptoms are mostly absent and this is so especially in the younger age groups. Symptoms usually begin gradually from the teens onwards and present as an intermittent dull ache in the low back. This is present on walking and standing and increases in frequency. At a later stage, pain can develop in the buttock and thighs and later still a unilateral sciatica develops. Often a protruded lumbar intervertebral disc is present in addition and if the sciatica is accompanied by other neurological disturbances, the possibility of spondylosis should be considered.

The treatment of spondylolisthesis is initially conservative and in the minor degrees of slip a rigid lumbo-sacral support is often sufficient. However, in many cases, surgery is required and the unstable spine is fused.

SCIATIC PAIN

The majority of pain in the low back is produced by a cause which can be diagnosed. Most of these will be due to prolapsed lumbar intervertebral discs of one type or another. However, a comprehensive differential diagnosis would consist of a very large list indeed as there are many conditions which produce sciatica, or pain in the lumbo-sacral region. Without producing such a long list, some of the causes can be mentioned. They can be extrinsic or intrinsic and if extrinsic can be from disease in the central nervous system, the gastro-intestinal system, the female reproductive system, or the genito-urinary system. If the cause is intrinsic then the condition is one which may involve the vertebra directly or indirectly and will include congenital abnormalities such as spondylolisthesis, infectious diseases, neoplasms, and degenerative diseases.

Another thing to remember is that there may be more than one of these conditions present at the same time, as often, in addition, a primary condition produces changes in the central nervous system.

The physical examination of these patients should be exhaustive with particular attention paid to the neurological signs, to the presence of postural alterations, to spasticity of painful muscles, and to the distribution of the pain itself. Sciatica is not always due to serious disease and can be produced by simple superficial lesions of the fascia as in the myofascial syndromes.

When all the examinations have been carried out, when all the investigations have been performed, and when no obvious cause for the sciatic pain or lumbo-sacral pain is produced, a diagnosis of idiopathic sciatica or lumbago may be cautiously made.

Initially, conservative treatment with physical therapy, bed rest with or without traction, and exercises is adopted. A firm bed is helpful and when the patient is mobilised, a back brace can be applied for a few weeks.

Analgesic drugs and other drug therapy to relieve pain and muscle spasm is used throughout treatment.

Usually these measures help to speed up the normal recovery but sometimes lumbo-sacral pain and sciatica of unknown origin gradually change into a chronic condition. These are some of the most difficult patients to treat because they are impossible to treat. If the cause of the condition is unknown and the symptomatic treatment fails, the medical practitioner has little to offer except supportive treatment in its fullest sense and such symptomatic therapy as is indicated.

INTRACTABLE PAIN FOLLOWING MULTIPLE LUMBAR OPERATIONS

One of the commonest and most difficult problems that a Centre for Pain Relief has to deal with is the patient who has had multiple operations on his lower spine and has intractable residual pain of more or less severe degree.

The history can vary in many ways but a typical one would be a patient who starts off with a disc lesion which is removed at operation and he may or may not be relieved of his pain at this stage. If the pain is not relieved he is often explored again within a short time, and following this, in which more disc material may be removed, he settles down. In both these cases in a shorter or longer period, usually a year or more, pain recurs, often in a similar fashion to that on the first occasion and once again he is explored and probably a disc removed from a different level to that on the first occasion. Following this, pain is only partially relieved and radiculogram reveals no prolapse. After a variable interval, sometimes of years, he returns with pain of an intense degree and a myelogram shows a typical rat-tail appearance of the conus showing fibrosis around the lumbar and sacral nerve roots, or a radiculogram demonstrates similar features and in either case, no significant prolapse is present.

It is possible at this stage for the patient to be explored once more and nothing is found except that one or more of the nerve roots is bound down in scar tissue. These may be freed and perhaps covered with silastic sheet. If the patient is fortunate this is where surgery stops, but in some countries patients may be treated with further laminectomies.

When this stage is reached, treatment should be symptomatic: analgesics, heat, physiotherapy, orthopaedic appliances if there is foot drop, and supportive measures to keep the patient active and if possible, gainfully employed. Such measures as epidural blocks and facet blocks are tried and injections into spastic muscles.

Occasionally, remarkable results have been seen from acupuncture, hypnosis, faith healing, alpha feedback, and other methods which can all be reasonably tried.

In the Liverpool Centre for Pain Relief the dorsal column stimulation has been found to be of value in phantom limb pain and in some of the chronic back pains of the type being considered. A complicated work-up of various techniques to see which patients will respond to this treatment is carried out and culminates in the temporary implantation epidurally of wire electrodes. In this way, the patient can test, over a period of time, whether or not the dorsal column stimulation technique benefits him.

Moreover, it must be mentioned that patients who have had chronic pain of this type for many years can develop other conditions. Intraspinal tumours, malignant tumours with secondary spread, neuropathies, and even another true disc protrusion.

Finally, when it is believed that movement plays a large part in producing the pain, a spinal fusion can be considered as a last resort.

RADIOLOGICAL INVESTIGATIONS

Straightforward radiographs of the bony spine, that is, the antero-posterior and lateral views will show many abnormalities. The presence or absence of a normal curvature, and the alteration in normal joint and intervertebral space is readily seen. The presence of osteophytes and changes in vertebral shape can be observed, and such abnormalities as a Klippel–Feil syndrome cannot be mistaken.

In addition to these, oblique views may well be valuable to distinguish more definitely whether the spinal foramina are normal in shape or are narrowed by osteophytic outgrowths.

Often the presence of a disc lesion can be suspected by sclerosis of the vertebral end plates, by narrowing of the disc space, and by the presence of gas in these spaces. Nevertheless, it is important to know whether or not there is an actual protrusion of disc material into the spinal canal and also if this protrusion presses upon nerve roots. Until fairly recently, the use of an oily solution such as Myodil (Iophendylate B.P.) was injected intrathecally and the theca was outlined by this opaque material and observed on X-ray plates. Indentations into it would show the presence of tumours and whether they were new growths, spondylotic bars, or retropulsed discs. This method was, and is, particularly useful in finding out how much space there is around the spinal cord in the dorsal and cervical regions. However, for lesions below L2, a new method of using a water soluble radio-opaque dye (Dimer X) is now used and this will outline the nerve roots as they pass from the cord to the dural sleeve through the foramen. Abnormalities of the nerve root position is more easily seen in this method and is particularly suitable for deciding whether or not a prolapsed disc impinges on the root. The great advantage of this method is that using a water soluble dye ensures it is eventually absorbed into the blood stream and no foreign substance is left inside the theca.

REFERENCES

BRADLEY K.C. (1974) The Anatomy of Backache. *Aust. N.Z. J. Surg.* **44**, 3, 227-232.

BULL J.W.D. (1948) Rupture of the intervertebral disk in the cervical region. *Proc. roy Soc. Med.* **41**, 513.

CLOWARD R.B. (1964) Cervical chordotomy by the anterior approach. Technique and advantages. *J. Neurosurg.* **21**, 19-25.

KITE W.C. JR., WHITFIELD R.D. & CAMPBELL E. (1957) The thoracic herniated intervertebral disc syndrome. *J. Neurosurg.* **14**, 61-67.

LOGUE V. (1952) Thoracic intervertebral disc prolapse with spinal cord compression. *J. Neurol. Neurosurg. Psychiat.* **15**, 227.

SPURLING R.G. & GRANTHAM E.G. (1949) The end results of surgery for ruptured lumbar intervertebral discs. *J. Neurosurg.* **6**, 57.

FURTHER READING

BRAIN, LORD & WILKINSON M. (1967) *Cervical Spondylosis and Other Diseases of the Cervical Spine.* Heinemann, London.

NORTHFIELD D.W.C. (1973) *The Surgery of the Central Nervous System.* Chapter 22. Blackwell Scientific Publications, Oxford.

MATTHEWS J.A. & REYNOLDS D.A. (1977) 'The management of low back pain'. Chapter 14. In *Recent Advances in Surgery*, No. 9. Ed. Selwyn Taylor, Churchill Livingstone, London.

Chapter 7
The Treatment of Cancer Pain

THE ANTERO-LATERAL CORDOTOMY

The most effective methods of relieving the intractable pain of Cancer involve destruction of one or other of the conductive nerve pathways. There is a marked difference in effectiveness of the various nerve pathway sections, and certain of these are generally acknowledged to be more useful practically than others. It is not really difficult to see why this is so. The nearer the ablation, partial destruction, or damage is to the receptor organ which signals the presence of painful stimulation, the more effective will be that procedure in relieving the sensation of pain. As a corollary the further away from the receptor that pain pathway is destroyed the less effective does that particular method become, because study of the anatomical pathways of pain show that the further one progresses from the periphery to the cerebral cortex the more branching of, and modulation to, the pathways occur. In other words it is difficult to destroy a multiplicity of pathways.

The previous statement, like all blanket pronouncements, is not strictly correct, nevertheless there is a large measure of truth present. What is implied is that there will be an optimum position where ablative procedures can be made to produce long-lasting effects with adequate pain relief. When other factors are added in, such as producing the required lesion safely and quickly without too much strain on the patient's physical or mental condition, the antero-lateral cordotomy has obvious advantages.

These are, first, that this method is anatomically and physiologically sound. Given that our knowledge of the anatomical pathways of pain is correct, and that the physiological effects of sectioning these pathways are also correctly known, then sectioning these pathways has certain definite results. If there are variations from the normal then these can be explained on the basis of known variations in the anatomy or in the physiological response. Such is the case with the cordotomy. Pain nerve fibres enter the spinal cord at the posterior nerve root, ascend, or sometimes descend, for a variable number of segments and then cross to the other side of the spinal cord to take up position in the antero-lateral quadrant. Sometimes the pain pathway is called the spino-thalamic tract, but it must be clearly understood that the various operations of cordotomy do more than section the spino-thalamic pathway. There is destruction of a much wider region of the spinal cord which involves other known tracts, and also the spino-reticular fibres which form the bulk of it.

The result of sectioning the antero-lateral quadrant of the spinal cord is to produce freedom from the sensation of pain on the opposite half of the body and limbs. This depends on the level of section and when complete the alteration of sensation extends from anus (sacral five) to four or five spinal segments below the level of the destruction. The sensations of heat and cold have nerve pathways which travel in the antero-lateral quadrant and thus these sensations are also ablated following the section. In some patients there is a noticeable difference in the sensation of touch (on the opposite side of the body), after a cordotomy, but in most this is minimal and in some there is no alteration to the usual simple tests.

It has to be remembered that the whole procedure of the antero-lateral cordotomy, whichever particular method of performing this is used, depends on a reasonably normal cross-over of pain fibres in the spinal cord. This cross-over is said to be of the order of 90 per cent crossing and 10 per cent not crossing, and thus it can be seen why section of this tract produces analgesia on the opposite side of the body. There are well-documented cases where this type of cross-over does not occur, in fact, quite the reverse seems to be present and a section of the antero-lateral tract under direct vision at operation has resulted in analgesia developing on the same side of the body. In these patients the normal cross-over has not occurred and it is reasonable to assume that only 10 per cent of pain fibres cross, while 90 per cent do not cross. Following on from this it would also seem reasonable to expect that there would be intermediate variations of say, 80–20 per cent, or 70–30 per cent and so on. Variations of this type might account for some of the failures following what appears to be a satisfactory cordotomy. They might also account for the early fading of an initially satisfactory level.

Thus the second and third advantage of the antero-lateral cordotomy are concerned with the fact that this type of surgery gives reproducible results, which are reasonably long-lasting, and that unexpected results can be simply explained.

The fourth advantage is that the period of surgery, stress, and blood loss is not excessive and that even in patients who have advanced malignant disease one can expect to have a reasonable mortality. Of course this is not such a simple matter as might be thought as mortality does not depend on a single factor. It does, however, depend to large extent on two factors. These are the surgical operation involved and the physical condition of the patient at the time of surgery. Perhaps mention should be made of the unspoken third factor, that of the skill and dexterity of the surgeon but this involves considerations of a different type to those developed here. Mortality depends on the criteria used to include or exclude patients of a particular physical state. Thus a decision to have a limited selection or a very wide selection of patients can vary the mortality rate from 4 to 25 per cent. In addition there will be a variable morbidity.

Morbidity is the fifth consideration. The problem is an anatomical one and stems from the fact that the surgeon in the usual posterior approach to the spinal cord is at a disadvantage as the antero-lateral tract is positioned anteriorly. In other words the surgeon advances towards the spinal cord and having gone through skin, muscle, and vertebral bone, and having opened the dura has the posterior columns directly in view. To obtain sight of the antero-lateral quadrant the cord has to be rotated one way or the other. If both sides of the spinal cord are to be sectioned then the cord has to be rotated first one way and then the other. The technique of performing this is described most adequately in the surgical textbooks but briefly, the dentate ligament at the required level is released from the lateral dural wall and the free end is clamped by a fine mosquito forceps. This is then used to lever the cord round by rotating it until the antero-lateral quadrant comes into view. This quadrant of the spinal cord is then sectioned to a predetermined depth with a fine knife blade. All possible measures are taken to ensure section of all the nerve fibres in this area of the spinal cord and a sharp hook is usually passed through the cut to destroy any remaining uncut fibres. The wound is then closed.

There can be a considerable morbidity involving all modalities, including position sense and co-ordination, power, bladder function, and respiration. This depends to some extent on the level at which the cordotomy is performed, and whether it is a unilateral or bilateral one. It is possible to avoid some of these complications by carrying out a bilateral cordotomy in either two stages with a time interval between, or to make the sections on each side of the spinal cord at two different levels. The complications cannot be avoided entirely but they do clear up in time. However, in patients with a reduced expectation of life before surgery, and who have a further reduction in their expectation of life because of the surgery, a third reduction due to recovery from the morbidity of the operation may convert what was originally a reasonable operation for the patient concerned into an unreasonable one. Variations of the basic operation have therefore been sought ever since Spiller proved that pain is related to the intact spino-thalamic tracts (really to intact antero-lateral quadrants of the spinal cords). He demonstrated this on a patient who was shown to have tuberculomas in both anterior quadrants of the spinal cord at post-mortem, and who in life had lost the sensations of pain and temperature in the lower half of the body. Work on animals confirmed this and in 1912, Spiller and Martin reported a cordotomy carried out on a human being, the surgeon concerned was Martin.

It is obvious that if only one cordotomy, i.e. a section of one antero-lateral quadrant is required the rotation of the spinal cord is reduced and therefore the morbidity will also be reduced, and this in fact applies in practice. Methods are therefore used which tend to reduce or eliminate the rotation of the cord. They involve approaching the spinal cord either from the lateral aspect or anteriorly. In the latter case the approach is as in the Cloward operation for the removal of a cervical disc. A hole is drilled through the body of the vertebra from the front, the dura is exposed and incised thus bringing the antero-lateral quadrant into direct view. This exposure is somewhat limited but little rotation of the spinal cord is required and morbidity is said to be reduced. Whether rotation of the spinal cord produces direct injury to the cord or affects the blood supply to the cord is unknown. It may well be there is some element of both.

Some aspects of the complications following a cordotomy can be mentioned briefly at this stage particularly those referring to power, bladder function, and to respiratory function. Nathan showed that following unilateral surgical cordotomy there was often a period of loss of motor power which usually recovered. If at a later stage the other side of the spinal cord had a cordotomy performed on it then not only was there the possibility of weakness from the second cordotomy but the initial weakness reappeared.

A unilateral cordotomy does not usually produce any urinary problems unless these were present before the surgery. Bilateral cordotomies on the other hand were said to produce urinary problems invariably. This statement is not accepted by all authorities (Crue).

Bilateral cordotomies performed below the cervical 5 vertebral level do not produce respiratory difficulties except as part of the general motor weakness that develops. However, bilateral cordotomies carried out at the cervical 1–2 vertebral level may produce profound respiratory changes. In particular if high bilateral levels of analgesia have been produced a peculiar type of apnoea may result known as the 'Ondine' syndrome, where the patient can breathe voluntarily without any difficulty but loses all or part of the ability to breathe involuntarily. Thus the patient is at risk when they go to sleep as they tend to stop breathing and die. This only happens in a proportion of the cases and it is said can be forecast by allowing the patient to breathe 5 per cent carbon dioxide when susceptible patients do not have the normal doubling of tidal volume (Rosomoff).

There are other types of surgical tractotomy than the one so far described at spinal cord level. Only a little higher in position than the C_1–C_2 cordotomy is that at the cervico–medullary junction (Hitchcock). At this position is the decussation of the pyramids where the motor fibres are intermingling as they cross from one side to the other of the spinal cord. These fibres are anteriorly situated so that the anatomy of the various bundles of nerve fibres is different to that lower down the cord. As the motor fibres are anterior the fibres carrying the sensations of pain and temperature are posterior to these and more laterally placed. Further because the upper cervical pain fibres cross over a rather restricted length of spinal cord they almost form a decussation of their own. By ablating the area where they cross it may be possible to produce analgesia of both sides of the neck, and if one or other antero-lateral tract (in its posterior position) is ablated analgesia over the opposite half of the body and limbs is possible. In addition the descending trigeminal tract and nucleus at this level is still more posterior and lateral and ablation of one or other of these will also produce analgesia in the trigeminal distribution. Because of the anatomical arrangement of the nerve fibres in this region of the spinal cord the approach has to be from the posterior surface through the white and grey matter at the level of the cervico–medullary junction to those tracts, more anteriorly situated, which are to be destroyed. It is obvious that this cannot be performed by normal methods of surgery, and it is carried out by a stereo-tactic needle method. This technique has promise but is not in general use.

Other operations at higher levels which have been used in the past, but are not in favour now, are methods of sectioning the spino-thalamic fibres in the brain stem. A section of this tract can be made at the level of the base of the superior colliculus in the mesencephalon. In this method the auditory fibres in the lateral lemniscus are also destroyed but in unilateral cases there is no auditory deficit as sound is transmitted bilaterally. However, if this operation is performed bilaterally complete nerve deafness results. Another disadvantage of this operation is that the analgesia tends to wear off in a short time and there is a high level of dysasthesiae.

A much more effective and acceptable operation is to destroy the spino-thalamic fibres at a level a few millimetres below the obex. If the incision is made at this level, damage to the vestibular and restiform bodies tends to be avoided.

Finally mention must be made of stereo-tactic methods of destroying thalamic nuclei in the relief of pain. The actual technique of performing the thalamotomy is now well understood and described, and is carried out at many Centres. When used for pain the usual thalamic nuclei destroyed are those near the mid-line and in particular the Centre Median. However, the disadvantages of the thalamotomy in the relief of pain is, first, that it is a complicated method requiring much skill and patience, and secondly, that the analgesia produced by a unilateral thalamotomy tends to wear off in a relatively short time, 6–12 weeks. If a further period of relief is required the thalamotomy can be converted to a bilateral one. A thalamotomy which is bilateral from the beginning will last rather longer than twice the length of time a unilateral one will last. This method is particularly useful to relieve the pain due to inoperable malignancy in the head and neck.

When ablative methods are used there is an optimum level where the analgesia produced is effective, lasts a reasonable length of time, does not have too great a morbidity or mortality, and can be carried out in a reasonable time. This level seems to be somewhere in the spinal cord. Here the nerve fibres subserving pain are gathered into compact bundles which are accessible and if destroyed give reliable and reproducible pain relief. There is no doubt that the surgical cordotomy was the most effective method of relieving the pain of cancer that was developed up to 1963, when Mullan introduced the concept of the percutaneous cervical cordotomy. The surgical cordotomy was not as effective a form of treatment as it might have been solely because it was not used very much, and when it was used tended to be used late. Under these circumstances the surgery involved reduced the life expectancy of the patient concerned. In any case these patients often had had one or more major operations due to their primary condition and neither they nor their medical advisers were interested in further surgery.

Probably the most important statement that can be made about the surgical cordotomy is that the quality of the pain relief is excellent. When a cordotomy is carried out properly and all the nerve fibres have been sectioned the pain relief provided is complete and profound, and there is no, or little, loss of the sensation of touch.

PERCUTANEOUS METHODS OF ANTERO-LATERAL CORDOTOMY

From the remarks made in the previous section the disadvantages of the surgical cordotomy in its various forms can be seen. In the mid 1960s

Mullan used a new approach to the problem of destroying the antero-lateral quadrant which avoided most of the disadvantages of the surgical methods.

Radioactive method

The first alteration in technique was to avoid open surgery by the use of a closed method. This consisted of inserting a needle intrathecally from the lateral approach, at the level of the C_1–C_2 vertebrae. This was carried out under local anaesthesia with an X-ray technique. The needle was inserted in such a way that the tip of the needle pressed into the posterior surface of the vertebral body, below the odontoid process, where it was anterior to the antero-lateral quadrant of the spinal cord. This needle tip was not usually accurately placed in the mid-line but was to one side of it and it was possible to determine how far the needle tip was from the mid-line by means of X-rays. The next stage was to insert a radioactive-tipped probe down the spinal needle, this being Strontium 90 in Mullan's technique. The length of probe tip from which the radioactive Strontium radiated was known from previous measurements and it was possible for the radio-therapist to calculate the dose of radiation that could be given to the antero-lateral quadrant of the spinal cord in a given time and from this to work out how long an exposure was needed to produce destruction of this quadrant. To give a dose of radiation it was only necessary to push the radioactive probe down the spinal needle till it was jammed against the vertebra, and then withdraw the spinal needle enough to uncover the active portion of the probe tip. This was left exposed for the calculated time, when the probe was sheathed by the spinal needle once again, and then removed.

In this method pain relief did not occur immediately but gradually as the tissues of the antero-lateral quadrant were disrupted progressively. The time involved was of the order of one week but could be speeded up by giving a larger dose. There were great disadvantages in using larger doses as the lesions produced spread deeper into the cord as time went by. This had two results, first, as the sensory arm area was further away from the radioactive source than the leg area pain relief occurred first in the leg region and then in the arm, having spread up the body in dermatomal order. Secondly, as far as motor power was concerned the leg was affected as the dose of radiation increased. Thus if pain was to be relieved in the arm a larger dose of radioactivity had to be given, and in due course this produced weakness and eventual paralysis of the ipsilateral leg. Indeed if the dose of radiation was too large and the patient lived long enough the weakness would spread to the opposite side.

Thus for practical purposes the radioactive-tipped probe method was used for pain in the lower limb. For this purpose the method was most successful, and once the initial X-ray films and calculations were made no further manipulation of the needle or patient was required. Within the limitation of the method it was quite acceptable for ill patients, particularly for those who were not expected to live above two months. The danger of a progressive paresis existed beyond this time.

Direct current method

The disadvantages of the radioactive method are fairly obvious. The attack on the antero-lateral quadrant is indirect and there is no real control over the extent of the lesion produced. Further, the lesion should develop over a shorter period of time and any unwanted effects should be reversible. Rather surprisingly it is possible to obtain all these advantages but only at the expense of an increase of operative time. The method selected by Mullan was to use a direct electrical current to disrupt the cells of the antero-lateral quadrant electrolytically.

The method is basically very simple and similar to that of the radioactive method. The spinal needle instead of being placed anteriorly to the cord is pointed directly at the antero-lateral quadrant and an electrode is inserted down this needle until its tip is embedded in the tissues of the antero-lateral quadrant. This quadrant is disrupted by passing a direct electric current through the electrode, and the disruption can be monitored by the developing analgesia on the contra-lateral body and limbs. There are, of course, a few problems that need to be overcome, the most important being how to aim the electrode so that it can be inserted into the antero-lateral quadrant, which is approximately 5 by 7 mm. The problem is resolved very easily by using the dentate ligament as a reference line and measuring from that. The dentate ligament is, as its name implies, dentated with a continuous attachment to the spinal cord and intermittent attachments to the lateral dura. These attachments are regular and ideally the ligament is continuous, but in practice this is not necessarily so. The ligament may have holes in it, or have a complete section missing, or only be partially developed.

As far as the anatomy of the spinal cord is concerned, there is a definite arrangement in relation to the dentate ligament. It must be remembered that this relationship is the 'normal' or 'usual' one but it is not an absolute one. The antero-lateral quadrant for the most part lies in front of the dentate ligament, and the motor tract (corticospinal) lies for the most part, posterior to it. In addition the antero-lateral quadrant is, to some extent, segmented in that the sacral and leg pain fibres lie close to the ligament, the abdomen, thorax, arm, and cervical fibres lie successively more anteriorly. In fact, the lowest sacral fibres often lie somewhat posterior to the dentate ligament, close against the motor fibres to the lower limb. Thus, if the lowest sacral pain fibres require to be destroyed there may well be a degree of unavoidable motor weakness developing as well. However, this should be minimal and should not last.

The first necessity of this operation is to see the dentate ligament in relation to the spinal cord. This is done by inserting the spinal needle into the theca and obtaining cerebro-spinal fluid into which is then injected an emulsion of a radio-opaque material. The globules of this emulsion settle on the dentate ligament and as the patient is lying in the dorsal position, a lateral X-ray film will show up the globules lying on the dentate ligament, and thus the ligament itself, as a line running along the spinal cord (see Fig. 2). The emulsion is made up by shaking 3 ml Iophendylate B.P. (Myodil, Pantopaque) with 6 or 7 ml saline, and 5–10 ml sterile air (air drawn through sterile cotton wool). The mixture is not critical and many workers use cerebro-spinal fluid instead of saline as the proteins give a better emulsion which tends to last longer.

Usually, not only is the dentate ligament seen but also the anterior border of the spinal cord, or rather the spinal cord at the level of the anterior rootlets as they exit from the spinal cord. Some of the emulsion is held up on these nerve roots and form another more anterior line along the spinal cord. These 'lines' can be seen for some minutes on an image intensifier until the myodil emulsion drops away posteriorly on to the posterior theca, and in this position sometimes into the skull. This description is of a 'good' X-ray film and this can only be produced if the tip of the spinal needle is positioned anterior to the dentate ligament so that the injected emulsion which is heavier than cerebro-spinal fluid drops on to the ligament. Thus, if the spinal needle is placed posterior to the ligament the Myodil emulsion can only outline the dentate ligament if the injection pressure is sufficient to drive the fluid posterior to the spinal cord and then anteriorly along the opposite lateral wall. The best that can be hoped for under these circumstances is that a relatively faint line of emulsion will be seen along the ligament which can then be used as a target when the spinal needle is withdrawn and reinserted. If there is no mark of any kind to aim at then the needle must still be withdrawn and reinserted at a more anterior position. The dentate ligament can be estimated to be 10 mm posterior to the posterior surface of the vertebral body when the head and neck is in a neutral position. This, of course, is an average measurement and will also vary depending on the position of the head and the neck.

One fairly obvious point that can be made is that the effectiveness of the Myodil emulsion in showing the dentate ligament depends not only on a satisfactory emulsion being formed and injected but on the degree of cervical lordosis. It is clear that a patient with a marked cervical curve will tend to have the emulsion shed rapidly from its initial position on the dentate ligament, whereas a patient who has no or little cervical curve, as in cervical spondylosis, will retain the emulsion for a much longer period. This will make the procedure easier. There is one other factor of importance. A straight cervical spine means not only that the dentate ligament is straight but also that the antero-lateral quadrant is straight and therefore it is easier to insert an electrode into it.

The electrodes used can be of various materials but Mullan (1965) used an alloy of platinum 70 per cent and iridium 30 per cent. The diameter of 10/1000 inch will, after insulation by a simple coating method with an epoxy resin, allow the electrode to pass through a 22-gauge needle. The author found that this needle was too flexible and usually used a 20-gauge instead. If there is a big gap between the circumference of the electrode and the inner circumference of the spinal needle used there will be much leakage of cerebro-spinal fluid during the operation with the prospect of a severe spinal headache to follow. The tip of the electrode is not insulated over the terminal 2 mm and the point is sharpened.

The electrical apparatus used to produce the direct current is quite simple and can be easily produced by any electronic department. One such apparatus has been described (Mullan 1964). Such an apparatus should have three ranges, up to 200 μA, 500 μA, and up to 5 mA. The lower range is used in the initial stage to ensure that no rapid or unexpected effects are going to be obtained. Also switching on and off, makes and breaks the circuit and will stimulate motor fibres or nerve cells if the electrode tip is near them. In other words, it gives a crude indication whether the electrode is too posterior, or is actually in the cortico-spinal tract, by producing muscle twitches on the ipsilateral side of the body. This test is carried out with a current of 200 μA for a few minutes and if no analgesia or paresis occurs, the apparatus is switched to the next range for another two or three minutes. Finally, the highest range is used and the current gradually increased to about 2 mA while monitoring the gradually increasing hypoalgesia and eventually analgesia. Motor power is also monitored during this period. An adequate lesion and therefore analgesia will develop in about twenty minutes which is a rather long time compared with the twenty seconds or so of the radio-frequency method which is described next. Nevertheless, because the lesion develops slowly it is an exceedingly safe method. If untoward effects develop the current can be shut off; and the patient returned to the ward in the confident expectation that the unwanted effects will have disappeared by the following day. The procedure can be attempted again a few days later.

The direct current method was supposed to be a safer procedure if the electrode was the anode as it was believed there was less chance of haemorrhage developing when the lesion degenerated. Using the currents described above, this effect may have been exaggerated and many lesions have been made safely with the electrode as the cathode. There is no doubt that it is safer to use a smaller current for a longer time than a larger current for a shorter one, whatever the polarity of electrode.

The final comment on this method which has been superseded by the radio-frequency method is that it provided a very safe way of producing a lesion in the upper cervical cord without side-effects. Its one disadvantage was the length of time it took to produce a satisfactory lesion and the stress this placed on an ill patient.

Radio-frequency method

In 1965 Rosomoff on the one hand and Mullan on the other, began using a radio-frequency electrical current to produce a lesion in the antero-lateral quadrant of the spinal cord. This method used the heat produced from the passage of this type of current through the tissues. It was in effect, a low-powered diathermy current similar to that used in surgery for cauterisation of blood vessels. A completely different type of lesion generator was required than that used for the direct current method but no different to those in use for many years in stereo-tactic procedures on the brain. Because of the small area involved in the spinal cord and the widespread effects that were produced when coagulation was made in the wrong place, certain refinements were soon developed in the lesion generators.

The lesion generator, these machines are often multipurpose and used not only for the cervical cordotomies but also for brain lesions and in the radio-frequency coagulation method of controlling the pain of trigeminal neuralgia. There is often a switching mechanism so that a lower power range for cordotomies is available at up to 10 watts, and a much higher power suitable for the other purposes. There is one feature of these machines which should be considered of importance and that is whether they are constant current or constant voltage devices. The heat produced is a function of the current that passes through the tissues and as the resistance of the tissues rises as they are coagulated, increased power is used to keep the current constant in a constant current device. Thus, more heat is produced and a dangerous situation may arise when the tissues boil. This can and does produce an explosion inside the cord which is an exceedingly dangerous procedure as the tracking of the steam produced is completely fortuitous. It is necessary for the lesion generator to be of the constant voltage type which means that as the temperature of the tissues rises, and the resistance rises, the current falls. Modern machines contain safety devices preventing this particular danger. This merely underlines the care that has to be taken in all the phases of the percutaneous cordotomy. The penalty for failing to do this is, at the very least, a failed cordotomy and at the worst, a paresis for the patient. It should also be stated that provided care is taken and no lesion made until the operator is sure that the electrode is in the correct position, a satisfactory and safe lesion will be produced.

There are usually two other features of note in the modern lesion generator. The first is of use when the electrode is being inserted into the cord initially. At this stage it is important to know that the tip of the electrode has not been advanced too far into the cord and this information can be provided by a measurement of the resistance of the tissues through the electrode. This is called the *impedance* of the tissues and is high when the resistance to the passage of an electric current is high, and low when it is reduced. If a continuous measurement of impedance is made as the electrode is being inserted into the spinal needle the impedance measurement goes through four phases. First is an infinite impedance before the tip of the electrode makes contact with the cerebro-spinal fluid, and is a measurement of the impedance in air. Next the impedance drops to a very low value (about 200 ohm) as the electrode tip enters the cerebro-spinal fluid. Here it is in contact with a salt solution of low resistance. Shortly after this the impedance rises slightly which signifies that the tip of the electrode has entered the cord tissue and the resistance has an intermediate value. Finally, as the bared end of the electrode is completely buried in cord tissue the impedance suddenly rises to about 800 ohm or more. This final rise varies from patient to patient and there is no constant value for it. However, the end point is quite obvious in all patients. Often the patient will appreciate a sharp pain in the neck when the electrode is finally pressed home.

It is not necessary to have an impedance meter as in most cases there is an appreciable resistance to the insertion of the electrode tip and this can be detected by the surgeon's sense of touch. However it is a better and safer procedure using a measurement of resistance as it prevents the electrode being pushed too far into the cord. An impedance meter is a convenient but sophisticated method of measuring resistance and this can be done just as easily if the lesion generator is equipped with an ammeter. An ammeter

measures current and current depends on resistance thus the ammeter
reading gives just as much indication of the resistance of the tissues as an
impedance meter except that ammeter and impedance meter give inverse
readings. When an ammeter gives a low reading it is because the resistance
is high and under the same circumstances an impedance meter will read high.
Conversely, when the resistance is low the ammeter shows a high reading
and the impedance meter a low one. Thus, as the electrode is inserted into the
spinal needle an ammeter will show a very low reading in air approaching
zero. Then as it enters the cerebro-spinal fluid the reading reaches its highest
level and this gradually falls as the tip is inserted into the cord. There is
a final fall when the whole of the exposed end is inserted.

The second feature is the provision of *stimulation facilities*. These are
extremely useful to ensure that the electrode is in the correct portion of the
spinal cord before coagulation is carried out. Two frequencies of stimulation
are normally provided, 2 hertz and 100 hertz; 2 hertz tends to stimulate
motor fibres and nerve cells and when the electrode is in the normal correct
position in the antero-lateral quadrant of the spinal cord, the tip of it is near
or in the anterior horn. During stimulation testing 2 hertz is usually used
first and if the voltage is gradually increased up to 10 volts (two to three
usually being sufficient) pulsing of those muscles that take impulses from
the C_1–C_2 region of the anterior horn occurs. The important feature is that
no pulsing occurs in any other muscles and certainly not in the arm, body,
or leg. If this does occur it signifies that the electrode tip is near or in the
cortico-spinal tract and must be moved. If it is not moved then paresis will
result on coagulation. The pulsing that occurs does so on the ipsilateral side
of the body to the electrode as at the C_1–C_2 level the motor tracts are not
crossed. This is not an absolute statement as the decussation of the pyramids
(the motor decussation) is normally completed at this level but very occasionally this decussation takes place over more segments and therefore
extends lower. Also the motor fibres to arm and leg tend to be somewhat
separate and the crossing of the fibres of the one occurs somewhat lower
than the other. For this reason it is also most important to test for motor
stimulation.

A similar test is then carried out using 100 hertz. The voltage used at
this frequency is about one-tenth of that used for 2 hertz, the average being
about 0·3 volt. It can go up to as much as 1·0 volt. Stimulation at this frequency
tends to affect the sensory tracts more than the motor, and this is shown by
the patient feeling sensations on the contralateral side of the body to the
electrode. These sensations can be of many kinds; of pain; discomfort; hot
or cold; sensations of a wind blowing on the skin, again either hot or cold;

or of indeterminate sensations of electricity or pins and needles. Sometimes the patient cannot even describe the sensation except that it is there and is like no sensation that has ever been appreciated before. These sensations are usually referred to the skin and are very definitely on one side of the body. At the lower stimulation voltages they are often confined to a small area of the body or limbs, and this extends and widens as the power increases.

The sensation appreciated depends to some extent on the position of the electrode in the antero-lateral quadrant. When this is peripherally situated and near the dentate ligament the sensation is referred to the leg and adjacent areas, when it is near the anterior roots the sensation is referred to the chest or arm. Why thermo-sensations are sometimes felt is a matter of opinion. These sensations can occur alone as a 'pure' sensation of heat or cold, or, for example, can take the form of a hot or cold pain or a hot or cold wind. It would seem logical to postulate that there are places in the antero-lateral quadrant where there is a preponderance of thermo-fibres. They must be in close proximity to fibres carrying pain as coagulation is usually most successful when there is an element of thermal sensation present as well. In fact, the author has only known one failure to produce excellent analgesia when the sensation reported on stimulation was of a cold wind. This is also the experience of Mullan.

It has been suggested that the pain fibres lie in a predominantly super-ficial position and in a layer underneath them lie thermal fibres. There is, of course, much intermingling of these various fibres. Deeper in the cord lie autonomic fibres and fibres carrying sensation from the deeper structures and the viscera. If the electrode is pushed into the cord tissue it may penetrate to these layers and this may be reflected in the patient reporting sensations of a peculiarly distressing nature, referred to the mid-line, often to lungs or abdomen, but 'deep inside'. The X-ray studies mentioned later will show when the electrode has gone too deep.

The lesion. The purpose of using a lesion generator is to make a lesion of a particular size in a particular place. The place where the lesion is made depends on the accuracy of the positioning of the electrode and on the skill of the operator. The lesion has a particular shape depending on the shape of the electrode. Usually the electrode is made of thin wire of one kind or another, and of a diameter between 10/1,000 and 20/1,000 of an inch. The exposed portion of the electrode controls the length and width of the lesion and is normally 2 or 3 mm. Under these circumstances the lesion is barrel-shaped with the length dependent on the longest measurement of the exposed portion, and the width approximately two-thirds of this. The size of a lesion depends on the power of radio-frequency current that is passed through the length of exposed electrode. There is a limit to this size which depends on two factors. One is due to the resistance of the tissues increasing as the lesion progresses, and thus limiting the amount of the current that will continue to pass. Secondly, is the heat dissipating ability of the cord tissue surrounding the exposed electrode, which in part depends on the speed with which the lesion is made, i.e. the power used. Thus if the lesion is attempted with too low a power the heat produced is conducted away so quickly that an adequate lesion cannot be produced. On the other hand, if the power used is too great then so much heat may be produced that it cannot be conducted away and the tissues tend to boil rather than coagulate, and may explode. If this happens there is no way of determining the direction the exploding steam will take and the lesion-making procedure becomes extremely hazardous. Obviously there is an optimum level of current which will provide a constant size and satisfactory lesion.

Each lesion generator must be standardised so that it is known what size of lesion is produced by a given current. Again there will be variations of size in a given patient because the impedance of the tissues varies a little from patient to patient. A complete and maximum lesion will involve the whole of the antero-lateral quadrant of the spinal cord at the C_1–C_2 level, i.e. a lesion of 7×5 mm will be needed to destroy completely the whole of the quadrant. A lesion smaller than this will normally be quite adequate, say 5×4 mm. If it is known that a lesion of this approximate size is produced by say, 50 mA in 30 seconds, then the size of the lesion can be controlled during the coagulation process in one of two ways. The power used can be kept constant, say 50 mA, and the time varied, beginning with 5 seconds, then $7\frac{1}{2}$ seconds, 10 seconds and so on. Alternatively, the time can be kept constant, say at 30 seconds and the power varied, beginning at 15 mA, then 20 mA, 25 mA, and so on. In between each increment of either power or time, depending on the method used, the power of the ipsilateral muscles are tested and the level of analgesia developing on the contralateral side is also checked.

It is most important to realise that the safety of the whole procedure depends on a meticulous attention to detail and that no part of the stimulating tests before coagulation or motor power tests and analgesic level tests during, or in between coagulation, can be omitted without danger. If any of these tests suggest that the position of the electrode is incorrect then it will need moving. When it is moved the complete series of tests must be carried out again. None of the tests can be omitted, the whole series must be worked through in order. Disaster will result if any of the tests are not performed. It must also be borne in mind that the anatomy of this region of the spinal cord is not fixed in the sense that it is exactly the same in all patients. It is not, it is variable. This does not mean that an anomaly is present, but merely that this particular patient has one of the normal variations. This normal variation may be such as to make it impossible to carry out the percutaneous cordotomy procedure without danger, and in this case the procedure should be abandoned.

Anatomy

The relevant portions of the spinal pathways that are of most importance in relation to the percutaneous cervical cordotomy are on the one hand, the pain pathway in the antero-lateral quadrant of the spinal cord, and on the other, the cortico-spinal descending tract. As far as the gross anatomy of the cord is concerned the dentate ligament approximately divides the antero-lateral quadrant from the posterior quadrant. The former contains sensory tracts and the latter contains the descending cortico-spinal motor tract.

Under normal circumstances the sensory fibres are anterior to the motor fibres. This is not always the case as very rarely the decussation of the pyramids does not occur at the usual level above C_1–C_2 and occurs either partly at this level or even lower down the spinal cord. Also this variation may occur in part or in whole, and in very rare circumstances may not cross at the normal pyramidal level or even at all. However, what is important from the point of view of carrying out a percutaneous cordotomy is the relation of the various fibres at the C_1–C_2 spinal level. It is obvious that if any of the anatomical variations already mentioned occur the decussation of the pyramids either does not take place at all, or takes place to a partial degree only, and then the normal arrangement of the pain fibres anteriorly and the motor tract fibres posteriorly does not exist. In fact, the motor fibres can remain anterior and the pain fibres can be posterior.

Under the same conditions, the fifth nerve nucleus and its tract descending in the upper cord may not be in the usual position but may be in the same situation it is in the medulla. The importance of stimulation studies under these circumstances cannot be overestimated. If the motor fibres are anteriorly situated then an electrode in the normal position 1–2 mm anterior to the dentate ligament will be among motor fibres and the stimulation test will show pulsing of the body or limb musculature. This pulsing will be either contralateral or ipsilateral depending on whether there is no, partial, or complete cross-over, and whether there is not, partial, or incomplete, adoption of the normal posterior position at the C_1–C_2 level.

One type of anomaly which is very rare is a rotation of the spinal cord itself, inside the bony spinal canal. This is an abnormal anatomical arrangement. If it is present then not only will the X-ray appearances be most peculiar, but the stimulation studies will also be bizarre.

So far, only abnormal or unusual arrangements of the motor fibres have been mentioned but there can be corresponding abnormalities on the sensory side. It has been mentioned earlier that there are well authenticated cases where a surgical section of one antero-lateral quadrant has been followed by analgesia on the same side of the body as the section itself. These cases are rare but most neurosurgeons who have been concerned with performing the surgical antero-lateral tractotomy know either at first hand, or from one of their colleagues, of a case where this has occurred. Thus, it is not unusually rare and when carrying out a percutaneous cervical cordotomy it is as well to test both sides of the body and limbs in the early stages of the developing coagulation lesion, to check whether a patient with one of these abnormal cross-over cases is on the table.

PERCUTANEOUS CERVICAL CORDOTOMY— TECHNIQUE

It needs to be emphasised that the physical technique of carrying out a percutaneous cervical cordotomy (P.C.C.) is not difficult in the majority of patients. Unfortunately, dexterity in inserting spinal needles and electrodes is not enough for success, as it is the stimulation testing and lesion making that produce complication free results. Under no circumstances can any stage of the particular technique adopted be omitted. If a repositioning of the electrode is required, the full routine series of tests must be carried out. If any of these are left out to speed up the operation, or to save the patient some tension, or through laziness on the part of the operator, then sooner or later complications will arise. Probably sooner than later. Persistence in carrying out the stimulation tests, and checking the analgesic level and motor power, both during and after each increment of coagulation is most important. The number of 'steps' in the series of coagulations should be adhered to as it is most unwise to 'jump' one or more of these. It may be thought that the author is emphasising this particular feature of the P.C.C., but it is the care taken with the features mentioned that provides the high safety and success rates in this method of pain relief.

Premedication

The patient has to remain reasonably still while in position on the operating table. It is not so much that the body and limbs should be at rest, as that the head should not move. A slight rotation, tilt, or other movement of the head on the neck will make an enormous difference to the image intensifier or other X-ray. If the patient finds that maintaining the position becomes uncomfortable and shifts position only very slightly, a less than optimal appearance results. Therefore, adequate premedication is a necessity but care must be taken not to over-medicate. Ideally, the patient should be so depressed during the preliminary stages when the spinal needle and the electrode are placed in position, that they do not remember this happening. At the same operation and about thirty minutes later, they should be capable of responding to questions in a sensible and coherent fashion. In the majority of cases this is impossible without the use of intravenous analeptics, or narcotic antidotes. A lesser degree of premedication is therefore used, whereby the patient will either doze in a very light sleep during the early stages of the procedure, or be awake throughout it. In the latter case they should be relaxed and comfortable.

Any premedication suitable to the operator can be used; there is no merit in any particular combination of drugs. Usually the operator values the method with which he has had the most experience, and in general this is the best way to decide on the drug or combination of drugs to be used. The author uses the standard Neurolept analgesia by means of Phenoperidine, and Haloperidol. Other combinations are used at times such as Droperidol and Fentanyl, but phenoperidine has advantages as it lasts about one hour and is usually sufficient to cover the complete procedure. It is given intravenously in doses of not more than 1 mg for a 60 kg person and the drug is assessed after fifteen minutes and further small increments given as required. If caution is not used with the drug, the patient may become too drowsy to respond to questions and the whole purpose of the premedication is lost.

When the percutaneous cordotomy lasts longer than the usual forty-five minutes, and goes on beyond one hour, the patient becomes restless as the premedication wears off. It is possible to give more phenoperidine at this stage and this can work very well, but there is the possibility of depressing the patient a little too much at a critical stage of the operation. A very useful drug at this point is Pentazocine (Fortral) given by means of small increments starting with 20 mg and continuing with 10 mg until sedation occurs. This drug attains its maximum effect within five minutes, has only mild respiratory depressant effects, and at the same time provides a satisfactory degree of sedation. It is a narcotic antagonist.

At times a patient is in so much pain or is so mentally disturbed by their condition that they cannot be treated in this fashion. Under these circumstances the percutaneous cordotomy in the early stages must be conducted by means of anaesthetic 'sleep'.

The patient is premedicated as for Neurolept analgesia, and then in addition receives Brietal (Methohexitone) in small increments. These produce sleep and in between the doses the patient is allowed to wake, move, and even say a few words. It is not difficult to arrange for the patient to breathe 50 per cent nitrous oxide/oxygen (Entonox) during this period which deepens the sleep and increases the time between the injections. When the nitrous oxide/oxygen mixture is withdrawn, wakening occurs rapidly. The simplest method of arranging this is by means of disposable nasal catheters with the nasal tubes extended somewhat so that they pass deep through the nares. They should be well lubricated with one of the analgesic gels or creams.

This type of patient control means that there may be a period of disorientation during the recovery phase, when the patient may try to move. It may be necessary to restrain the patient during this phase until they realise exactly where they are, and what is required of them. A little time spent before the operation informing the patient what is going to be done, the type of anaesthetic that will be given and what it will feel like when they start to awaken will prove valuable.

The author is inclined to think that not enough use has been made of this method in the past, but this is anaesthesia of a highly skilled character. Further, in the Rosomoff technique, which is a more rapid method than the one normally used by the author (taking about thirty minutes in the hands of Rosomoff himself), there is no need to advocate the use of anaesthesia.

Position during percutaneous cordotomy. This will depend on the type of cordotomy that is to be carried out. In the Rosomoff technique where air is the contrast used, the patient is placed in a position which will keep this air from escaping into the skull. The head is flexed on the cervical vertebrae and the lower vertebrae are raised anteriorly compared to the upper ones. A very simple way of placing the cervical vertebrae into position is by means of a small inflatable pad placed under the shoulders, which can thus be raised or lowered at will. If the head is too flexed it will be difficult to see the odontoid process in the antero-posterior view, as the base of the skull or the naso-maxillary region will mask it.

The patient's head is fixed in a head holder, and this can be of a very simple type such as that advocated by Mullan, or can be of complex type such as that made by the Owl Company of Toronto. There are two ways to use these manufactured head holders. The head can be held between the head rest posteriorly and the padded forehead support anteriorly, or instead of a forehead support, there are two eye pads which fit over the eyes and actually restrain the patient from moving at all. The latter is the method used by Rosomoff, where it is necessary as the spinal needle is gripped in a micromanipulator, and once the electrode is in position any movement of the head or neck invites a transection of the spinal cord. When the spinal needle merely rests loosely on a micromanipulator the danger is not so great.

Local anaesthetic injection

The actual local anaesthetic solution used is of no great importance but probably Marcaine $\frac{1}{2}$ per cent (Bupivacaine) without adrenaline should be used as it lasts beyond the time taken for the cordotomy.

Rosomoff places his initial local anaesthetic solution level with the estimated anterior border of the spinal cord, between C1 and C2. A thin metal rod with side markings on it is used. This is placed in the X-ray image intensifier beam and moved until it is seen in the C1–C2 space. The injection is then made in the correct position by lining up the side markings with the required point of injection. Rosomoff also varies the brightness control on the image intensifier with the room darkened and in most cases can distinguish the anterior border of the cord in this fashion. The spinal needle is then inserted accordingly. The author has been unable, as a routine, to use this manœuvre though on occasion has been convinced the cord edge was seen.

The relationship between the tip of the mastoid process and the space between C1 and C2 can be noted or a small 25-gauge needle used for the initial injection can be left in the skin and seen on the image intensifier as a marker (Figs. 16 and 17). The Rosomoff technique injects along a line level with the anterior border of the spinal cord as already mentioned, and then the spinal needle is inserted along this line until it penetrates the dura. The Mullan technique which relies on seeing the dentate ligament outlined by radio-opaque Myodil (Iophendylate B.P.), injects the local anaesthetic and inserts the spinal needle more posterior than that of Rosomoff. As mentioned, the dentate ligament lies about 10 mm posterior to the posterior edge of the vertebral body (Fig. 18).

There are three possible dangers in the injection of local anaesthetic

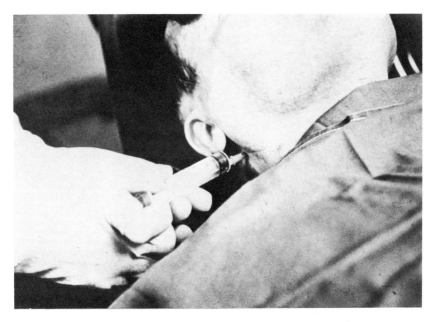

FIGURE 16. Local anaesthetic injection.

solutions in this region. First, and particularly if the injecting needle wanders anteriorly towards the body of the first vertebra, there can be a direct injection into the vertebral artery. The results of this are immediate and temporarily devastating. The patient loses consciousness, stops breathing, goes blue, and may fit. The treatment is to maintain a good airway and to oxygenate the patient. This is best done by means of a face mask and Magill rebreathing circuit with oxygen, but any method of respiratory resuscitation can be used. Within five minutes the patient is breathing normally and in another five, talking coherently. In the few cases where this occurred to the author the operation could continue within twenty minutes. This problem presented during the first 100 cases or so (and not since) so is presumably due to lack of experience or lack of care.

Secondly, there can be an injection into the epidural space and the production of epidural anaesthesia. This can only arise if the quantity of anaesthetic solution injected is large. If it is no more than $\frac{1}{2}$–1·0 ml then danger from this inadvertent injection cannot result. In fact it is normal practice to inject a little solution into the epidural space to provide a certain degree of analgesia in the upper cervical nerves during the procedure.

Thirdly, there is the injection made into the anterior venous plexus or the subarachnoid space. In either case it is so relatively easy to detect

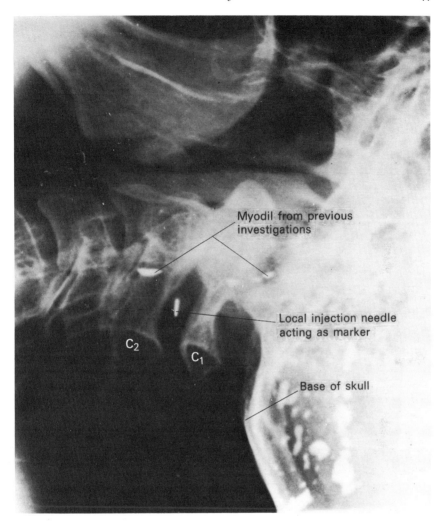

FIGURE 17. Hypodermic needle acting as marker.

whether blood or C.S.F. can be withdrawn through the needle that this problem should never arise. The danger would be if a subarachnoid injection were made using enough anaesthetic solution to produce a total spinal anaesthetic. The treatment of this is to support respiration artificially, then to withdraw C.S.F. and thus the local anaesthetic solution, and to have a slight Trendelenberg tilt to prevent hypotension. It might be necessary to use hypotensive drugs to maintain the blood–pressure. These measures continue until the total spinal wears off.

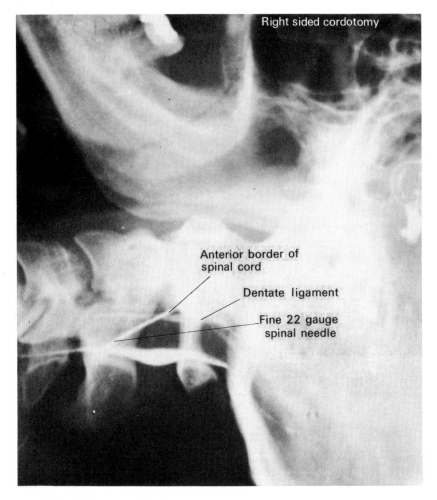

Right sided cordotomy

Anterior border of
spinal cord

Dentate ligament

Fine 22 gauge
spinal needle

FIGURE 18. This is an optional stage. Using a fine spinal needle (22-gauge) to inject myodil emulsion and show up dentate ligament before inserting the large 18-gauge spinal needle which carries the electrode.

Insertion of the spinal needle. As mentioned previously, there are two 'lines' on which the spinal needle can be inserted depending on whether it is aimed at the anterior border of the spinal cord or anterior to the dentate ligament. A sharp 18-gauge thin-walled spinal needle is usually used, and is first measured from hub to tip. There are many types of electrode but whichever type is used, it is arranged so that the electrode as a whole projects a known distance from the sharp tip of the spinal needle (see Fig. 19). This is usually 4 mm but may be more or less on occasion. Also the terminal

2 mm of the electrode is bared and the tip is sharpened. There is a locking device which makes sure that the projection of the electrode from the spinal needle once set cannot be altered.

Insertion of the spinal needle is made from the lateral approach between C1 and C2. Insertion is continued until, on the antero-posterior image intensifier view, the tip of the needle lies mid-way between the medial

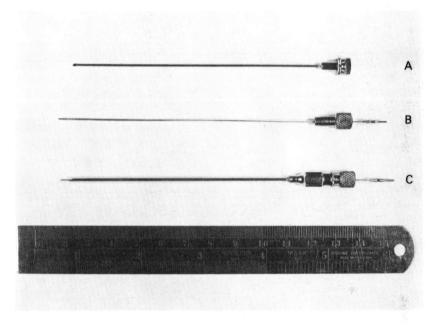

FIGURE 19. Proprietary cordotomy needle with built-in stop. (A) Stylette. (B) Electrode. (C) Spinal needle with electrode inserted.

border of the pedicles on the lateral side, and the lateral border of the odontoid process on the medial side (see Fig. 20). It should be noted that the average width of the interpedicular distance as demonstrated on X-ray films is 3·5 cm. Thus if the distance between the tips of the mastoid processes is measured, either approximately with a ruler, or accurately with calipers and 3·5 cm subtracted, halving the residual amount will give the distance from skin to lateral dural wall. This is the penetration through the tissues the needle has to make before C.S.F. is obtained, and is approximately correct.

If the needle is very sharp there is no problem in advancing it through the tissues of the neck, which can be very tough at times. If the tissues are difficult to penetrate it may be easier to advance the needle by 'screwing' it

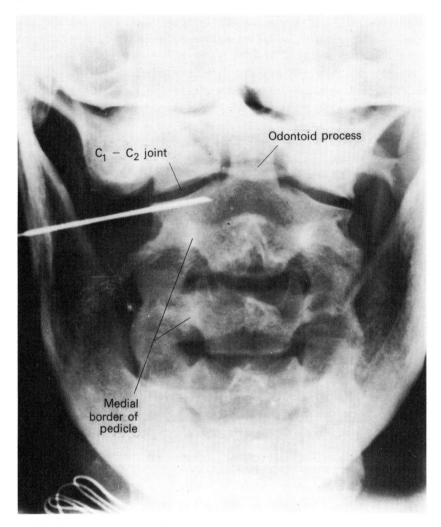

FIGURE 20. A–P view through open mouth.

through the tissues. A much more delicate control of its insertion through the dura can be obtained in this way. It should not be forgotten that the question as to how much further the needle has to go before penetrating the dura, or any question as to how far it has gone after penetrating the dura, can be resolved merely by viewing the odontoid process in the anterior-posterior view with the mouth open (see Fig. 20).

If the spinal needle is directed too anteriorly it may actually miss the dura or push it out of the way as it is thicker and tougher anteriorly than elsewhere. The needle tip will enter the venous plexus which is present anteriorly and blood will drip slowly out of the hub. If this happens the needle is withdrawn almost to the skin and reinserted. There is a temptation when inserting the needle to push it in too far (2–3 cm) before looking at the image intensifier screen. A better method is first to penetrate the skin a centimetre or so, enter the muscles, and observe the line of the needle. In particular whether its path is central between C1 and C2. Of course, the weight of the hub will cause the hub to drop and the needle tip to point much too far anterior at this stage. The needle is advanced a few millimetres at a time, viewing between each movement and correcting the direction. Eventually the dura is penetrated at the correct level depending on the method adopted. Alternatively the micromanipulator support can be raised to support the spinal needle at the correct height and on the correct line during insertion.

There is one point of great practical value. Often there is a small venous plexus outside the lateral dura and in a slow and careful insertion of the needle blood will be obtained at a depth where C.S.F. may be expected. All that needs to be done is to advance the needle a few millimetres more and the distinctive penetration of the dura will be felt and C.S.F. obtained.

It is possible at this stage for the spinal needle to penetrate the spinal cord. This has happened to the author on seven known occasions (approximately 1 per cent of cases). In four there was no observable alteration in sensation or motor power. In the other three there was a well marked and complete Brown Sequard syndrome. Removal of the spinal needle showed some blood in the C.S.F. and then return of power and sensation beginning about ten minutes after withdrawal. Within thirty minutes movement has returned and was of fair power though by no means normal. Sensation to pin prick was slower to return but was normal by the following morning in two cases. In the other case although motor power had returned to normal, loss of pin prick occurred over most of the dorsal region which became less dense in the course of the following week, finishing up as hypoalgesia. It so happened that this patient was being treated for a carcinoma of the lung invading the mid-thoracic wall and an excellent practical result was obtained. Presumably the spinal needle had been aimed very correctly at the thoracic pain fibres and the cutting edge of the spinal needle had cut or damaged enough pain nerve fibres to give this result. This particular patient had a most satisfactory result which lasted fourteen months, the pain then recurred.

There is a corollary to this mishap which is that if the spinal needle penetrates the cortico-spinal tract, presumably there could be permanent

motor damage. Further, the reason that in the other four cases there was no
obvious damage at all may be that it requires a certain depth of penetration
to produce pressure effects preventing function. Alternatively, if the needle
penetrated anteriorly, it might have been too far anterior to affect either
sensory or motor fibres.

Once the spinal needle is inserted to the correct depth, its hub is placed
on a micromanipulator (see Fig. 21). In the Mullan technique it rests on the
elevator, in the Rosomoff it is gripped by it. In either case by raising or
lowering the hub of the spinal needle the tip can be directed posteriorly or

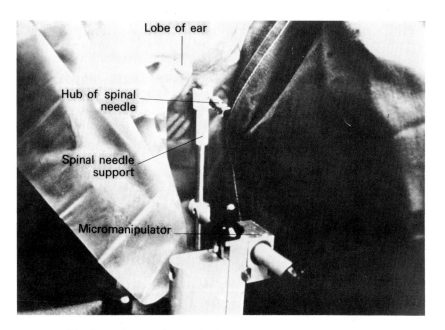

FIGURE 21. Needle resting on micromanipulator.

anteriorly respectively. A movement of about 3 mm at the tip seems possible
in this way and this represents a movement of the aim from the dentate
ligament to the anterior horn region of the cord.

In the Mullan technique if fibres concerned with pain in the lower half
of the body need ablating, the spinal needle is aimed 1 mm or so anterior to
the dentate ligament. If fibres in the thoracic or cervical region are to be
destroyed the aim is 2–3 mm anterior to the dentate ligament. Also because
of the curve of the spinal cord, a deeper penetration is necessary as the
surface of the cord is further away anteriorly.

In the Rosomoff technique 10 ml of sterile air (i.e. air drawn into the syringe through sterile cotton wool) is injected. The lateral view on the image intensifier will then show the anterior border of the spinal cord, usually along a length of two vertebrae at least. The edge of the spinal cord seen anteriorly in this fashion is not the true edge of the spinal cord but is somewhat posterior to it. The spinal needle is aimed 3 mm posteriorly from the apparent anterior edge and here will produce maximum analgesia in the lower half of the body. A direction more anteriorly will tend to centre on the thoracic level. The spinal needle can be directed as far posteriorly as it will go, relying on the dentate ligament to prevent movement too far posteriorly when the leg and sacral fibres will be maximally affected.

In the Mullan technique, an emulsion of Myodil is made as mentioned previously (p. 132). Holding the syringe vertically the top 1–2 ml of the supernatant fluid is discarded after the various layers settle out as it is said to be more irritant than the rest of the solution. The remainder is re-emulsified and 1–2 ml is injected. This will outline the dentate ligament, the anterior border of the spinal cord, and the posterior dura (see Fig. 18). On rare occasions some of the emulsion will cling to the spinal cord posteriorly and gravitate to the most dependent, i.e. posterior part, and this also shows up as another thin line on the lateral X-ray. Sometimes if the patient is not exactly square to the X-ray tube, or if the spinal cord is not quite square inside the bony canal, both dentate ligaments will be seen, it is easy to distinguish these by a slight rotation of the head on the neck while using the image intensifier when one dentate ligament will move posteriorly and the other one anteriorly. If the head moves to the left, the left ligament is the one that descends and vice versa.

In the Mullan technique it is relatively easy to see where the electrode is to go and therefore easier to aim the spinal needle 1–2 mm anterior to the dentate ligament for the lower pain fibres, and slightly more anteriorly than this if the upper pain fibres are required.

When the spinal needle is aimed in the correct direction the electrode is inserted down the needle as far as the 'stop' will allow. The pia mater membrane is surprisingly tough at times and sensitive and often the patient will feel a sharp pain momentarily but this wears off in a minute.

Electrode insertion is the key to the whole technique of percutaneous cordotomy, since if the electrode is not properly inserted into the spinal cord a correct lesion cannot be produced. Further, unless there is confidence in the situation of the electrode, no reliance can be placed on the stimulation studies which are carried out through this electrode.

The problem is two-fold. First, is the depth of the penetration of the exposed 2 mm portion of the electrode into the spinal cord tissue correct?

The second concerns the whole question of whether the electrode has been placed in the correct area of the antero-lateral quadrant to produce the required lesion.

The depth of penetration is decided by using lateral and antero-posterior X-rays viewed on the television screen of the image intensifier. The lateral X-ray will show the direction of the electrode, through the needle, in relation to the dentate ligament which is outlined with Myodil. As the Myodil emulsion tends to drop past the dentate ligament over a period of about ten minutes, it is useful to take a lateral X-ray film for reference purposes as soon as a satisfactory demonstration of the anterior border of the cord, and/or dentate ligament is obtained. The antero-posterior X-ray will show the odontoid process in relation to the medial tip of the electrode. As a fairly rough and not too inaccurate indication the centre line of the odontoid process may be taken as the centre line of the cord. This is not strictly true as the spinal cord is not held rigidly; there is a certain mobility both antero-posteriorly and laterally. The stimulation studies mentioned later are also an important part of the technique for deciding when the electrode is correctly placed.

The electrical impedance method for inserting the bared tip of the electrode into the cord tissue up to its insulation and no further (see p. 135), gives great accuracy.

If the electrode is inserted up to the stop and there is no marked rise in impedance the tip either has not reached the pia mater or, more likely, has not penetrated it. The spinal needle–electrode combination is slowly pushed in a further millimetre or so until the impedance does rise. It is then in a correct position and this is checked by X-rays (see Fig. 22).

The question as to whether the electrode tip has been placed among the pain fibres is an anatomical one. Unfortunately, there is controversy over the arrangement of pain fibres in the antero-lateral quadrant. The author uses a model where the fibres carrying pain are arranged in a thin layer about 3 mm thick, from the dentate ligament to the exit of the anterior root. Some thermal fibres are intermingled with these but are also, to some extent, in a thin layer deep to the pain fibres. The author believes that on occasion the pain fibres are arranged in a tight bundle but usually there is a segmental arrangement, with the lower dermatomes near the dentate ligament and the upper ones near the anterior root.

If this concept of the arrangement of the pain fibres is approximately correct then there is no need for the electrode to penetrate the spinal cord deeper than 3 mm, and in normal circumstances 2 mm will be enough. The electrode, as previously stated, is insulated except for the terminal

2 mm which is bared, and sharpened for easy penetration of the cord. The best points are provided by electrolytically etching the terminal few milli- metres by means of an electrical current. This tends to be a tedious process and suitably etched electrodes can be obtained commercially at reasonable cost. They are sold in matched sets with a spinal needle. Alternatively, simple electrodes can be made very cheaply in any ordinary hospital laboratory, by using 1/1000 inch stainless steel piano wire covered with

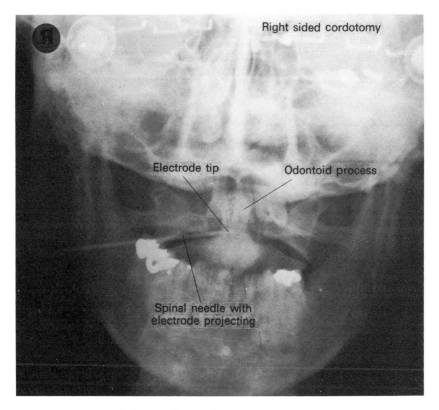

Right sided cordotomy

Electrode tip

Odontoid process

Spinal needle with electrode projecting

FIGURE 22. Electrode tip inserted into cord.

a polythene sheath of suitable internal diameter. The polythene sheath is heat shrunk on to the wire in a hot air oven (about fifteen minutes at about 65 °C, the exact times and temperatures are not critical). A sharp point is then put on the tip of the electrode by means of a fine rotating grindstone. Sometimes the electrode is coated with very fine insulating material by means of an epoxy resin, or a length of wire can be covered with teflon by commercial processes.

Stimulation studies

Once it is known that the electrode is properly inserted into the spinal cord, the position of the electrode as seen on the check X-rays is correlated with the results of stimulating the nerve fibres of the cord, or its grey cells. If the stimulation is carried out at 2 hertz the motor fibres and cells are more likely to be stimulated than the sensory fibres. The opposite holds good when the rate of stimulation is 100 hertz. The stimulation used is of the order of 3 msec square waves at up to 10 volts for the 2 hertz stimulation, the usual value being about 2 volts, and up to 1 volt for the 100 hertz stimulation, the usual value being about 0·2 volt. The 2 hertz voltage required is roughly ten times that for 100 hertz stimulation.

It is important to realise this point as usually the motor stimulation test at 2 hertz is used first, followed by the sensory stimulation at 100 hertz. If one forgets to switch the power from high to low in those lesion generators which provide such a control, the patient will get such a surge of sensory stimulation that it may quite literally lift them off the operating table. Any gross movement of the patient when the electrode is in position is dangerous and the author has heard of one death occurring from this cause. The patient developed an immediate quadriplegia.

The technique of stimulation testing is, first, to make sure that the patient understands what is to be done. He is told about the procedure quite explicitly and in detail. He is also told of the sensations that may be felt and movements that may be noticed. The patient is told not to worry about these as they are caused quite deliberately by the operator. Then slowly the voltage is turned up, the machine having been set to 2 hertz. At around 1·5 volts the trapezius on the ipsilateral side of the electrode usually starts to pulse if the electrode is in an approximately correct position. There may be a more or less vigorous contraction of the small muscles of the head which cause a slight turning movement. These movements are due to stimulation of anterior horn cells.

During this stimulation period the patient's arms, hands, legs, and feet are exposed so that any movement in them can be seen immediately. This is one of the crucial tests in the whole operation, as it shows whether or not the electrode is located in the motor cortico-spinal tract. This tract is uncrossed at this level so it is the ipsilateral body or limbs to the electrode which are affected. It is important to distinguish permissible movements in the arm caused by the trapezius pulling it up from above, and the unwanted active pulsing of, say, the biceps or triceps muscle.

Any pulsing in upper or lower limbs or body will require the electrode to be moved anteriorly away from the cortico-spinal tract. This will mean withdrawing the electrode, altering the position of the spinal needle and reinserting the electrode. It will then be necessary to carry out the impedance measurement and the full series of stimulation studies. Each time the electrode is moved, however many that may be, this routine series of tests is performed.

These tests are not routinely used in some methods of performing the percutaneous cordotomy. The author believes that full use should be made of them so that the technique of the percutaneous cordotomy can be converted from an art to a science.

Some difficulties may arise with the motor stimulation at 2 hertz. Although rare sooner or later an operator will get a patient with an abnormal decussation of the pyramids at the C1–C2 level, so this should be suspected if consistently abnormal motor movements result on 2 hertz stimulation. It is possible when a lower than usual decussation takes place that stimulation of the motor fibres may produce pulsing of the muscles on the contralateral side. A quick check of the antero-posterior X-ray should show whether the electrode has crossed the cord and is stimulating the contralateral side directly. It is a useful routine to measure the length of the spinal needle in the preliminary stages, and when the tip of the needle is properly placed mid-way between the odontoid process and the pedicle to measure the skin to hub distance. Admittedly this distance varies a little as the local anaesthetic solution absorbs, but it does not vary by more than a millimetre or two, and it can be checked from time to time to see if the needle has been pushed in or dragged out a little.

If the electrode is on the correct side of the cord and contralateral pulsing of muscles occurs, then an anomalous arrangement of the fibres at this level is present. It is reasonable under these circumstances to abandon the procedure. Before abandoning such a patient, especially if the pain is due to inoperable cancer, it might be reasonable to make a search for the sensory fibres by gradually and deliberately moving the electrode anteriorly from the dentate ligament to the anterior border of the spinal cord. This is carried out at the lowest possible dermatomal level, i.e. as near to C2 as possible, which allows the maximum distance for decussation to be complete. At each position stimulation studies would be performed. If sensory fibres were found a small test coagulation in the fashion described later could determine whether it was reasonable to continue.

A second anomaly on stimulation may occur when the trapezii on both sides pulse. This is due to the electrode being placed centrally in the cord with just enough of the bared portion of the electrode on each side to provide stimulation on that side. A slight withdrawal of the electrode by withdrawing the spinal needle from the skin can be checked by means of the skin to hub measurement as described previously. On occasion when the electrode is too far on the contralateral side and stimulation at 2 hertz produces pulsing of muscles on the contralateral side, gradual withdrawal produces a progression from contrapulsing, to bilateral pulsing, to ipsilateral pulsing.

Other strange sensations can be produced by 2 hertz stimulation, such as a contracting sensation in the pharynx, or a tightening in the chest. It is usually due to the electrode being too deep and approaching the mid-line. Unusual sensations of mid-line type are mostly produced by stimulation at 100 hertz.

Once the stimulation test at 2 hertz is correct then one moves on to the stimulation test at 100 hertz, remembering that the voltage used is one-tenth that used at 2 hertz. The voltage is gradually turned up from zero and at about 0·2 volt some sensations come through. Usually these are on the contralateral side of the body, but can be mid-line or ipsilateral. If the sensations reported are ipsilateral then, just as in the 2 hertz stimulation when it appears on the 'wrong' side of the patient, penetration of the electrode to the opposite side of the cord has to be checked. If it is too far then it must be withdrawn. During withdrawal the stimulation sensations will change first to bilateral sensations and then to unilateral ones again, but this time on the opposite side to the one they started on.

It must not be forgotten that occasionally, but not very rarely, a patient presents who has uncrossed pain fibres at the C_1–C_2 level. In this type of patient sensation will occur on stimulation at 100 hertz on the 'wrong' side consistently, and all the evidence from X-rays and physical measurements will confirm this. Before moving the electrode to the opposite side of the spinal cord it is just as well to do a small coagulation and check where the area of analgesia develops. If it develops on the 'wrong' side then indeed this patient has an uncrossed pain tract.

On occasion the patient reports sensation on the ipsilateral side on stimulation with 100 hertz but all the measurements and X-rays show that the electrode lies on the ipsilateral side. Sometimes the patient reports sensation on both sides of the body with the electrode very definitely on the ipsilateral side. Again a small cautious coagulation will determine where analgesia develops. Bilateral sensation can occur with an anteriorly placed electrode.

Coagulation is carried out by the method described on page 138. The actual lesion made is barrel shaped because it is made with an electrode which is relatively narrow compared to its length. It is approximately two-thirds as wide as it is long, and it will be longer than the exposed length of electrode used depending on the R.F.C. power.

Suggestions on likely currents and times are provided for commercially produced machines, but otherwise they have to be standardised before use. In those countries where it is permissible, lesions can be made in the brains of small animals, using variable times and currents. The animal can be killed and the brain examined, post-mortem to determine which parameters gave the most satisfactory lesions. In countries where there are anti-vivisection laws a less satisfactory method can be used.

The author has found that the best test material under these circumstances is a piece of fresh liver. Any animal liver can be used, for instance, in India goat liver proved satisfactory. The liver lies on saline-wetted gauze resting on a metal plate which is connected to the indifferent terminal. The electrode is connected to the active terminal and is inserted into the liver, either into the surface edge or deeper in according to preference. If inserted into the surface it must have the insulation flush with the surface and all the bared portion of the tip buried. A current is passed through the electrode of an order which is expected to give too great a lesion, say 50 mA for sixty seconds. The production of heat may be too great and crackling and steam are produced. If this type of lesion were made in the patient, a steam explosion would result in the cord with unknown and uncontrollable results. Next time make a lesion of half this, say 50 mA for twenty-five seconds. If a lesion is made without the crackling or popping noises denoting steam then this could possibly be suitable. A scalpel blade is used to cut down on to the lesion, the aim being to split it through the middle. The lesion will show up as a greyish area. Measurement of the width and length will give a rough idea of its size. It must be remembered that the effective lesion will be wider and longer than the grey area and an allowance should be made for this. If desired, microscopic sections can be prepared and will give a more accurate estimate of the damage produced and its extent. In this fashion a number of lesions with differing power and time are prepared, and an estimate made of the lesion each produces. From these it is not difficult to choose a range which can be used in the patient in safety. The principle is to start low with parameters which are unlikely to produce any lesion at all, and then increase from that, carefully testing all the time for developing analgesia or motor weakness.

Safety measures during lesion production. In some techniques testing is carried out between coagulations, in others during coagulation, and in others, a combination of both these. The author uses the latter technique. The whole basis of testing between coagulations is to assess the level of analgesia produced on the contralateral side to the electrode, and also any diminution in motor power developing in the musculature on the ipsilateral side. Analgesia is detected by pin prick and multiple pricks are made rapidly at intervals at about 2 cm extending over the body and limbs. Before coagulation is begun test for pin prick on both sides of the body, and also test the motor power on both sides. It is also sensible to test both these again after the electrode is inserted into the spinal cord, because when the electrode is in a good position the mere pressure of it in the cord may affect function which appears as analgesia. Similarly if the electrode is placed too near, or in, the cortico-spinal tract some motor weakness may develop.

Immediately after the first small coagulation, testing for analgesia and for motor weakness should be carried out on both sides of the body and limbs to see where they develop and in case the patient has an anomalous arrangement of nerve fibres. Once analgesia develops on the contralateral side without any noticeable motor weakness there is no need to continue testing both sides.

Motor power in between coagulations is conveniently tested by asking the patient to raise the extended leg off the operating table. This checks the power of the lower limb, while the upper limb is tested by asking the patient to grip two or three of the operator's fingers.

Motor power during coagulations is observed by asking the patient to hold the arm up in the air. Some estimation of the power of the leg is obtained by bending the leg at the knee, and in addition pointing the toes up at the ceiling so that only the heel rests on the table. Any weakness either of arm or leg is shown up fairly rapidly by the arm or hand drooping, or the leg tending to wander laterally with an inability to keep the toes dorsi-flexed.

Procedure during lesion production. There are two basic techniques in the production of lesions. In the early Rosomoff method the electrode was placed in the correct position and coagulation proceeded. Nowadays stimulation studies are also available before coagulation. This technique produced analgesia beginning at the lowest dermatomes. This was not invariable but it did happen in a very high percentage of cases. Presumably the method of inserting the spinal needle on a line level with the upper border of the spinal cord, and then re-directing it towards the dentate ligament for insertion of the electrode places the electrode at the anatomical situation where the pain fibres are arranged in overlapping layers, much like the skins of an onion. Thus the initial coagulation will destroy those fibres in immediate contact with the electrode and analgesia of the ankle results. As coagulation continues more layers of pain fibres are destroyed, and as these are arranged in somewhat segmental fashion the analgesia spreads up the body from below upwards. It is most important to test ipsilateral motor power and contralateral analgesia as they develop in between each coagulation which is carried out by using a fixed R.F.C. and varying the time (see p. 138).

When the level of analgesia lies several segments above that required, the final coagulation is repeated three times. This ensures that all the fibres at that level are destroyed and helps in maintaining the level of analgesia in the future. The Rosomoff technique does not specifically use an impedance measurement to detect when the electrode is in a satisfactory position. However, the lesion generator is fitted with an ammeter and this means that there is a measurement of current when the lesion is being made. This, in effect, is a measurement of the resistance of the tissues and is observed during the Rosomoff technique (personal communication, 1975). There is no doubt that this method is by far the quickest in producing a satisfactory lesion with analgesia to the required level. It is done by a meticulous attention to detail and the cutting out of all frills. Each operator will have to decide whether to forego the stimulation studies and specific impedance measurement, or to keep these and have a method which takes longer (about half as long again). The author's preference is for the use of stimulation studies, and the longer period of time.

The second technique, based on the method of Mullan, first demonstrates that the electrode is in the correct position in relation to the antero-lateral quadrant before coagulation. The electrode is inserted and penetration is known to be complete by an impedance measurement. This is followed by stimulation studies. Only if these are correct, as described previously, will the operator go on to a coagulation. During the coagulation the patient has the ipsilateral arm and leg raised in the air as previously described. This enables the patient's power to be observed during the coagulation. If weakness develops then the arm or leg, or both, will show this and coagulation is immediately stopped and the situation reviewed. In between coagulations the power is also tested, but in addition, sensation is tested for developing analgesia by monitoring the developing contralateral analgesia with pin prick. This analgesia, unlike that which usually develops with the Rosomoff technique, can begin at any level of the body or limbs. As the electrode is usually aimed just in front of the dentate ligament the analgesia tends to develop more in the lower half of the body initially than in the upper. The initial coagulation is made using the minimal level indicated for the particular lesion generator used. It is usually of the order of $2\frac{1}{2}$ or 5 seconds at 25 mA. This power, 25 mA, will be much less than that required for a full lesion of the antero-lateral quadrant. After a few coagulations are made at the lower power the situation is reviewed. If a lesion develops as shown by analgesia, then coagulation can continue on this lower power, and if analgesia to the desired level can be obtained in this way, all well and good. If not, then the power is raised, say to 35 mA and the time starts again at $2\frac{1}{2}$ seconds. If necessary the power can be raised to higher levels, but if no analgesia at all develops with an R.F.C. current of medium size and average duration of about 10 seconds or so, then the electrode is in an incorrect position. An anomalous arrangement of pain fibres is rare and therefore any difficulty in obtaining analgesia must be regarded as being due to the operator. It is most likely that if any anatomical variation is present it will show up during the stimulation study phase. Wherever the initial development of analgesia occurs, then succeeding more powerful lesions (either in current or time) will extend the initial analgesic area, but this area tends to be the centre from which the final lesion develops. Thus if the initial analgesia appears on the body at T9 level, succeeding lesions may extend this further so that it finishes at an area of T3 above and L3 below. If the pain is mainly felt in the perineum and sacral dermatomes this will be an unsatisfactory lesion. It must be extended, therefore, to include all the lower dermatomes, and it may well be that the final lesion, if it retains its symmetry, will extend from C5 to S5. On some occasions the lesion will develop in one direction only. This is most satisfactory if that is the direction the operator wishes it to go, but not quite so satisfactory if it is the wrong direction.

The reasons for this are not certain but it is possible to make a few reasonable guesses. There may be a difference in the electrode, in that one side may not be as good at conducting the current as the other. This may be due to a film of insulation which may adhere during the sterilising process. It may be due to an asymmetric coagulum forming during production of the lesion. It can be due to the presence of a relatively large blood vessel on one side of the electrode which thus conducts the heat away too rapidly to allow the formation of a lesion in that direction. There may be other anatomical differences present in the spinal cord which produce this effect; for instance, the pain fibres in the region of the electrode might not be arranged symmetrically. Under these circumstances it is worth rotating the electrode through 180° and repeating the last lesion in case the sheltering is due to the electrode.

Differences in lesion production between the Rosomoff and Mullan techniques are obvious. It is relatively easy to understand why the Rosomoff method provides a rising level of analgesia up the body as lesion production progresses, as an acceptance of the arrangement of pain fibres in the antero-lateral tract in overlapping onion-skin fashion will account for this. It is intrinsic to the method of performing the Rosomoff technique that the spinal needle is initially inserted on the line of the anterior border of the spinal cord, and is then directed posteriorly towards the dentate ligament. Thus the needle and therefore the electrode must enter the tissues of the spinal cord at right angles to the surface.

If one accepts the above explanation then there is no truly satisfactory accounting for the type of analgesia development that occurs in the Mullan technique. As mentioned above the analgesic centre of development can occur anywhere in the body and then spreads out from this. However, in some patients the analgesia develops widely from the beginning. In fact, occasionally, the mere insertion of the electrode and the pressure it produces in the spinal cord is sufficient to produce this type of widespread analgesia. In the Mullan technique the spinal needle is inserted along a different line than the Rosomoff one. In general terms it lies along a more posterior line roughly level with the dentate ligament. The personal technique of the author involves an oblique insertion of the spinal needle from a level below the dentate ligament at the skin to an insertion into the dura anterior to the dentate ligament level. Thus the intrathecal portion of the needle is anterior to the dentate ligament. Before insertion of the electrode the hub of the needle is raised so that the spinal needle is aimed just anterior to the ligament. The general direction of the spinal needle at this stage is either horizontal, or still oblique sloping from posterior to anterior from without inwards. Thus the electrode when it is inserted into the spinal cord does not do so at right angles but probably more obliquely.

In the Mullan technique favoured by the author, occasionally during stimulation tests the patient reports a sensation of a cold wind on one or other part of the contralateral body or limbs. Usually this sensation is felt over a wide area but occasionally is confined to a smaller region such as the shoulder area or the leg from knee to foot. This sensation is always a good sign that a coagulation will give a good result. Often a very small coagulation will produce the most widespread analgesia involving the whole of the body, leg, and the medial arm. Usually the sacral dermatomes and the cervical dermatomes tend to be left out of this initial analgesia. Rarely a patient reports a sensation of warmth and not cold. This is also a good sign but coagulation under these circumstances does not produce the widespread analgesia that follows the sensation of cold. The reason for this is unknown but the fact that a coagulation of small degree can produce widespread analgesia, i.e. by a coagulation of small volume must mean that in some cases the pain fibres are concentrated into a small area, forming a definite bundle. On these occasions the antero-lateral quadrant as a whole must be relatively untouched.

This speculation is very interesting but does not advance our real knowledge of the pathways involved. It merely emphasises that under normal circumstances all anterior quadrant fibres are not destroyed and yet most satisfactory pain relief results for long periods of time.

Post-mortem results would perhaps decide the problem one way or the other but it is not easy to obtain the most interesting cords for section. In most cases when satisfactory relief of pain has been obtained in the inoperable cancer group of patients, they return home and eventually die, where they are lost as far as possible post-mortem material is concerned. In the Liverpool series of over 600 cordotomies, less than 10 per cent of post-mortems have been obtained and by the very nature of the patients dying in hospital the majority of these are patients with recent cordotomies. The over-all mortality is 6 per cent.

Mortality

Perhaps mortality should be discussed at this point lest the 6 per cent mortality mentioned in the previous paragraph is taken to indicate poor technique. Any patient dying in the first post-operative week is included in the mortality figures. What is important is the selection of patients because just as in the surgical cordotomy the surgeon's criteria for the patient to be admitted to surgery decides whether the mortality is almost nil or 25 per cent, so the same considerations (though to a lesser extent) hold good for the percutaneous cordotomy.

Selection of patients for the percutaneous cordotomy. The majority of patients presented for percutaneous cordotomy are those suffering from the intractable pain of inoperable cancer. Some of these patients are in the early stages of the disease when the criteria is to use a method which will relieve the pain until they die, and meanwhile will be so effective that the patient will be able to return to their previous work or family life. These patients are in such good general condition that a death is exceedingly rare. It is only in those patients who have inoperable cancer at an advanced stage and are pre-terminal that any appreciable mortality occurs. Even then it is mainly in those patients who have cancer of the lung with a poor lung function, and pain in the upper chest wall or in the arm. It also occurs in any patient requiring a bilateral high level cordotomy who has a poor respiratory reserve. Thus it is quite easy to avoid poor mortality figures for the percutaneous cordotomy merely by excluding these patients from the procedure.

In the Liverpool series no patient was refused the percutaneous cordotomy provided it was expected that they would live for at least two weeks.

In addition, the lung function was expected to be reasonable though this criteria was very elastic. Normally an FEV 1 of 1·5 litres was hoped for, but anything above 1·0 would be accepted provided the patient understood that their respiratory reserve would be diminished post-operatively for some weeks and perhaps permanently. As an FEV 1 of 0·7 represents the minimum amount of lung tissue that will keep the patient alive under basal conditions in bed something more than this must be regarded as the minimal requirements. On a few occasions the percutaneous cordotomy has been performed at the C1–C2 level for pain along the inner border of the forearm following a carcinoma of the lung with secondary spread, the patient having very poor lung function indeed. Either the lung on the affected side was useless for respiratory purposes or had been totally resected and there was also a reduction of respiratory function in the 'normal' side. In each of these cases the patient had given informed consent in the fullest sense of the word. They were told the prospect of death was high, about 20 per cent, but it was realised they were in very severe pain and the operator was prepared to perform the procedure if the patient wished to accept the risk. The patient's relatives were also informed as to the situation.

Benign conditions

In the Liverpool series most, but not all, of the patients who have a per-cutaneous cervical cordotomy are suffering from an inoperable malignant process. Thus the main disadvantage of the percutaneous cordotomy (or any cordotomy for that matter) is overcome as the patient does not live long enough for pain to recur. In the Liverpool series less than 10 per cent of the patients have a non-malignant condition. These are roughly split between post-herpetic neuralgia and intractable sciatica. There are two criteria used for selection. First, if the patient declares that he is suicidal because of the constant pain, and his medical adviser believes this to be a real threat and second, if the pain interferes with a young person earning a living and supporting his family.

In both cases the patient is told in detail the possible complications, and emphasis is placed on making sure he appreciates that the procedure can make him worse. This point is difficult to 'get across to the patient', who usually believes that it is impossible that he could, in any way, be worse. It is best explained by pointing out that he may get some of the complications without prolonged, or even any, benefit from pain relief. Even worse he may get pain relief but develop severe dysaesthesiae. The incidence of dysaesthesiae seems to be higher in the non-malignant group of patients

and may be a reflection of mental attitudes. Certainly, psychological testing for stability in particular, should be carried out on all non-malignant
patients before operation. Even then the decision must be made on clinical
grounds as long as the psychological profile is not grossly abnormal. In
general terms the author would advise great care before non-malignant
patients are treated in this way for their pain. These patients have a normal
expectation of life, they are around for a long time, and a large part of the
'grief' given to the author by his patients have come from this small group.

Nevertheless, some authorities have large lists of percutaneous cordotomies carried out on just the type of patient described above, with excellent
results. Rosomoff has a series of hundreds of percutaneous cordotomies,
most meticulously assessed and followed up. Many of these suffered from
non-malignant pain. He emphasises that the cordotomy procedure is
rapidly carried out, is usually effective, and can be repeated if necessary.
His complications in this group are comparable to the malignant group.
There can be no quarrel with the effectiveness of the cordotomy, merely that
results wear off in time. It may be that in the American setting there is more
pressure to return to work as quickly and effectively as possible, and to
remain there, than there is in England, where the social effects of being
out of work are not so profound.

Another feature is that in the United States of America there are many
patients who have had multiple lumbar spine surgery, of a type and frequency
which is quite beyond the experience in other countries. The only hope of
pain relief in these patients is to have either an ablative procedure on the
lines of the cordotomy or a Dorsal Column Stimulator implant.

Finally, it must be stated, that despite the objections raised above, the
results of the cordotomy on these non-malignant pain sufferers will be as
effective, with the same success rate, and with the same complication rate,
as in the malignant group. The long-term complication rate is increased
only because they live longer.

Success rate of the percutaneous cordotomy is high, and this is a reflection of the inherently sound nature of the operation. It is based on standard
anatomical and physiological knowledge and most failures should be put
down to operative failure and not patient failure.

In the author's experience about 5 per cent of patients are returned from
the operating theatre without any relief of pain at all. This, of course, is
a reflection of the experience of the operator. The figure of 5 per cent is in
relation to the last two hundred cases or so performed. It was much higher
in the author's early series.

This figure refers to patients in whom no lesion at all results and the patient is unaffected except that he also has a headache and neck ache from the attempted procedure. In addition to this group of patients there is a group where either an unsatisfactory level, or an unsatisfactory degree of analgesia is obtained. Also in addition will be a few extra patients where either an initial satisfactory level shrinks or the analgesia originally satisfactory, fades, or both occur, and pain relief becomes unsatisfactory.

It has to be remembered that there is no definite percentage of patients which can be said to be satisfactory as this percentage success rate drops steadily over a period of years. The most successful percutaneous cervical cordotomies are in the inoperable cancer group of patients and it is obvious why this is so. These patients do not live long enough for complications to develop or for analgesia to fade. Conversely patients with a normal expectation of life exhibit all the known complications of the cordotomy, whether or not it is performed by operative or percutaneous methods.

It can be then said that immediately after the percutaneous cordotomy the success rate is 95 per cent. The following day there will be some frank unsatisfactory results in that the analgesia is not at the required level or is not 'dense' enough. Often patients, who later prove to be unsatisfactory, can be picked out at this stage, as they show 'patchy' analgesia or there are complaints of tingling or pins and needles.

Patchy analgesia deserves a few words separately. During coagulation it is best to test the contralateral analgesic area of the body by pin prick most meticulously. At times a small area of normal or nearly normal sensation will be found in the middle of areas of analgesia. The most vigorous attempts to remove these areas should be made, especially if they are in painful dermatomes. If unsuccessful, pain will either be present in the post-operative period or will occur at some time in the future. It does appear that if normal pain fibres are left intact in an analgesic area then pain relief will not be complete.

It is usual for patients in whom there is no obvious motor weakness present at the end of the operation to develop weakness of varying degree in the seventy-two hours post-operatively. After this period the weakness speedily clears and the power returns to that present at the end of the operation. This is due to cord oedema and some operators give their patients corticosteroids for three days in reducing doses to mitigate the effects of this.

There is one other effect produced by oedema. Percutaneous cordotomies which should technically be failures, may be masked by this oedema. Just as loss of function in motor fibres can be produced by oedema so can loss of function be produced in sensory fibres. Thus a proportion of patients

will have their pain recur on or around the fourth post-operative day. However, once this period is over and provided there is no 'patchiness' a long-
lasting and satisfactory result can be predicted. There will still be some
percutaneous cordotomies which suddenly, and for no known reason, have
fading of analgesia or the development of patches of normal sensation.
These progress, at a faster or slower rate, until analgesia disappears and it
may be difficult to believe that there was any analgesia present previously.

For these reasons the criteria of pain relief used by different authorities
tends to vary. There is only one criteria from the patient's point of view and
that is that relief of pain should last until the patient dies. Even this criteria
is not entirely satisfactory as the length of time between cordotomy and
death depends on the stage of the disease, and good statistics can be obtained
by accepting only advanced malignant patients.

Rosomoff published a series where patients who had had percutaneous
cordotomies for inoperable cancer pain were followed-up until they died.
These figures show a steadily reducing number of patients surviving as time
went by, and concomitant with this was a steadily reducing success rate.
One of the benefits of the percutaneous cordotomy is that it can be repeated
without too much difficulty, and with a reasonable chance of reproducing
a previously successful result. The prospect of being successful on a second
occasion is high, but not as high as on the first. This is because there is
a certain amount of fibrosis and scarring produced by the first cordotomy
and if the electrode on the following occasion enters this area, the second
coagulation does not follow normal lines and a much higher current is
required. If this happens it is preferable to change the position of the needle
tip so that it points either more cephalad or more caudad.

Thus any figures given for the 'success' rate of the percutaneous cordotomy must vary, according to the factors mentioned above. Bearing this in
mind the Liverpool series obtains relief of pain, until the patient dies (in
cancer patients), of 78 per cent. The remainder all have residual pain at
some stage of their remaining life. About 8 per cent of patients have
residual pain of such mild degree that simple analgesic drugs of the aspirin
or paracetamol type are sufficient to provide relief. These are also regarded
as a satisfactory result. The final figure then is 83 per cent for good results.

It would not be true to say that the remaining 17 per cent are all failures
as about one-third of them have fairly good pain relief, good enough to
reduce the type of drugs they need from the addictive to the non-addictive
type. Their pain is not completely relieved but is so much improved that
they do not want any further procedure carried out.

This leaves 10 per cent of patients who require further treatment. Half of these usually refuse a repeat cordotomy, and most but not all of the 5 per cent who have repeats obtain good relief. The final figures are 88 per cent successful, 7 per cent helped, and 5 per cent failures. There is no other method of pain relief in the intractable pain of inoperable cancer which approaches these figures.

Complications of the percutaneous cordotomy are relatively few. In the unilateral ones with normal lung function complications are minimal. There can be motor weakness, urinary problems, loss of erection, dysaesthesiae, and ataxia.

Motor weakness

Some degree of this occurs in all patients following cordotomy. In the Liverpool series of over 600 cases, about 10 per cent of patients have no demonstrable weakness after seventy-two hours post-operatively, i.e. after the initial operative oedema has settled down. Forty per cent of patients have demonstrable weakness, but this is of an order which does not trouble the patients in any way. They will agree that the one leg (the ipsilateral one) is weak but still will not admit to this preventing them moving about in any way.

Another 40 per cent of patients appreciate there is weakness which can be demonstrated in the leg. Half of these (20 per cent) have no trouble walking about, and can carry on with their normal activities. They can walk on the flat and the straight quite easily, but they have to be careful when turning. The other 20 per cent can also walk about but do have to take care. They are conscious that their leg is quite weak, and there is a tendency for it to give way underneath them. Going up or down stairs can be a problem as the weak leg may not carry their weight. Nevertheless, they can manage.

The final category is the 10 per cent of patients whose leg is so weak that they cannot support their weight without the knee giving way. Of this group 8 per cent recover sufficiently in a month to be able to walk without a back splint, while the remaining 2 per cent do not recover.

These figures do not exclude those patients who have had a long period of bed rest before cordotomy, or who have had ambulatory difficulties due to their primary condition.

So far mention has only been made of weakness of the leg but weakness of the arm does occur. The arrangement of the motor fibres in the corticospinal tract is such that during the percutaneous cordotomy the motor fibres to the arm and hand tend to be sheltered relative to those of the leg. Thus although weakness of the arm and hand can usually be demonstrated if this is present in the leg, it is usually to a lesser degree. It is very rare indeed for a patient to have weakness of the arm and hand of a degree which prevents using it for eating. The author has known a few patients who had marked weakness of the arm without much in the way of weakness in the lower limb, but this is unusual.

Urinary difficulties do not occur in unilateral cordotomies unless there was some previous difficulty in the genito-urinary system. In the present series this was $1\frac{1}{2}$ per cent, rather lower than is given elsewhere. When they do occur they tend to recover to the pre-operative level.

Loss of erection has occurred in both old and young patients. It is not usually a problem with patients suffering a malignant condition as their libido has been reduced by the illness. It is, however, a complication which should be mentioned to all patients who are having a cordotomy for a non-malignant condition. It is surprising that a unilateral cordotomy will produce loss of erection but this has happened in three patients in the present series. In two cases in young men, in one, in a much older age group.

Dysaesthesiae occur in about 5 per cent of patients, and about 1 per cent suffer from this disability to a marked degree. Much higher figures are given by other authorities. Many patients who have had a percutaneous cordotomy will mention odd or strange sensations that are felt from time to time. These are usually perceived in the leg or arm and take the form of 'pins and needles' or 'electricity'. They are fleeting and do not occur regularly. After the cordotomy the patients are informed that during the cordotomy for relief of their pain the nerves have been altered and they will probably feel strange sensations from time to time. These are to be ignored as the patient is slightly different now, and these new sensations are part of the 'new pain-free patient'. A few words on these lines will prevent most patients from dwelling overlong on minor degrees of dysaesthesia. It is only when these sensations are frequent and there is an element of unpleasantness about them that the patients may feel that their previous pain was a lesser evil.

Ataxia, only two patients in this series have shown ataxia of marked degree. One in the lower limb and one in the upper. In both cases there was no doubt that loss of position sense without loss of vibration sense or alteration in tone occurred. In the lower limb case there was no loss of power but there was some weakness in the corresponding upper limb. In the upper limb case both ipsilateral limbs were weak. These conditions improved very slowly over a period of some months. The patients were then lost to our records.

Rosomoff records a much higher rate of ataxia with an equivalent high recovery rate.

Other sensations are unaltered with the exception of the sensation of touch. In the majority of patients after a percutaneous cordotomy the patient's ability to appreciate touch is slightly reduced. Some patients deny any alteration of sensation between the two sides.

Bilateral percutaneous cordotomy (see Figs. 23 and 24) has much more profound effects than a mere doubling of the complications occurring in the unilateral one. However, as this method of treating intractable pain tends to be used on the hopeless, advanced cancer patients, the complications can be reduced to three categories.

General debility is increased. A bilateral cordotomy interferes with autonomic nervous control to an extent that falls of blood-pressure occur. This combined with the stress from the cordotomy procedure itself, and a generalised loss of motor power and muscle tone may hazard the life of the patient. It should be emphasised that this will occur only in the immediate post-operative period and once this is past (say four days) the patient's condition should stabilise. Further, as it is usually patients with a physical condition too poor for surgery who have bilateral percutaneous cordotomies performed on them, a high risk can be accepted. This provided the patients and their relatives appreciate the risk involved.

The bilateral procedure should not be performed in one stage. There should be an interval of at least one week between the two sides. This gives the opportunity for any oedema and motor weakness to settle down.

Urinary retention occurs in a high percentage of patients having bilateral cordotomy in the Centre for Pain Relief. This does not occur in other series. The fibres controlling and initiating micturition are believed to be in the spinal cord near the lateral horn area, but there is no great certainty about this. One thing does appear to be certain and that is that wherever these fibres are, they tend to be damaged in any cordotomy, and to be bilaterally damaged in bilateral operations. Many of our patients needing bilateral cordotomy have already some urinary problems and are already catheterised (40 per cent approx.) and a further 20 per cent require catheterising after the bilateral procedure is completed. Recovery may occur in time.

Patients who have bilateral cordotomies are automatically catheterised after the second cordotomy and this is left in place for a minimum of four days. This is to allow any cord oedema to settle. A residual urine test is then carried out and if the residue is more than 100 ml, the catheter is replaced. If the residue is between 50 and 100 ml the catheter is removed and a residual test is repeated after one day. If the quantity has increased to above 100 ml a catheter is reinserted. If the catheter has to be replaced initially another residual urine is performed one week later, and then repeated at two-weekly

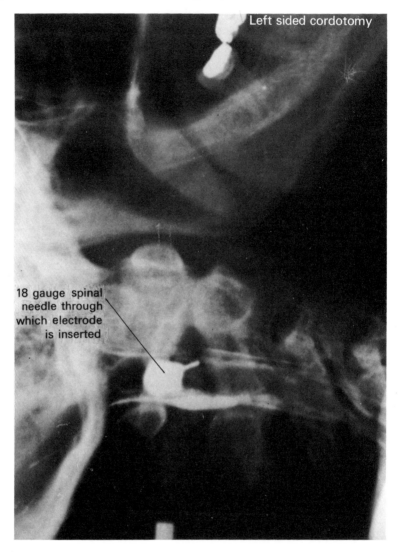

FIGURE 23. Left-sided PCC. Electrode directed caudad. (Cf. Fig. 18, same patient electrode directed cephalad), i.e. this is a bilateral PCC.

intervals while the patient is in hospital. It is repeated at one-monthly intervals after the patient has been discharged home.

Provided the expectation of life of the patient is reasonable a bladder neck resection may be worthwhile. In other cases where paraplegia from secondary spread has, or does result, an automatic bladder may develop.

Respiratory insufficiency can occur in unilateral cordotomy when the patient has poor lung function in general, or when the patient has pain from a spreading carcinoma of a lung and the cordotomy is performed on the normal lung side. In both cases there is a reduced motor activity on the side of the coagulation which is part of the post-operative motor weakness.

In addition to this there is a specific reduction in respiratory activity due to damage to ascending and descending respiratory fibres when coagulation occurs near the anterior horn cells at the C_1 to C_2 level. Damage to these pathways is most likely to occur when a high level of analgesia is required,

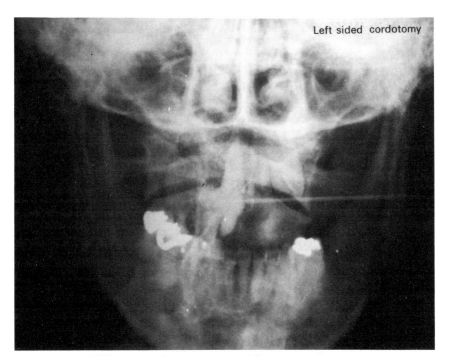

Left sided cordotomy

FIGURE 24. Second side PCC. (Cf. Fig. 22 same patient). Corresponds to Fig. 23.

i.e. when cervical pain fibres are destroyed as both they and the respiratory fibres occupy a position close to the anterior horn. The most obvious result of damage to respiratory fibres occurs when they are damaged bilaterally, and this tends to happen when bilateral percutaneous cordotomy produces a bilateral high level of analgesia.

Under these circumstances the condition known as the 'Ondine' syndrome may develop. In this the patient can breathe reasonably well while awake, but during sleep the respirations either become depressed or cease altogether. These patients may lose the ability to breathe involuntarily and the only treatment for the fully developed condition is for the patient to be intubated and placed on a respirator. In the Centre for Pain Relief the incidence of this condition has been 8 per cent over-all, with a mortality of 4 per cent.

Rosomoff believes that the incidence is 4 per cent and the mortality 2 per cent. If the patients are respired adequately they recover. He also states that he has not seen this condition develop when the level of analgesia has been below C_3. The author has seen this condition develop with analgesia at a lower level than this. However, Rosomoff has more experience of bilateral percutaneous cervical cordotomies than any other worker in this field.

Not every patient who has a bilateral cordotomy performed on him develops the Ondine syndrome. Those who are at risk can be distinguished (Rosomoff) by breathing 5 per cent carbon dioxide. Normal patients double their tidal volume at least while those at risk after bilateral cordotomy have no increase at all. Careful watch should be kept on patients distinguished in this way even to the extent of them spending the first three post-operative nights in an intensive therapy ward.

The condition does not necessarily develop on the first post-operative night but may first appear on the second or third. It usually appears during sleep when voluntary control of respiration is reduced. Warning signs are that the patient becomes restless and anxious, and may complain of difficulty in breathing. There are no other objective signs at this stage, but the patient may be in great danger from impending respiratory failure.

Over the past year the author has been carrying out more bilateral cordotomies than ever before. They are always performed on patients with inoperable cancer having bilateral pain, in whom the pain level on one side of the body is much lower than the other, or where bilateral pelvic pain exists in a patient with a fair expectation of life. The technique in these patients is to carry out the first cordotomy on the side contralateral to the highest level of pain. When this cordotomy is carried out, care is taken to take the level of analgesia only three segments or so above the level of pain. As long as this analgesic level is no higher than $C6$ or $C7$ the second side cordotomy can be performed with a certain equanimity. The second side is the one treating the low level pain, and even if a much higher cordotomy than desired is inadvertently obtained there should be no respiratory problems of the Ondine type as the first side is low enough to avoid this (see Figs. 18, 22, 23, and 24).

Problems arise, of course, when too high a level is obtained at the first cordotomy and if a decision is made (with the patient's informed consent) to go ahead with the second side a very cautious and careful coagulation should be carried out. The second cordotomy should be abandoned if the correct level cannot be obtained.

Avoidance of bladder and respiratory complications is a possibility as long as it is realised that bilateral cordotomies will always produce some bladder disfunction, and that bilateral high analgesic level cordotomies will frequently produce respiratory difficulties as well. In other words the problem can be resolved by either using another method of pain relief entirely, or by combinations of a unilateral cordotomy with another method for the second side.

The combination method works satisfactorily for both urinary and respiratory problems. In the case of urinary problems a cordotomy is carried out on the side of the worst and most widespread pain. Say this is performed on the left side for pain on the right. This will leave the patient with pain in the left of the body or leg, and an intrathecal injection of alcohol or phenol used on the left side of the spinal cord will relieve this pain. Both the lesions produced, one by the cordotomy and one by the intrathecal injection, are on the same side of the spinal cord and there should be no permanent urinary disability. There may be some, temporarily, for a short time due to the intrathecal injection.

As far as respiration is concerned as long as only one cordotomy is performed at a high level there will not be any difficulty except where there is a reduced respiratory capability already present.

The anterior cordotomy

The above statement that 'bilateral cordotomies will always produce some respiratory problems', only holds good for cordotomies performed at the upper cervical level at C1 to C2. This fact has been known by neurosurgeons almost since the time of the first cordotomy in 1912. Most cordotomies carried out surgically are at the upper dorsal level and these have no problems with respiration.

The percutaneous cordotomy has brought much benefit to patients, in that patients who are too ill for the surgical method can have the percutaneous one. This provides an effective cordotomy without a surgical incision. However, the necessity of carrying out the percutaneous cordotomy at the C1 to C2 space is not absolute. The spinal cord can be reached by two other approaches.

One is posteriorly, as in the Crue or Hitchcock methods, but no great advantage is gained here as they are both performed between the C1 to C2 vertebrae or between the base of the skull and C1.

The other is from the anterior approach through an intervertebral disc. Practically, this means through the disc spaces of the lower or middle cervical vertebrae. As there is no great benefit to be gained by using upper cervical discs the C5 to C6, or C6 to C7 space is used. The target in this method is exactly the same portion of the antero-lateral quadrant as in the higher C1 to C2 approach. A spinal needle is inserted intrathecally via a disc space (Fig. 3), aimed at the antero-lateral tract, and an electrode is passed down it and entered into the cord tissue. Stimulation tests are performed and eventually the antero-lateral quadrant is coagulated with relief of pain contralaterally beginning some segments below the level of coagulation.

As the level of this coagulation is below the respiratory fibres, and in particular below the outflow of fibres to the diaphragm through the phrenic nerve, there is no danger of the Ondine syndrome developing. There is, however, one serious problem the spinal needle when it enters the disc space is gripped by the disc material. Thus once the spinal needle is in the disc it cannot be manœuvred. It must be aimed on the correct line to reach the target point in the antero-lateral quadrant before it enters the disc material, and this is not an easy procedure. It can be done by hand in a trial and error fashion but this takes some time to carry out safely. At the Centre for Pain Relief a stereo-tactic frame is used to guide the spinal needle into the target. It was designed by the Bio-Engineering Unit of the University of Salford, is still being improved and works well. Even so, with the initial insertion of the spinal needle carried out under anaesthetic sleep, it still takes a minimum of twice the time taken by the C1 to C2 cordotomy.

An additional method to those described above for avoiding the complications of the bilateral percutaneous cordotomy at the C1 to C2 space is thus available. A C1 to C2 cordotomy can be performed to relieve pain on the side of the body where the level of pain is the highest, while an anterior cordotomy can be performed at a lower level to relieve pain on the other side of the body. This arrangement will produce problems with micturition, but there will be no danger to respiration.

Undoubtedly, this method of relieving bilateral pain would be used more frequently if there was a simpler way of carrying out the anterior approach cordotomy.

REFERENCES

CRUE B.L., TODD E.M., CARREGAL E.J.A., WRIGHT W.H. & MALINE D.B. (1970) Posterior approach for high cervical percutaneous radiofrequency stereotactic cordotomy. In *Pain and suffering—selected aspects*. Ed. B.L. Crue, Chapter 5. Thomas, Springfield, Illinois, U.S.A.

GANZ E. & MULLAN S. (1977) In *Persistent Pain—modern methods of treatment*. Ed. S. Lipton, Chapter 2, page 21. Academic Press, London and New York.

HITCHCOCK E. (1969) An apparatus for stereotactic spinal surgery. *Lancet*, 1, 705.

HITCHCOCK E. (1970) Stereotactic cervical myelotomy. *J. Neurol. Neurosurg. Psychiat.* 33, 224.

LIN P.M., GILDENBERG P.L. & POLAKOFF P.P. (1966) An anterior approach to percutaneous lower cervical cordotomy. *J. Neurosurg.* 25, 553.

LIPTON S. (1968) Percutaneous electrical cordotomy in relief of intractable pain. *Br. med. J.* 2, 210.

LIPTON S., DERVIN E. & HEYWOOD O.B. (1974) A stereotactic approach to the anterior percutaneous electrical cordotomy. In *Advances in Neurology*. Vol. 4. Ed. J.J. Bonica. Raven Press, New York.

NATHAN P.W. (1963a) Results of antero-lateral cordotomy for pain in cancer. *J. Neurol. Neurosurg. Psychiat.* 26, 353.

NATHAN P.W. (1963b) The descending respiratory pathways in man. *J. Neurol. Neurosurg. Psychiat.* 26, 487.

MULLAN S., HARPER P.V., HEKMATAPANAH J., TORRES H. & DOBBIN G. (1963) Percutaneous interruption of spinal pain tracts by means of a strontium 90 needle. *J. Neurosurg.* 20, 931.

MULLAN S., MALLIS M., KARASICK J., VAILATI G. & BECKMAN F. (1965a) A reappraisal of the unipolar anodal electrolytic lesion. *J. Neurosurg.* 22, 531.

MULLAN S., HEKMATAPANAH J., DOBBIN G. & BECKMAN F. (1965b) Percutaneous intra-medullary cordotomy utilising the unipolar anodal electrolytic lesion. *J. Neurosurg.* 22, 548.

MULLAN S. & HOSOBUCHI Y. (1968) Respiratory hazards of high cervical percutaneous cordotomy. *J. Neurosurg.* 22, 291.

MULLAN S. (1971) Percutaneous cordotomy. *J. Neurosurg.* 35, 360.

OWL INSTRUMENTS LTD., 4634, Yonge Street, Willowdale, Ontario, Canada.

ROSOMOFF H.L., CARROLL F., BROWN J. & SHEPTAK P. (1965) Percutaneous radiofrequency cervical cordotomy technique. *J. Neurosurg.* 23, 639.

ROSOMOFF H.L. (1969) Bilateral percutaneous cervical radiofrequency cordotomy. *J. Neurosurg.* 31, 41.

ROSOMOFF H.L. (1971) Percutaneous cervical cordotomy for intractable pain of benign origin. In *39th Annual Meeting American Association of Neurological Surgeons*.

TAREN J.A., DAVIS R. & CROSBY E.C. (1969) Target physiologic corroboration in stereotaxic cervical cordotomy. *J. Neurosurg.* 30, 569.

TENICELLA F., ROSOMOFF H.L., FEIST J. & SAFAR P. (1968) Pulmonary function following percutaneous cervical cordotomy. *Anaesthesiology*, 29, 7.

THE INJECTION OF ALCOHOL INTO THE PITUITARY FOSSA (MORICCA'S OPERATION)

Hormone therapy in the treatment of cancer was established in the last century. Cancers of the breast, ovaries, testes, and prostate gland are the most likely ones to respond to treatment and there are various directions which this treatment can take. Castration, i.e. removal of ovaries or testes is a relatively simple measure, but although it may work for a time the effect wears off as other tissues in the body secrete the specific male and female hormones.

Another method lies in the use of antihormones, or in the use of androgens in females and oestrogens in males. All these have disadvantages, some of them quite distressing, such as the masculinisation of a young female.

Steroids produce remissions in some patients but rarely are these effects long lasting but following the availability of steroids in the early 1950s, the operations of adrenalectomy and subsequently hypophysectomy were used in cancer treatment and particularly in cancer of the breast. Adrenalectomy involves a major abdominal operation, and the surgical hypophysectomy is equally massive. Further, the modern tendency is to avoid escalating the operations to which the patient is subjected by carrying out the initial oophorectomy by radiotherapeutic methods, followed by hormone medication and chemotherapy and later, hypophysectomy is considered.

Hypophysectomy can be performed by open operation through the cranium, or by a trans-nasal, trans-sphenoidal, or ethmoidal approach. These latter methods are much less traumatic but there are even simpler methods of destroying the pituitary gland. These are carried out by implanting radioactive particles into the pituitary fossa. The radioactive implant is inserted through a wide bore needle, which is progressively placed in position first through the nose, then the sphenoid sinus, and on into the pituitary fossa. The radioactive material usually used is Yttrium, in the form of Yttrium 90 which is a beta-ray emitter.

This method of Yttrium 90 implant carries as good a prospect of relief and remission as the formidable surgery of adrenalectomy or hypophysectomy and is tending to be used instead of these surgical methods. Naturally, these methods are not used in isolation but radiotherapy of conventional type, and chemotherapy, may be used concurrently in a patient having, or who has had, a hypophysectomy.

One of the difficulties found in these patients is the number and variety of the complications that can occur. To use the term 'complications' is not strictly correct as many of the problems facing the patient and his medical advisers, after say a hypophysectomy, are not complications in the true sense but consequences of the destruction of the pituitary gland. For instance, a diabetes insipidus is not uncommon, it is expected to occur, and will occur after removal of the pituitary secretion controlling reabsorption of fluid into the body. This then is a consequence of the operation and is not a complication.

It is common knowledge after hypophysectomy for widespread cancer, either locally at the primary site, or at a distance at secondary sites, that pain from the tumour is also relieved. This certainly happens in the hormone dependent tumours but what is surprising is that on occasion this relief of pain is rapid. For instance, a patient having a hypophysectomy for dis-seminated and painful cancer, by one of the methods mentioned above, may be pain free on waking from the anaesthetic. This is most encouraging when it happens but would appear to be pain relief of a different order, or by a different mechanism, to the gradual relief of pain which often happens after a hypophysectomy.

The percutaneous cordotomy mentioned in another chapter of this book is one of the most valuable methods of relieving the intractable pain of cancer that is available, but it does not offer any prospect of regression of the tumour unless this occurs spontaneously. Hypophysectomy does offer such a possibility, and with it the prospect of relief of pain, and this relief will occur at all the sites where the tumour is present. If relief of this kind is to be widely available an easily applied method of destruction of the pituitary gland is required. Such a simple and easily applied method has been worked out by Moricca (1974, 1977).

CHEMICAL HYPOPHYSECTOMY

Moricca calls this method of ablating the pituitary gland 'pituitary adenolysis' or 'chemical hypophysectomy'. The author calls it the 'pituitary injection of alcohol'. It does not matter what it is called, or how it is performed, because the method is effective in the relief of pain in inoperable cancer. An added benefit is that the method can be adopted for the active treatment of tumours, to produce regression.

Originally the method of pituitary injection of alcohol was devised as a simple way of carrying out destruction of the pituitary gland without major surgery or using complicated apparatus. The requirement of this method was that it should also be repeatable, perhaps many times, without hazard-ing the life of the patient. In 1963 Moricca began the development of his technique, which has progressed to that described later.

This early technique came from the observation that pain due to hormone dependent tumours can sometimes be relieved with hormone additive therapy, but is more likely to be relieved by hormone subtractive therapies such as orchidectomy, ovariectomy, adrenalectomy, and hypophysectomy. It was decided to suppress pituitary function and alcohol was chosen as the neurolytic agent. In this way it was hoped that the method would be available even in the poor-risk patient with advanced malignant disease who was too ill for major surgery. These hopes have been realised.

Naturally over the years the technique has altered and writing recently Moricca stated that 'pituitary adenolysis constitutes a non-traumatic and easily performed technique. It does not require special equipment, is absolutely inexpensive, and can be repeated without any technical limitations and with insignificant clinical contra-indications. In addition it controls with a single block, diffused, unbearable cancer pain.' The author believes this statement to be broadly true though his own results are not as good as those of Moricca. This statement is also broadly confirmed by a number of other workers in the intractable pain field, who have begun to use this technique (Madrid, Katz, McEwan).

Technique

This is basically very simple. A needle some 12·5 cm long, not counting the hub (see Fig. 25), is inserted through the nose, traverses the sphenoid sinus and is directed so that it rests against the floor of the pituitary fossa. A small E.N.T. hammer is then used to tap it through the bone and on into the pituitary fossa itself. 100 per cent alcohol is then injected down the needle into the fossa, while ocular movements and pupillary responses to light are monitored. If these become abnormal in any way the injection is terminated at that point.

During the injection the blood-pressure is also monitored and if it begins to rise the injection is again terminated, a lumbar puncture is performed and an intrathecal injection of hydrocortisone made. This injection spreads up the spinal theca to the cerebro-spinal fluid in the brain by means of barbotage. The purpose of this injection is to avoid the possibility of a pituitary apoplexy producing a serious rise in blood-pressure. In the Liverpool series the blood-pressure has not been monitored for this purpose.

The above is a very limited statement of the method of pituitary injection of alcohol, and each particular section will now be expanded in more detail.

The needle is not really a needle, it is a fine trocar and cannula. The gauge is variable, and in fact it is wise to have these 'pituitary needles' in a number of gauges so that a stronger one can be used if the bone is denser or thicker than normal. In the first few initial cases the author used a standard trigeminal needle normally used for injecting the gasserian ganglion. This needle of about 18-gauge was too thin for the average bone, but although tending to bend, an adequate injection was made in the first few cases. However, one patient with rather denser bone than the average could not be injected as this needle could not penetrate the bone. In the light of further experience this was unusual as bone of this density is experienced infrequently at the rate of about one in forty cases or so. A needle gauge of about 16 is suitable for most circumstances, but one heavier than this may be required for denser bone. These needles are manufactured locally, of stainless steel, and the hub is screwed to the shaft for added strength. There is one important feature of any needle used for a pituitary injection, namely

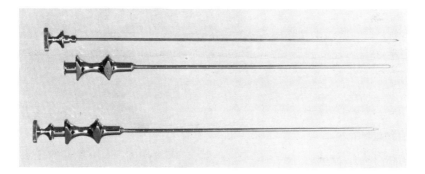

FIGURE 25. Pituitary trocar and cannula.

the internal volume. The needles used by Moricca have an internal volume of only 0·15 ml while those manufactured for us are 0·3 ml. The smaller quantity is advantageous as the effects of the injection will start that much quicker, and if the operation has to be abandoned for any reason there is less chance of further alcohol entering the pituitary fossa. In addition, at the end of the injection when the stylette (really the trocar) is reinserted before removal an extra increment of 0·15 ml is acceptable whereas one of 0·3 ml is not. In the latter case the trocar is inserted in a number of stages, say three, thus pushing alcohol in 0·1 ml increments into the pituitary fossa.

Near the hub a number of concentric marks at 0·5 cm intervals, ten in number, provide a visual aid if the position of the needle needs to be advanced or withdrawn. Apparently in the original models Moricca had concentric rings along the length of the needle but this only provided a source of weakness.

Image intensifier

The operation is carried out quickly and easily using an image intensifier. It is necessary to arrange it so that two views can be speedily obtained, the lateral and the antero-posterior (see Figs. 32 and 33), and of these the lateral is used more frequently. In fact, the antero-posterior view is only used in the initial stage when it is most important to be sure the trocar and cannula lie in the mid-line, as it rests against the floor of the pituitary fossa and before it is tapped on into the fossa itself. The pituitary fossa is rather wider than would appear from its shape in the lateral view, but there is still not much space available if the trocar is to be placed accurately. The most important feature during its insertion is that in the antero-posterior view the tip of the trocar is lying in the mid-line, when from the lateral view it is seen to be resting against the floor of the pituitary fossa.

From the lateral view the direction of the trocar can be kept under frequent review, first, to ensure that penetration from nares to sphenoid sinus occurs at a level suitable for onward progression into the pituitary fossa. Sometimes the trocar will enter the stoma between nares and sinus and if this is in a suitable position the pituitary needle can be placed against the pituitary fossa without any trauma at all. If the stoma cannot be entered or is in an unsuitable position then the needle must be lined up with the posterior clinoid processes and the bone hammer used to penetrate on the correct line.

It is an advantage to aim the trocar at the posterior clinoid process (see Fig. 35). The technique is to hammer the cannula and trocar in gently until they will go no further. The tip of the trocar is then against the posterior clinoid process, or preferably, a little caudad to it. The trocar projects from the end of the cannula about 1 mm or so and when it is withdrawn the cannula is not against the bone but is either in the pituitary gland, or against the pituitary gland, or in the space surrounding the gland. It can be readily understood that the cannula can be in many positions in relation to the apparent position of the pituitary gland as seen by the appearance of the pituitary fossa on the lateral X-ray view, and this has a bearing on the destruction of the pituitary gland. When regression of tumour is desired in hormone-dependent tumours, complete destruction of the gland is required and is more likely to occur if the alcohol injected at different times is deposited at different positions in the gland. A record must therefore be kept of the appearance in the lateral X-ray film of the position of the cannula tip each time an injection of alcohol is made. Not only this but a corresponding antero-posterior X-ray film will show the cannula tip in relation to the width of the pituitary gland.

The volume of alcohol injected varies with the size of the pituitary fossa. An estimation of this can be made by the radiologist expressed in cubic millimetres. An average volume would normally receive a volume of 1 ml of alcohol unless ocular signs appeared. If no ocular signs appear then the volume may be increased to 1·5 ml and the extra alcohol deposited in a different position. A total volume of 1·0 ml should be placed in two situations, but an exception to this would be if a direct injection into the gland occurred. This would be shown, when after placing the cannula in a correct position as shown by X-ray, the injection of alcohol needed more pressure than usual. Also after each injection of, say, 0·1 ml, a reflux of alcohol would occur. This would be evidence that the cannula was placed within the substance of the pituitary gland itself and, with the exception of any leaking back along the track, all the alcohol would spread through the planes of the gland and maximum destruction of the gland would occur under these circumstances. The injection of alcohol is made with a 1·0 ml syringe of the tuberculin type which allows very small increments of alcohol to be injected and thus increases the safety of the procedure.

The pituitary fossa as shown on a lateral X-ray film is relatively small but there is no difficulty in distinguishing that the cannula can be near the anterior clinoids, near the posterior clinoids, or in the mid position. Also in the anterior and posterior positions an upper and a lower situation of the cannula can be seen depending on whether it is near the base of the fossa, or is near the diaphragma sellae. In the central portion of the fossa three divisions can be made, an upper, a middle, and a lower. There are thus seven divisions that can be made quite easily from the lateral view. Using the antero-posterior view it is possible to distinguish whether the cannula is central or to one side or the other. In other words three divisions can be made. Thus to be meticulous 7×3, i.e. twenty-one positions for the cannula can be distinguished. The only purpose of these records is for future reference, so that if on the first injection of alcohol the cannula tip was placed low, near the posterior clinoid process, and on the left side, on the next occasion an attempt would be made to place it somewhere anteriorly and preferably on the right side. As it is usual to make at least two deposits of alcohol with each penetration of the pituitary fossa, one at the maximum distance within the fossa, and one at the nearest point of entry, a record of two positions is made each time. This is a useful record to keep. The shape of the pituitary gland is not the globe that is usually imagined. It is olive-shaped with the long axis coronally placed, and it is much larger than would be expected from the lateral X-ray film alone.

The operation of pituitary injection of alcohol is a short procedure, in the average case it takes about fifteen to twenty minutes from start to finish. The patient is in a neutral dorsal position with the head supported on a radio-translucent portion of the operating table. The image intensifier swings round the head to provide the lateral and antero-posterior views as desired. The operator stands at the head of the table with the patient's body stretching away down it. In this way the operator gets the best opportunity of keeping, and seeing, the needle in the mid-line. The operator can either stand within the curve of the swinging arm of the image intensifier, with the body of the machine in line with the table but behind him, or the machine can be placed to one side of the table. Whichever position is used a radio-opaque lead apron is worn, or an equivalent protective system adopted. In addition, care is taken to make sure the hands are out of the X-ray beam when viewing occurs. It is surprisingly easy to get into very bad habits in this respect. As in the percutaneous cervical cordotomy the best safety method is to have the image intensifier controlled by someone other than the operator, with instructions that the beam is not to be switched on if any part of the operator is in the beam.

The patient can be conscious or unconscious, and each method has its disadvantages and advantages. There are the obvious advantages with the unconscious patient of having no problems of movement, or expressions of pain during the operation. One great disadvantage is that the patient is unable to report on any alteration of visual acuity, double vision, or alteration of visual fields. However, it can be done safely if the anaesthetic given is a very light one, so that the reflex activity of the pupil to light is preserved, and if the injection of alcohol is made cautiously and in small increments while testing for the light reflex in between each injection.

The safest method is to have the patient conscious during the injection (Figs. 26 and 27), but in almost all cases the patient will complain of severe headache shortly after, or during each increment. Even with powerful pre-medication of the neurolept type, the patient will complain. If a series of alcohol injections of the pituitary gland are planned, the painful headache produced by the effect of the alcohol on the dura may preclude completion of the series. To avoid this pain the author made a preliminary injection of 1 per cent lignocaine, using this cautiously in divided doses with no increment larger than 0·5 ml and the total volume no more than 2·0 ml. Tests were carried out to detect diffusion of the local anaesthetic agent out of the pituitary fossa to important structures. In particular if it spread on to the cranial nerves producing ocular palsies the pituitary injection could not be carried out. In practice no patient developed any ocular paresis beyond a temporary dilatation of the pupil, lasting a few minutes. This quantity of

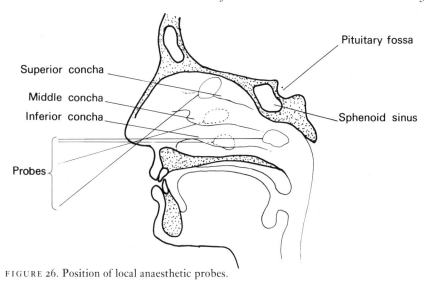

Pituitary fossa

Superior concha

Middle concha

Inferior concha

Sphenoid sinus

Probes

FIGURE 26. Position of local anaesthetic probes.

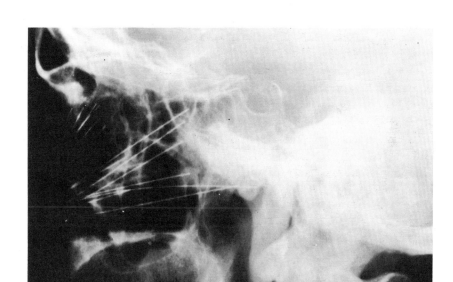

FIGURE 27. Lateral X-ray, probes in position.

local anaesthetic solution will reduce the pain that is felt but does not remove it in the majority of cases. There was no doubt in the minds of some of our patients, who had pituitary injections with and without a preliminary injection of local, that the local injection made a considerable difference to the amount and severity of the pain suffered. There is one very valid criticism made of this technique concerning the diluting effect the local anaesthetic solution must have on the alcohol. Whether there is a difference in the quality of tumour regression, or relief of pain cannot now be answered by the author as this method is no longer used by him. The series of cases, where it was so used, was not large enough to determine this question. For what it is worth the author does not think it made any difference.

Previous to the present method of using a general anaesthetic, complete with cuffed endotracheal tube, pharyngeal pack, and facilities for controlling respiration if necessary, Moricca used a short-acting intravenous anaesthetic during the placing of the pituitary cannula into the pituitary fossa. Once the bone work had been done the patient was allowed to wake up. This procedure was repeated during the injection of the alcohol and the testing of the pupillary responses to light. If great care is thought to be essential then this method could be used and the patient allowed to recover consciousness in between injections.

The present method of a continuous, but light, general anaesthetic with testing of the light reflex, works very well as long as no further alcohol is injected if a previously active pupil becomes sluggish, or a sluggish one does not react. There is no doubt that the safety margin is reduced when a general anaesthetic is given and the section on complications will illustrate this.

The records of the patient having an injection of alcohol into the pituitary fossa must be collected meticulously, not just for the period of the injection but also before and after this period. Any investigations, such as a hormonal survey must be completed, and in particular the records relating to the position, size, and shape of primary and secondaries; the presence of glands; adherence to skin; and X-rays in the case of bony and lung metastases should be collected. If the injection is for regression of the tumour then these records are absolutely essential. Unexpected regression sometimes occurs in tumours which are regarded as non-hormone dependent.

The purpose of the injection can now be mentioned conveniently. Moricca devised this technique originally as a simple and relatively easy way of ablating the pituitary gland in hormone-dependent tumours. This did two things. In certain patients regression of the tumour occurred for a shorter or longer period, and when growth of the tumour recurred the injection could be repeated with the prospect of another regressive response.

The second benefit occurred whether or not regression took place. This was relief of pain which was independent of regression. It was noted, and has been confirmed in the Liverpool series, in some patients with dreadful pain over wide areas of the body, that an injection of alcohol into the pituitary fossa was followed by immediate relief of the pain. In the majority of patients suffering from pain, relief does occur but over a period of days.

This raised the question as to what process was producing the relief of pain. It was fairly certain that regression of tumour occurred due to reduction or removal of pituitary hormonal influences, but it was not possible to be sure that the pain relief observed was solely due to this cause. In fact, it looked highly unlikely. The speed of action of the alcohol in producing pain relief in those patients mentioned above suggests a nervous system action and not a hormonal one. As the hypophyseal region is one where nervous, and hormonal influences are very much in combination this idea is not far fetched, and will be discussed later.

The anatomy of the pituitary gland is straightforward (see Figs. 28, 29, and 30). The hypophysis or pituitary body is oval in shape and lies in the fossa or sella turcica of the sphenoid bone. It is covered by a fold of dura mater, the diaphragma sellae, which has a central opening through which passes the infundibulum or pituitary stalk. The infundibulum (a part of the hypothalamus) connects the anterior part of the tubercinereum to the posterior lobe of the pituitary body. In its upper part the infundibulum is hollow, containing a diverticulum of the third ventricle.

The long diameter of the pituitary gland is transversely situated, and the gland consists of two parts, an anterior and posterior lobe.

The internal carotid artery lies in the carotid groove on the lateral aspect of the body of the sphenoid bone. It does, in fact, lie within the cavernous sinus, where its course is first upwards between the lingula of the sphenoid and the posterior petrosal process of the sphenoid, then forwards to the anterior clinoid process, and then upwards medial to the anterior clinoid process. Here it pierces the dura mater of the roof of the cavernous sinus and enters its cerebral path. The abducens nerve lies on the lateral side of the artery in its cavernous sinus pathway.

The optic nerves, chiasma, and tracts have close relations with the pituitary fossa of the sphenoid bone. Anterior to this fossa is the tuberculum sellae, and on this rests the optic chiasma. Anteriorly the optic chiasma is joined by the two optic nerves, and posteriorly is in relation to the tubercinereum and the infundibulum. It is thus closely related to the floor of the third ventricle. Passing backwards from the optic chiasma are the two optic tracts, which ultimately divide into lateral and medial roots.

Arteries   Nerves

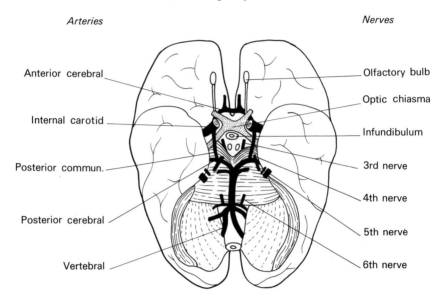

Anterior cerebral ————————————————————————— Olfactory bulb

————————————————————————— Optic chiasma

Internal carotid ——————————————————————————— Infundibulum

Posterior commun. ————————————————————————— 3rd nerve

————————————————————————— 4th nerve

Posterior cerebral ——————————————————————— 5th nerve

Vertebral ——————————————————————————————— 6th nerve

FIGURE 28. Base of brain.

Oculo-motor nerve
Trochlear nerve   Sella turcica
Ophthalmic nerve   Abducens nerve
Maxillary nerve   Internal carotid artery

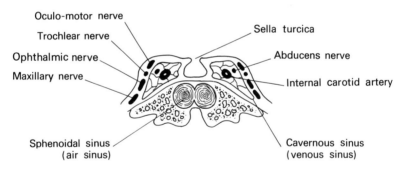

Sphenoidal sinus   Cavernous sinus
(air sinus)   (venous sinus)

FIGURE 29. Sella turcica, coronal section.

The arrangement of the efferent fibres from the retina to the brain is well known, but is briefly mentioned here. In the optic chiasma there is a rearrangement of these fibres, whereby efferent fibres from the temporal half of the retina of the same side, and those from the nasal half of the retina of the opposite side join and form the optic tract of the same side. This arrangement means that the nasal fibres cross in the optic chiasma. Not only is there a rearrangement with regard to the laterality of vision but also a corresponding arrangement of fibres in a horizontal fashion.

In addition to the optic nerve, the infundibulum is in fairly close relationship with a number of the cranial nerves. The third nerve pierces the dura mater forming the upper and outer wall of the cavernous sinus in front of the posterior clinoid process of the sphenoid bone. The fourth nerve pierces the dura mater a little behind the posterior clinoid process of the sphenoid bone and lies lateral to the third nerve, and then crosses the outer wall of the cavernous sinus. The fifth (trigeminal) nerve has sensory roots and a small motor root, and occupies the cavum trigeminale (Meckel's cave) where the sensory roots form the gasserian ganglion. The first and second divisions of the trigeminal nerve lie in the outer wall of the cavernous sinus. The opthalmic nerve lies below the fourth, and the maxillary nerve below the ophthalmic.

The sphenoid bone contains the sella turcica in its superior surface. It is a large bone taking part in the formation of the anterior, middle, and

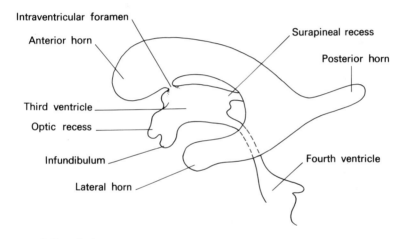

FIGURE 30. Ventricular system.

posterior fossae of the base of the skull. It also takes part in the formation of the nasal fossae, a point of particular importance in relation to carrying out the injection of alcohol into the pituitary gland. It is the body of the sphenoid bone which is of interest in this procedure, as within the body are two large cavities, the sphenoidal air sinuses which have openings on their anterior surfaces. These two air sinuses are separated from each other by a septum, which is rarely mid-line and may be incomplete. These sinuses are usually loculated and can be extensive. They are lined with mucous membrane, continuous with that of the nasal fossae. Each side opens, above and behind the superior meatus, into the spheno-ethmoidal recess.

The sphenoidal air sinuses thus surround the sella turcica below and on all sides. As long as the body of the sphenoid contains air cells anteriorly and below the sella turcica a needle can be inserted from the nasal fossa, through the sphenoid sinus to the base of the sella turcica. If the sphenoid air cells have not formed normally and dense bone is present instead, then the operation of pituitary injection of alcohol cannot be performed. Fortunately this lack of development rarely happens in a complete form, more usually a partial development occurs and only the anterior portion of the sphenoid sinuses is pneumatised. This will often allow the pituitary needle to be inserted along the correct line.

The physiology of the pituitary gland or hypophesis is well defined at the present time but details of its actions are constantly under review. The action of the pituitary gland must be considered in relation to the hypothalamus which controls it.

The hypothalamus is a part of the forebrain which lies in the floor of the third ventricle. It is the main centre co-ordinating nervous and endocrine activity, and has three functions. It controls the production of releasing and inhibiting hormones, and thus the activity of the anterior lobe of the pituitary gland; it influences the hypophysis by means of the process called neurosecretion; and thirdly, it controls activity of the autonomic system. It must also be realised that the hypothalamus has fibre connections with many other regions of the central nervous system, and although these connections are not known in detail, it is known that they are widespread both afferent and efferent. Nerve fibre tracts connect the supra–optic and para-ventricular nuclei of the hypothalamus with the posterior lobe of the pituitary gland, and the remaining nerve cells in the hypophysis control the anterior pituitary gland.

The median eminence is the name given to that part of the tubercinereum (the inferior surface of the hypothalamus) near the pituitary stalk. In the median eminence are capillaries, which are in contact with nerve endings of the hypothalamus. These form long portal vessels, which pass down the pituitary stalk and form secondary capillaries around the secretory cells of the anterior lobe. They are also some short portal vessels, which also supply the anterior lobe. The arterial blood supply of the posterior lobe of the pituitary gland is quite separate from that of the anterior lobe.

The anterior pituitary gland is controlled by neurohormones which are produced in the hypothalamus, and stored in the hypothalamus until required. They are transmitted to the anterior lobe of the pituitary along the hypophyseal portal system. These neurohormones are both of releasing (i.e. stimulating), and inhibiting types and control the release of the anterior pituitary hormones. The releasing hormones also control the synthesis of hormones.

The posterior pituitary gland is controlled in a different fashion. The nervous connections from hypothalamic nuclei to the median eminence and thence to the pituitary stalk and the posterior lobe have already been mentioned. These structures form another storage and secretory mechanism.

Of particular importance in relationship to the pituitary injection of alcohol is the fact that the posterior lobe of this gland secretes the anti-diuretic hormone (A.D.H.), while the anterior lobe is concerned with growth hormone (G.H.), and adreno-corticotrophin (A.C.T.H.). There are, of course, many others but growth hormone may be important in the regression of malignant tumours, and replacement therapy for a diabetes insipidus, or reduced steroid secretion may be necessary.

Selection of patients is no problem as, provided the patient is not moribund, there is little risk attached to the operation apart from a number of rare possibilities. In practice there is no difficulty in selecting patients as there is little selection. In the percutaneous cordotomy selection depends on whether or not the patient will live two weeks. The pituitary injection of alcohol needs slightly more than this minimal criteria. There is, however, one absolute contra-indication and that is the presence of infection in the nose and especially in the sphenoid sinus. The possibility of carrying infec-tion into the pituitary fossa and thus producing a meningitis is a very real one. An antiseptic solution is used by Moricca to swab out the nasal mucosa and thus sterilise it. After the operation the nose is plugged with ribbon gauze soaked in the antiseptic solution and this is left in position for twenty-four hours at least. If there is much in the way of haemorrhage from the nose post-operatively the pack may be left in for a longer period.

At the Centre for Pain Relief, on the advice of the oto-rhinolaryngologist associated with this work, no swabbing of the mucosa beforehand is carried out, nor is a pack inserted post-operatively except temporarily to control haemorrhage. Packs are never left in position for very long. It is the opinion at the Centre that swabbing and packing defeat their purpose by increasing the risk of infection.

Another absolute criteria would be the presence of a solid sphenoid sinus. These are extremely rare but there is the more frequent, but still rare, presence of a sphenoid sinus which is only pneumatised in its anterior portion. In most cases it is possible to insert the pituitary cannula through the nose in such a way that it can enter the open portion of the sphenoid sinus on a line that will permit entry into the pituitary fossa but it may be necessary to distort the vestibule and alae of the nose considerably to get on to this satisfactory line. A lateral X-ray will show whether this is feasible or not. A general anaesthetic may be advisable for this type of patient.

Apart from these two contra-indications all patients with intractable pain from spreading or multiple centre cancer pain can be treated, and without doubt this is the method to use in hormone-dependent tumours, where pituitary ablation would normally be used. In the case of hormone-dependent cancer this method of pituitary injection of alcohol is used on three occasions in the first two weeks, if the patient's condition will allow it. Thereafter further injections will be necessary, one at about one month after the first group, and again after three months. The condition of the patient will be reviewed regularly from then on in relation to regression and freedom from pain, and further injections may be required. In these hormone-dependent tumours the use of the pituitary injection of alcohol, i.e. the destruction of the pituitary gland, is for therapeutic purposes and must be pursued vigorously.

In the non-hormone-dependent tumours where the problem is one of control of intractable pain, the procedure is as above except that if pain relief occurs after the first injection the procedure is stopped, and only repeated if, and when, pain recurs. There is some validity in the argument that all patients with pain and widespread cancer should have the series of injections, as according to Moricca some of the so-called non-hormone-dependent tumours do respond to pituitary ablation. In other words, non-hormone dependency is only relative, some hormone-dependent tumours being far more sensitive than others.

The type of patient who is particularly suitable for the pituitary injection of alcohol is, first, where there are multiple bony secondaries, or multiple lung secondaries with severe pain which has not responded to other measures of cancer control. In this group of patients there is bilateral pain present, or if it is not present at the time of the injection of alcohol it is expected to develop. The percutaneous cervical cordotomy is by far the best method of relieving pain of unilateral distribution in dermatomes below the level of C5. It can under certain circumstances be used bilaterally with some difficulty and some possible complications. However, in bilateral pain, for sheer ease of performance, combined with a fair success rate, the pituitary injection is better. It may well be the only method which can be used in the very ill patient.

The second group of patients where the pituitary injection should be used is in those patients who have known hormone-dependent tumours. This dependency is known by their previous response to one of the hormone control methods. Also the injection can be used empirically on all patients who have cancer of the breast or prostate when these have not responded to hormone control previously. A proportion who have not responded before will respond to the pituitary injection, and for this reason alone it is worthwhile performing it, apart from the pain relief it will provide.

A third group is where there is pain in the pelvis or lower limbs in tumours which are not normally regarded as hormone-dependent, such as head of pancreas or bladder, but where the problem is to find a method of relieving bilateral pain without affecting control of micturition.

Fourth, is the group of patients who have been failures in all other methods of cancer control, or pain relief, and another approach is required.

Anaesthesia for this operation is straightforward and can be of many types. As mentioned before a short-acting general anaesthetic can be given intravenously during the insertion of the pituitary cannula, and also during the injection of alcohol. In the former procedure the hammering of the cannula through bone can be distressing and painful, in the latter severe headache develops.

As an alternative to the short-acting anaesthetic, a standard general anaesthetic can be given, but the safety of the operation depends on the presence of pupillary light reflexes and any general anaesthetic given must be very 'light'. In fact, an anaesthetic so light that the patient coughs on the tracheal tube, or moves, occasionally is what is necessary for this particular method.

There is a third method of anaesthetising the patient during this procedure and that is to use a local anaesthetic both to the nasal mucosa and to the dura at the base of the brain (see Figs. 26 and 27). Anaesthesia to the nasal mucosa is most effective, and if carried out in the way described shortly will not only provide pain-free insertion but also reduce haemorrhage to a minimum. Local solutions to the dura are only partly effective.

The anatomy of the nerves supplying the nasal mucosa is complicated by their number but is nevertheless straightforward as far as carrying out the application of the local anaesthetic solution is concerned (see Fig. 26). The upper nasal branches of the spheno-palatine ganglion traverse the spheno-palatine foramen and supply the mucous membrane of the superior and middle concha, the upper and posterior part of the nasal septum, and within the posterior ethmoidal sinus.

The lower nasal branches arise from the greater palatine branch of the spheno-palatine ganglion in the greater palatine canal. Through foramina in the perpendicular plate of the palatine bone they supply the mucous membrane over most of the inferior concha, and the middle and inferior meatus.

The posterior part of the roof of the nasal cavity and the adjoining septum is supplied by branches from the nerve of the pterygoid canal. The anterior and upper part of the septum is supplied by the septal branch of the anterior ethmoidal nerve. Also the lateral branches from this are distributed to the anterior parts of the inferior and middle conchae.

The mucous membrane of the nasal septum is also supplied from the spheno-palatine ganglion by the long spheno-palatine nerve, which crosses the roof of the nasal cavity and then descends on the septum.

The upper nasal branches of the anterior dental nerve supply the mucous membrane of the front of the inferior meatus, and the near-by floor. The infra-orbital branch of the trigeminal supplies the vestibule.

The main artery of the nasal cavity enters through the spheno-palatine foramen with the long spheno-palatine nerve, and the upper nasal branches of the spheno-palatine ganglion itself. It is the spheno-palatine artery and is a branch of the maxillary. The mucous membrane of the nose is very freely supplied with blood vessels but these are superficially placed and can be reached easily, as can the nerves, by surface application of suitable anaesthetic solutions.

Thus the application of local anaesthetic containing a vasoconstrictor, or the use of a cocaine solution which provides both combined, at four specific areas of the nasal cavity, produces anaesthesia of the mucous membrane, constriction of all vessels supplying the mucous membrane, and shrinkage of the mucous membrane itself.

As shown in the diagram (Fig. 26) the four places are at the spheno-palatine foramen; under the inferior turbinate; under the middle turbinate; and in the roof, on the line of the insertion of the pituitary cannula.

The use of a vasoconstrictive substance is useful even when a general anaesthetic is given as it cuts down the bleeding that occurs. The method adopted for application of the local anaesthetic solution is by means of flexible thin wire probes, which have a small pledget of cotton wool at the end. These are manœuvred under the middle and inferior turbinates, posteriorly against the wall over the spheno-palatine foramen, and into the roof. Usually two probes are placed in each place and left for fifteen to twenty minutes. Both nostrils are usually probed as it is not certain from the X-rays which side will provide the best entry. X-rays will show deviation of the septum and loculation of the sphenoid cavity.

It is not usually difficult to place the probes under the inferior turbinate, unless the level of the inferior turbinate is below the nasal vestibule. Usually the main problem is in those patients who have inflamed and 'soggy' mucous membrane which fills up the space under the inferior turbinate making it difficult to place the probe.

A similar problem exists in relation to the middle turbinate, but here the problem is due to the shallowness of this space, which may not retain the probe when this is placed correctly.

Remember that absolute anaesthesia of the nose is not necessary, as surgery is not being performed. Only an approximation to the anaesthesia necessary for surgery is required, and if the probes are placed approximately in position satisfactory anaesthesia will result. However, although it is the upper portion of the nasal mucosa, at the point of entry of the pituitary cannula, which is important, if the whole procedure is being conducted under local anaesthesia it is helpful to the operator and kinder to the patient when the whole of the nasal mucosa is anaesthetised.

When inserting the probes, they are first dipped in the anaesthetic solution, and then touched to a piece of gauze to remove the excess solution. This is particularly important if the anaesthetic is one of the cocaine solutions. It is permissible to provide a quick superficial anaesthesia by swabbing over the entire mucous surface with one wet probe, before the more accurate placing of the probes begins.

Complications from the local anaesthetic method of performing the pituitary injection of alcohol are due to the patient moving or to reaction from absorption of the local anaesthetic. The problem of movement is dealt with by proper sedation, and that depends on the personal preference of the operator. At this Centre neurolept sedation was chosen, and as stated previously was combined with an injection of up to 2 ml of 1 per cent lignocaine, given in divided doses through the pituitary cannula, to relieve the pain during the injection.

The actual method of anaesthesia adopted depends on the seriousness with which the dangers of ocular palsy, alteration in visual acuity, and visual defects, are viewed by the operator and whether he feels these can be adequately overcome by pupillary reactions when the patient is anaesthetised. The view of the author is that general anaesthesia is safe and necessary in view of the frequent number of pituitary injections that may be needed. This method of performing the injection is not without some risk, but so far it is a reversible risk. It can also be mentioned that Moricca has a large experience, running into two thousand injections at least, without much in the way of complications and with excellent results. Also the results in relatively small series of patients from a number of different centres, suggest that Moricca's operation works well in other hands and the author, for one, accepts it as a useful advance.

The light reflex is the safety factor on which this operation depends and an examination of the anatomy on which it is based is well worthwhile.

The light reflex consists of a constriction of the pupil when light enters the eye. The size of the pupil is due to a balance between the parasympathetic fibres from the oculo-motor nerve, which relay in the ciliary ganglion, and the sympathetic fibres from the upper two thoracic cord segments, which relay in the superior cervical ganglion, and then follow the internal carotid artery. Constriction of the pupil is produced by stimulation of the parasympathetic, while stimulation of the sympathetic produces dilatation. This simplistic arrangement is not thought to be the whole picture but is quite sufficient for the present purpose.

The efferent limb of the light reflex is from nuclei in the mesencephalon, via the oculo-motor nerve, to the ciliary ganglion where the post-ganglionic parasympathetic fibres arise. The short ciliary nerves complete the pathway to the sphincter of the pupil.

The afferent limb in the reflex arc is thought to be to the tectal area from the superior colliculus, the superior quadrigeminal brachium, and the optic nerve. The central connections of this limb of the reflex arc must be bilateral as pupillary constriction occurs from light shone into one eye.

Thus when one pupil is dilated it is relatively easy to demonstrate whether the interruption of the reflex arc is in the afferent or efferent portion. If a light is shone into the affected eye the opposite pupil will constrict when the afferent pathway is intact, but the efferent pathway along the oculomotor nerve, ciliary body, or short ciliary nerves is damaged. If there is no reaction on either side when light is shone into the affected eye then the lesion is in the optic nerve, and this can be corroborated by shining light into the normal eye when both pupils will contract, the efferent pathway being bilaterally intact.

Partial lesions will produce a reduction in the size and spread of the reaction.

Bearing in mind the position of the optic nerves, the optic chiasma, and the optic tracts, in relation to the infundibulum, and the position of the patient, lying on their back during the actual injection of the alcohol, any lesion produced by the hypobaric alcohol can be expected to occur at the chiasma or more likely at the optic nerves.

If the pupillary light reflex is carefully monitored in between each injection of alcohol, and if the injection is immediately terminated when there is any alteration in the size of either, or both pupils, or when the rapidity of the alteration of the pupillary size becomes sluggish, recovery will occur.

Two other complications can occur following alcohol injection. The first is due to a bilateral partial or complete dilatation of the pupil. This occurs through damage to either the afferent or efferent light reflex arc (which can be distinguished as previously described). During the normal process of accommodation the pupil constricts, this occurs when a near object is looked at. It is accompanied by fixation of gaze and convergence of the eyeballs, and these movements are impossible or not easily performed when the pupil will not constrict.

The patient will, therefore, complain that they are not seeing as well as previously, and that they cannot read. The print appearing fuzzy to them. The distinction between these complaints due to inability to constrict the pupil, and those due to damage to the visual pathways themselves can be resolved by allowing the patient to look through a pin-hole opening. If the complaints are due to the size of the pupil this device should enable them to report normal vision.

The second complication is due to damage to one or other of the ocular motor nerves. If damage to one of these is complete then strabismus, diplopia, vertigo, and altered posture of the head will result. In the series from the Centre for Pain Relief in 155 cases, there has been no case of ocular palsy. This fact reinforces the value of monitoring the ocular reflexes during injection of the alcohol.

The technique of the operation has been mentioned but if the patient is conscious, or allowed to become conscious in between short spells of general anaesthesia then not only can the pupillary reaction be tested by shining a light into each eye successively, but also the reaction to accommodation. The actual size of the pupil is seen by observation and by direct enquiry the visual acuity is checked. When a general anaesthetic is used throughout the operation the visual acuity cannot be checked and great care is necessary between increments of alcohol. The patient is kept as 'light' as possible and only the light reflex and size of the pupil can be monitored.

In the total of 155 cases in this series all three types of anaesthesia previously mentioned have been used. With the one difference that under the present method of continuous light general anaesthesia a lower volume of alcohol is injected, there has been no difference in the complications.

Initially, the quantities of alcohol used were based on those used by Moricca and went up to 1·7 ml for those patients with large pituitary fossae. In the recent cases under light general anaesthesia not more than 1·0 ml is injected at any one operation. It has been felt that under general anaesthesia the ocular and pupillary reflexes are sluggish and that it was wise to limit the amount of alcohol injected each time. It is significant that Moricca uses smaller quantities of alcohol nowadays than in his early series.

The method of observation of the pupils is to observe them closely over two to three minutes after each increment of alcohol. If there is no change another increment is injected. Each increment is of 0·1 ml bearing in mind that the cannula has to be filled with alcohol before any enters the pituitary fossa. The observations involve both pupillary size and reaction to light and of the two the size of the pupil is the more easily seen. If either of them alters and does not revert to normal within five minutes the procedure is stopped at that point and repeated at a later date. If it does return to normal another cautious injection can be made but if the reaction is abnormal on a second occasion no further injections are made.

When this operation is carried out under local anaesthesia the visual acuity of the patient is tested in addition. This must be tested before the operation to obtain the normal parameters for that patient. One of the problems occurs with patients who are short-sighted and are not wearing their glasses, and another is with the patient who does not quite understand what is expected and gives a long blow by blow account of their ocular history over the past twenty years. The author has not felt that much has been lost by not being able to check visual acuity during a general anaesthetic. All patients who have had any post-operative visual defect produced by the operation have had a dilated pupil at some stage of the operation. So far none of these defects mentioned later have been permanent.

During the injection of alcohol under local anaesthesia alone the patient in most cases (but not all) will complain of a feeling of pain and fullness behind the base of the nose, and as the injection of increments proceeds, pain in either the temporal or frontal regions. This pain can be relieved in large part in most people and completely in some by injecting a small quantity of local anaesthetic solution, such as 1 per cent lignocaine, as previously mentioned.

When the patient is to have this injection of local anaesthetic into the pituitary fossa, it is done in increments of not more than 0·5 ml observing the pupillary size for two to three minutes between each injection. In all injections of either alcohol, local anaesthetic solution, or radio-opaque Iophendylate (Myodil) the cannula lumen has to be filled first and no effects can be obtained until this volume has been filled. Similarly at the end of the injection, and this particularly applies to alcohol when the trocar is inserted prior to removal of the cannula, inserting the trocar will push more alcohol down the cannula. If the operation has been terminated because of an untoward reaction then no further alcohol should be injected, and the cannula should be removed without the reinsertion of the trocar. Also towards the end of the operation when all is going well, allowance has to be made for the final amount of alcohol that will be injected into the pituitary fossa merely by inserting the trocar. If the internal volume is 0·3 ml, then the trocar must be inserted in three stages so that no alcohol of more than

0·1 ml is injected at any stage of the operation. There is no point in carefully injecting 0·1 ml throughout the operation for safety and then injecting 0·3 ml at the end. There is, of course, a place for individual variation here and my impression is that Moricca, while injecting the same total volume, injects slightly larger increments more rapidly.

Inserting the pituitary cannula is straightforward. Before doing this the cannula and trocar should be checked that they are a good fit, and that the cannula and trocar are matched. The trocar gets blunted by use and needs sharpening from time to time which shortens it, and eventually the corresponding cannula has also to be shortened. If the wrong cannula and a normal length trocar are matched the trocar projects to a dangerous degree. To avoid this problem those cannulas used at the Centre are all the same length. All our trocars and cannulae are interchangeable and are discarded and not shortened. It is also important that these instruments are changed from time to time as the metal gets fatigued and may break.

If the cannula does break outside the nose it can be easily removed with any instrument that will provide a secure grip. Our only problem has been when the hub and needle tubing separated during removal from rather dense bone. However, if the tubing broke off in the nasal fossa then a suitably thin instrument would be necessary for removal. If it broke off in the sphenoid sinus while still penetrating the pituitary fossa a neurosurgical opinion might be necessary to decide whether to leave it or not. If it can be seen easily then its lumen could be blocked with bone wax to prevent cerebro-spinal leak. Otherwise it can be left quite safely for many days, the patient being given antibiotic cover with two tablets, twice a day, of Septrin. At this Department of Medical and Surgical Neurology patients with a head injury and a cerebro-spinal rhinorrhoea are placed on this regime for many weeks.

The image intensifier is used constantly while the cannula is being inserted, both in the lateral view and occasionally in the antero-posterior. The latter to make sure the cannula will be inserted in the mid-line. The direction of the cannula in the lateral view is inferior to the posterior clinoids. If it is aimed too posteriorly it may glance off the floor of the pituitary fossa and not penetrate it. If it is aimed too anteriorly it will penetrate below the anterior clinoids and may penetrate the fossa for a very short distance before penetrating the roof of the fossa (see Figs. 31–35). In normal cases this procedure will be repeated and it is best to place the cannula differently each time so that alcohol injections can be made at different places within the pituitary fossa. This will aid destruction of the gland. Unless the cannula is placed within the pituitary gland itself there is no resistance to the injection. As mentioned, if there is resistance to the injection the alcohol is placed in the gland without moving the cannula. The series of cases at Liverpool is not large enough to decide the question as to whether the subsequent pain relief is better if alcohol is placed in the gland or around it. If it is placed around the gland then some leaks through the opening in the diaphragma sellae, and should have action on the infundibulum and the associated near-by regions of the hypothalamus. Nor is it possible to

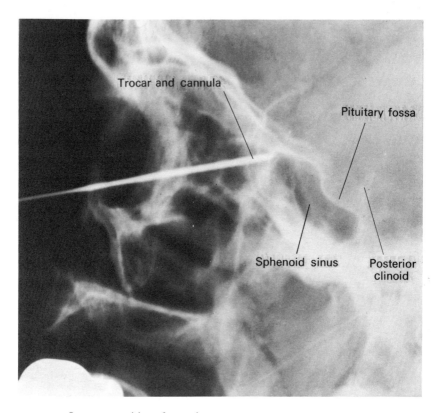

FIGURE 31. Incorrect position of cannula.

decide whether regression of tumour occurs more readily if the injection is made directly into the pituitary gland or not. Logically one would expect that pain relief should be associated with damage to nervous pathways and therefore injection of alcohol through the sella on to the hypothalamus or other nervous pathways, would be better. Conversely that injection into the pituitary gland would aid its destruction and therefore benefit tumour regression.

The Queckenstedt test is performed as soon as the cannula has been placed in position. The presence of cerebro-spinal fluid signifies that either the cannula is placed in the pituitary fossa but outside the pituitary gland, or it has penetrated through the sella and is in the middle fossa. These can be distinguished with the lateral X-ray view. If blood wells up the cannula then penetration of the pituitary gland has occurred or some damage to its

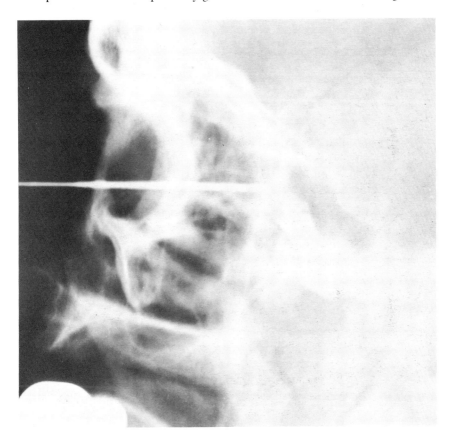

FIGURE 32. Correct position (lateral view).

surface, or to a small vessel entering that surface. Marked haemorrhage occurs from the carotid artery and this occurs if the cannula strays from the middle line and penetrates the sphenoid too laterally. It can also occur from an aberrant carotid artery which sometimes is present. If the carotid artery is penetrated the needle is moved. As long as the trocar is sharp so that it does not tear the artery the haemorrhage stops. With normal care this happens rarely; in the author's present series it has happened once. The entry into the carotid artery was quite dramatic; as the trocar was removed blood spurted out but did not pulse; the antero-posterior view with the image intensifier showed that the cannula was not mid-line. An X-ray plate was taken and gave more definition, showing the cannula was outside the pituitary fossa. In this position it can be in the cavernous sinus and haemorrhage can be either venous or arterial.

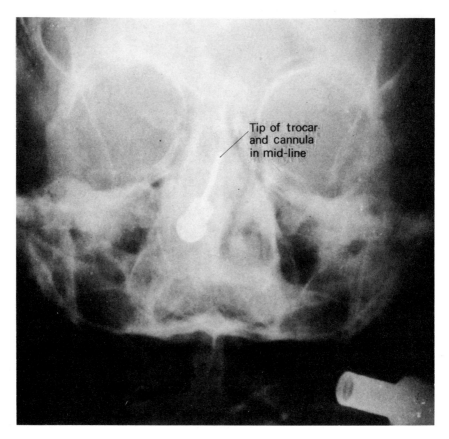

Tip of trocar and cannula in mid-line

FIGURE 33. Correct position, i.e. central (A–P view).

Complications

Bearing in mind what has been said previously about complications and consequences, what are regarded as the complications will be discussed first.

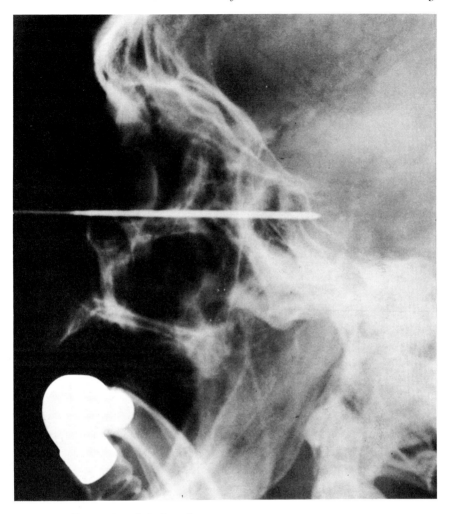

FIGURE 34. Penetration of pituitary fossa.

Mortality

In this series of 155 pituitary injections involving 92 patients there have been 7 deaths post-operatively. Five of these deaths have been ascribed as due to the method.

The cause of one was found at post-mortem. This patient had a closed sphenoid sinus which was full of pus. X-rays even when looked at with hindsight did not show any suggestion of this empyema. The pituitary injection was performed under local anaesthesia, and entry into the pituitary fossa and the injection of alcohol was uneventful. Pain relief was satisfactory but not complete. Some three days later the patient became pyrexial, developed a headache, and was diagnosed as a meningitis. Culture of cerebrospinal fluid suggested suitable antibiotic cover. The conditions did not resolve and it was thought that a leaking brain abscess was the cause. No abscess could be seen on angiography and there was a negative cranial exploration. The patient died before it was realised that the source of the infection was the sphenoid sinus discharging through the artificial stoma in the pituitary fossa which remained open.

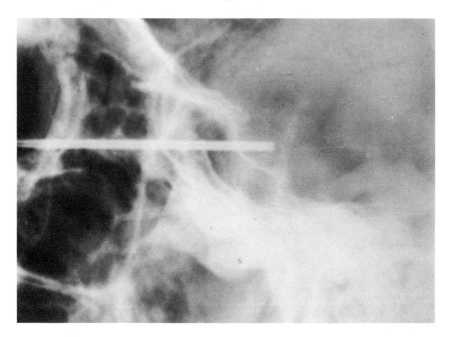

FIGURE 35. Cannula below posterior clinoid process.

One patient having had two pituitary injections of alcohol, and awaiting admission for the third, died suddenly and unexpectedly. She had been on large doses of steroids for her primary condition and had been having some problems with her respiration. These were thought to be due to the effects of long-term prednisolone on the interstitial tissues of her lungs. A post-mortem was not obtained.

The third patient was drowsy for a day or two immediately after the pituitary injection and this was thought to be a hypothalamic effect. The patient recovered from this and had about 50 per cent improvement in her pain. In a further week she gradually became drowsy again, and over a further week became comatose and died. She developed a deep venous thrombosis of one leg before this stage. At post-mortem there was no explanation for this course of events, and it was put down as a hypothalamic coma produced by the pituitary injection.

A fourth died of dehydration and electrolyte imbalance in a 70-year-old man. It was not realised at first that dehydration from a diabetes insipidus was such a dangerous hazard in old people. This death can be ascribed to the lack of urgent treatment.

The fifth and sixth patient deaths were similar in many respects to the third with the patient becoming increasingly drowsy with a fluctuating level. They developed coma and died. One of these developed a mild hemiparesis which partially cleared up after forty-eight hours and after a further forty-eight hours reappeared.

The seventh death is included for completeness but is due to poor selection of the patient, who died within forty-eight hours. The patient was not fit enough for the procedure and should not have had a pituitary injection carried out.

It must be remembered that many of the patients presenting for the pituitary injection have advanced malignant disease. It is not surprising, therefore, that some of these patients will die suddenly and unexpectedly from natural causes. A mortality of five deaths in 155 injections is not unreasonable (see Fig. 36).

Rhinorrhoea

This occurs in a few patients for an hour or two after the pituitary injection and then it stops. Five patients continued to drip for the rest of that day but were dry the following morning. Two patients had rhinorrhoea for twenty-four hours, one patient for three days, one for ten, one for six weeks. The latter was after the second injection. In this patient the cannula slipped into the pituitary fossa without any difficulty or use of the hammer, and it was thought it had entered through the original hole. On the first occasion there was no rhinorrhoea at all. The patient was kept in hospital, although quite active and pain free, and was placed on Septrin 2 tablets b.d. as described previously. The patient subsequently had a third pituitary injection without any further problems.

Presumably there may be a patient where the base of the pituitary fossa is composed of brittle bone. If this type of patient has a pituitary injection, the cannula and trocar may not perforate the bone cleanly and may shatter it. It would be likely that a rhinorrhoea would develop and be present for some time, and might even require a surgical repair. However, it

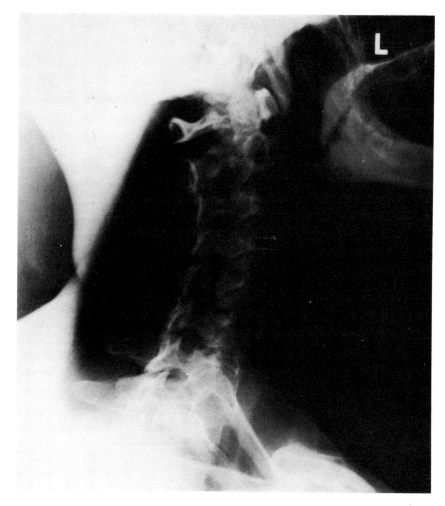

FIGURE 36. Cervical spine X-ray showing multiple bony secondaries. Patient died while awaiting second pituitary injection, having obtained over one year complete freedom from pain from the first.

is encouraging to remember the massive injuries that occur in head injuries, with tearing of the dura and severe rhinorrhoea, which heal off in time without surgical intervention.

Headache

This is a common complication following the pituitary injection. Usually in patients where the operation is carried out under local anaesthesia it develops immediately the first increment of alcohol enters the fossa, when it is described as a headache behind the eyes. Under these conditions it can occur when a very small amount of fluid has been injected and is probably due to a raised tension inside the pituitary fossa itself. Sometimes the first few increments are painless and as following increments spill over into the middle fossa, pain in definite areas will be described. These areas are one or other of the temporal regions or in one or both frontal regions. If no local solution has been injected before the alcohol this pain can be excruciating. By the time the injection is complete the patient will be describing a generalised headache with no definite focal point.

Patients who receive general anaesthetics recover from the anaesthetic with the generalised headache described above.

There are a few patients who do not suffer at all with the generalised headache, even when the procedure is performed under local anaesthesia to the nose alone.

Local anaesthesia to the pituitary fossa does modify the pain at the time of alcohol injection, but does not modify the subsequent headache.

In general terms patients who undergo the procedure under local anaesthesia alone are reluctant to undergo a subsequent operation using the same technique. Thus it is logical to use some form of general anaesthesia where this is at all possible.

Disorientation and lethargy has been seen occasionally for periods of two or three days. Lethargy has occurred without any apparent relation to the operation date. It has occurred over the first few days; towards the end of the first week; and even at the end of the second week. Where disorientation is concerned there is a definite relation with the injection, tending to occur in the first few days. Disorientation has been accompanied in all cases, except one, with lethargy. Once it has cleared it does not usually recur. Three patients already mentioned became disorientated, lethargic, went into coma, and eventually died.

It would appear that this effect is due to a direct action on the hypothalamic region of the brain. It is known that in malfunction of the hypothalamus, as occurs from pressure by tumours, obesity, drowsiness, polydipsia, polyuria, and alterations in body temperature control result. As will be seen all these consequences of the pituitary injection have been observed at one time or another. Glycosuria, alterations of sleep rhythm, appetite, and respiration, can also appear. This latter group, with the exception of glycosuria, has not been seen in the present series. Glycosuria has occurred rather fleetingly in the first few days.

Euphoria is commonly seen after the pituitary injection and in some cases for a considerable time afterwards. It is rather difficult to assess but it certainly occurs during the first days post-operatively, and in three notable cases lasted at least two weeks. One wife mentioned, three months after the pituitary injection, that her husband seemed to have stopped worrying about things since the operation and she did not think this was due solely to the relief of pain. As the patient had multiple secondaries throughout his body, lungs, and skull, it was impossible to decide whether this effect was due to the alcohol injection or to a leucotomising effect from the secondary tumours in the brain. From the way many patients behave shortly after the injection of alcohol, a leucotomising effect is possible. It does not occur in the majority of patients, and when it does, only to a minor degree for a short period. It might be related to alcohol spreading on to the under surface of the frontal lobes. If this were so there should be some relation between those patients developing euphoria, and those who have frontal pain when the operation is performed under local anaesthesia. In this series there is no correlation in this respect.

Diabetes insipidus is the commonest consequence following the pituitary injection of alcohol. It is unusual for it not to occur. There does not appear to be a relation between the development of diabetes insipidus and pain relief. As approximately 30 per cent of patients do not obtain pain relief, and as most patients develop diabetes insipidus, it follows that many patients with diabetes insipidus do not get pain relief. One of the consultant gynaecologists, whose patients received the pituitary injection of alcohol for relief of their pain, believed that they did not get pain relief unless they developed a diabetes insipidus. Further when the diabetes insipidus was controlled by pitressin (as Piton snuff) then the pain relief was not as satisfactory. This observation could not be confirmed.

In the author's observation pain relief has occurred when the patient has not developed diabetes insipidus. Pain relief has and has not continued after it had been initially produced in patients with and without diabetes insipidus. Pain relief does not usually develop immediately after performing the pituitary injection, but occurs gradually over two or three days. However, there are a number of patients whose pain does not improve for up to five days, and conversely some patients whose pain disappears immediately the injection has been performed. About one in seven patients respond in this immediate fashion.

For the purpose of the post-operative management of these patients, a diabetes insipidus is treated if the urinary output rises above $2\frac{1}{2}$ litres. In one patient it rose to 7 litres. The diabetes insipidus is treated initially by

Piton snuff or Desmopressin nasal drops (D.D.A.V.P.), from one to four times per twenty-four hours, depending on the volume of urine passed. If the patient is not distressed by the volume, can maintain hydration by drinking enough fluids, and has no or little alteration of electrolytes, then they do not need Piton snuff at all. They may be given one dose at night to prevent disturbance from waking to urinate.

Normally the diabetes insipidus gradually improves, in that the volume of urine passed decreases with time, and ultimately approaches the previous normal figure. Naturally a second or third pituitary injection tends to produce a marked diabetes insipidus again.

If a diabetes insipidus cannot be hydrated by mouth fluid balance will have to be maintained by intravenous drip. Fortunately this is rarely necessary and then only for short periods.

Mild cases of diabetes insipidus can be controlled by Piton snuff, which is posterior pituitary extract in powder form. It is given in measured amounts sniffed on to the nasal mucosa. The patient soon learns to regulate his own dose. A nasal spray of lysine vasopressin can be used containing fifty international units of synthetic 8-lysine vasopressin per ml (Syntopressin). This is useful in all but the most severe cases, as is D.D.A.V.P., which is an analogue of vasopressin having a long action. Chronic and severe cases that cannot be maintained in balance by the above methods can be given Vasopressin tannate in oil by deep intramuscular injection. It contains 5 pressor units per ml, a normal dose being $2\frac{1}{2}$ to 10 units, and in severe cases may need to be given twice a day. The dose is adjusted so that the urinary output is between 1200 and 1800 ml of urine per twenty-four hours. Vasopressin injection B.P. given in 5 to 15 unit doses intramuscularly is an aqueous solution useful for controlling these acute cases in the early stages.

Some patients with a mild diabetes insipidus are relatively insensitive to Piton snuff and then must use one of the other preparations. Fortunately this reaction is rare. Anti-diuretic-hormone (ADH) is a polypeptide and therefore is destroyed in the gut. It can be absorbed from the nasal mucosa, so in those patients not insensitive to it, this is the most convenient method of replacement.

Hyperpyrexia has occurred in a few patients, somewhat fleetingly, postoperatively. In the present series it has never reached more than 1·5 °C and has disappeared in two days. In view of the influence the hypothalamus has over temperature control there are bound to be patients who will react much more vigorously than this.

Hyperphagia is mentioned by Moricca as having occurred in his series which is markedly larger than this. Again it is a feature which has not been seen so far in the Liverpool series but it is expected to appear at some time.

Glycosuria has been seen fleetingly and, in the main, immediately post-operatively. It has not continued in those few patients where it has occurred.

Two complications stand out in importance in the whole series.

Ocular defects

The first of these complications was in a patient with a carcinoma of the rectum with an abdoperineal resection. He had severe pain in the pelvis, lumbo-sacral vertebrae, groins, and thighs. He needed catheterising in addition to his colostomy. He had a routine injection of alcohol 1·0 ml in divided doses carried out under general anaesthesia (method three later). During the injection of alcohol between each increment of 0·1 ml the pupillary light reflex was tested. He had needed heavy sedation pre-operatively and very little added general anaesthesia was required. A cuffed endotracheal tube was inserted under brietal and scoline, and anaesthesia continued with nitrous oxide, oxygen, a trace of halothane, and further increments of brietal as necessary. There was nothing untoward in the anaesthetic, the patient being kept light.

The pupils were sluggish to light and this was thought an effect of the narcotics given in the pre-operative period combined with the anaesthetic. From the start of testing the light reflexes the left pupil was less active than the right. This continued until 0·9 ml of alcohol had been injected when the left pupil was still reacting but more sluggishly than previously. The right pupil was also somewhat reduced in speed of reaction. A further 0·1 ml of alcohol was injected when the right pupil became more sluggish and the left one ceased to react. The injection was stopped at that point, and the patient returned to the ward.

Post-operatively, on the following day, the visual fields had marked defects. The left eye had a temporal visual field defect, while the right eye had an inferior altitudinal field defect. This suggested that the alcohol had damaged fibres bilaterally in the optic nerves. The patient had a devastating defect as although he had half his field of vision in each eye, and no loss of visual acuity, he could not read. His problem was that the combination of field defects made it impossible for him to scan across lines of print. He could read from left to right, but could not return his centre of vision to the left-hand side of the next line of print.

Gradually over the course of the next five weeks the patient's field defects improved, and at the end of this period he was able to read once again. Fortunately his pain, while not entirely absent, was very much improved, and remained at this improved level. The patient only needed D.F. 118 two or three times a day and sometimes only required one tablet at night. Previous to the pituitary injection he needed narcotics every two hours.

This patient did prove to us that if care was taken over the injection of alcohol by using small increments, and stopping the injection as soon as any gross alteration of light reflex was lost, any defect produced was reversible. The method was thought to be inherently safe, but that alterations had to be made to the technique to improve the safety factor. As this safety factor seemed to be related to observation of the light factor anything which gave an active reflex was to be encouraged. It was decided that pre-operative medication was to be kept to a minimum, even if this meant that the patient would be in pain. In practice this meant that the patient did not receive his last dose of analgesic or narcotic drug before the operation. Also that the general anaesthetic given should be designed to have the patient as light as possible, even to the extent of him moving or bucking on the tube. This type of movement was not desired but it was considered that it was safer in the pituitary injection of alcohol to err on the side of lightness. Since these ideas have been used there has been no further problems with field defects.

Hemiparesis

The second complication is included for completeness, but there is no certainty that it was due to the injection of alcohol. A woman of 45 having had a left radical mastectomy some seven years previously developed axillary and supraclavicular glands on the right side. Following this she had biopsy, radiotherapy, chemotherapy, and further radiotherapy to a secondary in one of the ribs under the old left mammary scar. On admittance she was in severe pain, and an X-ray of the chest showed multiple secondaries in all the lung fields.

Pituitary injection of alcohol was performed because of the widespread nature of her pain, and because there was always the possibility of regression with this method. Further the pain in her neck on the right side was at too high a level to be covered by a percutaneous cordotomy though this would have dealt with all her lower pain on that side. The pituitary injection was uneventful and within twenty-four hours there was a marked reduction in her pain, which became concentrated and confined to her right shoulder only and there was a marked reduction in her medication requirements. Because pain relief was not complete, and also because of the possibility of the tumour being a hormone dependent one, a second pituitary injection of alcohol was planned for one week later. During the sixth post-operative night she developed a right-sided hemiparesis. She was right-handed, had only the suggestion of slurred speech, and had complete paresis of arm and leg. By the following morning there was some movement of the fingers and over the next three weeks she made steady recovery. Power in her leg became sufficient to allow her to walk with some help. Her pain returned steadily until it was controlled by 10 mgm Dextromoramide B.P. (Palfium) every four hours.

Two days after the onset of paresis she had an angiogram for the possibility of a secondary or haemorrhage into a secondary. It was thought that the speed of onset precluded an abscess. Previous straight X-rays of skull had appeared normal. The angiogram showed no abnormality. There were no areas of infarction, no spasm of any blood vessels, no secondary tumours, no blood clot, and no aneurysm.

This hemiparesis could have little to do with the pituitary injection, arising through the patient's poor general condition. On the other hand it was impossible to dismiss the pituitary injection from any share of the blame, as the injection is made near to the carotid artery, and spasm could have produced this result. Considering that the paresis did not develop for six days this is unlikely. However, one real possibility is that damage to, or irritation of, the wall of the carotid artery, with or without spasm, could cause the formation of a mural clot. Embolisation of this at a later date could produce a hemiparesis of this type.

The consequences of pituitary injection of alcohol are concerned with damage in one form or another of the pituitary axis. In a number of our patients, investigations of their output of pituitary hormones pre- and post-injection have shown in all cases that there has been a diminution of all or some of these. In particular, notice must be taken if there is a diminution of cortisol production, or if thyroid function is depressed. Replacement therapy will be necessary only if the depression of function continues. It is surprising that within a month of an apparent destruction of the pituitary gland all its functions can be working satisfactorily.

Patients who are about to have a pituitary injection do not appear to need substitution therapy of the type that is given for other methods of ablating the pituitary gland. Here they are given prednisolone 2 mgm twice a day, from the pre-operative day for one month. Their free cortisol is then estimated if possible (most of them have returned home) and if reduced then a proper replacement regime is instituted. If salt deficiency occurs then fludrocortisone may be required, and if a hypothyroid deficiency appears then replacement in the form of thyroxine in small dose may be necessary.

In most cases no replacement therapy of any kind is needed. The most likely problem is that from diabetes insipidus and this has been discussed. Even with this most common of the consequences of the pituitary injection of alcohol, the need for replacement therapy dwindles with time. In only one patient was the requirement of Piton snuff during the day, and pitressin injection at night, unaltered after three months.

In the small number of patients who do require treatment for diabetes insipidus, it is mostly required at night to enable them to have an undisturbed night's sleep.

Pain relief

The patients comprising 70% of this group fall into three distinct treatments. Initially patients were treated by a single insertion, sometimes two insertions at the same time, of pituitary cannulae under local anaesthesia. No injection of local anaesthetic solution was made into the pituitary fossa, but there were injections of myodil (Iophendylate B.P.) an oily solution of radio-opaque material 0·2 to 1·0 ml. Sometimes fortuitously air also entered the pituitary fossa. Initially this injection of myodil was carried out to confirm to the operator that the cannula was indeed in the pituitary fossa. However, it was very quickly seen that injections of myodil did not remain in the fossa but spread along the pituitary stalk and along tracks around and towards the third ventricle. In fact, in some patients, the myodil was seen in the posterior portion of the third ventricle around the pineal recess (see Figs. 37–41). Accompanying the myodil could be seen small quantities of air.

This tracking of the myodil was a totally unexpected finding in a scheme for localising the position of the pituitary cannula by means of a visual aid system. It was at first a very frightening finding because if myodil could track to the third ventricle, then the much more easily diffusible alcohol could also do so. The potential hazard from this could be immense.

The next stage was to wonder if the pain relief obtained by this method depended on alcohol diffusing in this way. It was realised that this spread of myodil was seen in about one-quarter to one-third of the patients, all of whom had an injection of myodil into the pituitary fossa. It was also realised that in those patients who obtained pain relief most developed this over a period of a few days, but that there were a few, about one in seven, who obtained their pain relief almost instantaneously. The suspicion grew that the instantaneous relief of pain might have had something to do with the alcohol tracking. In other words, that the normal relief of pain depended on destruction of the pituitary gland, but that on occasion certain unknown

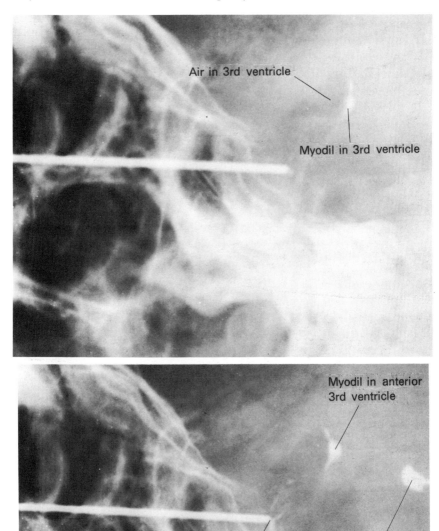

FIGURES 37–41. Lateral X-ray view showing myodil progressively spreading along the pituitary stalk, the third ventricle (anterior and posterior), and the fourth ventricle. Finally air appears in the lateral ventricle (anterior horn). FIGURES 37 (above) and 38 (below).

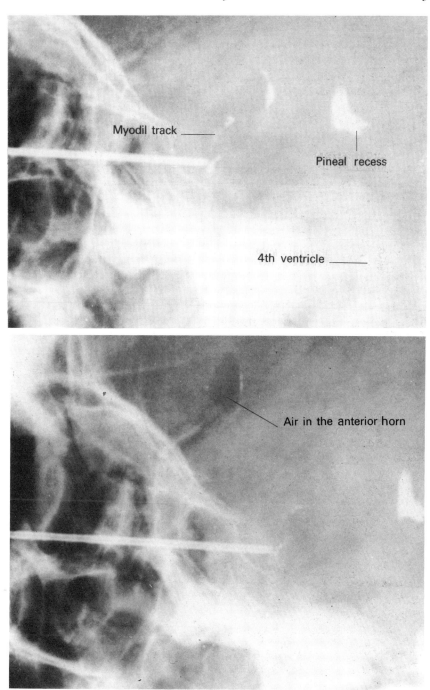

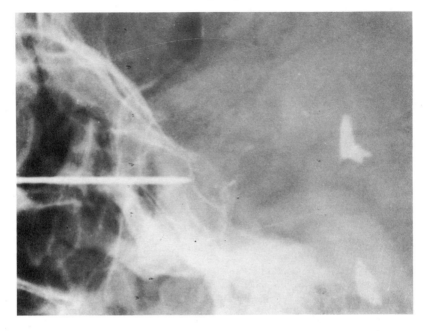

FIGURE 41.

pain pathways in the nervous system were destroyed, or interfered with, producing very rapid pain relief indeed.

In this initial group the amount of alcohol tended to be relatively high, between 0·8 and 2·0 ml, with the average around 1·3 ml. This was given through one cannula, but if there was any difficulty about this another cannula was placed through the opposite nostril, or the same one if that proved impossible.

There was a high incidence of minor visual problems. Some of these patients had bilaterally slightly dilated pupils for one week, and associated with this would be difficulty in reading, and a fuzziness of vision. In two patients this difficulty with reading remained after the pupils became apparently normal in size. There were no ocular palsies producing a strabismus, or diplopia. There were no visual field or macula defect. The method produced a relatively high initial relief of pain, but slowly most of these patients had a recurrence of the pain but not usually to the same severe degree. This is a small number of patients and these results only gave an indication of the value of the method.

The next group of patients (the second group) had treatment exactly like the first but an injection of 1 per cent lignocaine was made down the pituitary cannula before the myodil was injected and followed by the injection of alcohol. Some of these patients had an injection of sterile air either before or after the myodil injection. Certainly this addition of air to the technique increased the number of patients where either air, or myodil, or both could be seen in the third ventricle to over one-third of the patients. It did not seem to make any difference to the proportion of patients developing pain relief, either immediately or at a later stage. In this group the amount of alcohol was gradually reduced until the average dose was 1·0 ml or less. Although two cannulae were inserted at times, particularly when the pituitary fossa was larger than usual, this was not the usual technique. The patient was brought back for a further pituitary injection when pain recurred after initial relief. If the first injection produced inadequate relief, then the patient was offered another pituitary injection after two weeks.

The incidence of post-operative minor ocular morbidity decreased in this series and this was thought to be related to the reduction in the amount of alcohol injected at any one time.

After some fifty cases had been treated through this method there was an immediate success rate of 70 per cent with some pain relief. This effect wore off in time but when the pituitary injection was repeated at either the one- or two-monthly levels the success rate rose again.

These figures were most encouraging in the type of cancer pain conditions that were being dealt with, but they did not approach the success rate that was claimed by Moricca. They were undoubtedly useful and on these figures the method would continue to be used, and would be satisfactory to those surgeons, physicians, and radio-therapists who were referring their patient to the Centre for treatment. The figures were, broadly speaking, that one-third of the patients obtained excellent and long-lasting results, one-third were not completely pain free but had enough relief to change from addictive narcotics to non-addictive ones, and one-third obtained no relief at all.

Examination of the methods used showed that in the Moricca series the quantity of alcohol used was greater than in our second series of patients but not by much. But the frequency of pituitary injections was much greater in the Moricca series, and the tendency was for more needles to be used.

A third series of patients was therefore begun, continuing with the same amount of alcohol and the same number of insertions at any one time, as in the second series, but repeating the injections so that there were three in the first two weeks provided the patient's physical condition could stand it. A fourth injection was also to be carried out after three months. This schedule was to be adhered to for hormone-dependent tumours where the pituitary injection was not only used for pain relief but was also a specific treatment. If the injections were carried out for pain relief and there was no evidence of regression after three months, then further injections would depend on the response to pain relief.

So far this programme has been in use for less than twelve months so that not enough results are to hand to warrant an opinion as to its effectiveness. The personal estimation of the author is that the adoption of the method has increased the number obtaining complete relief slightly, and has also increased the number obtaining some but not complete relief. It has thus reduced the total number of complete failures.

The method of carrying out the pituitary injection operation is to insert two needles only if the pituitary fossa is noticeably enlarged, or there is difficulty in injecting through the initial cannula. No injection of local anaesthetic solution or myodil is made, but sterile air is injected to see if this will find a way into the third ventricle. The whole procedure is carried out under general anaesthesia in the way described earlier, as it was felt that repetition of the injections at this frequency would be refused by the patient if they had to suffer the dural pain under local anaesthesia.

Conclusion

To sum up, then, it can be stated without any doubt that the method of pituitary injection of alcohol will relieve intractable pain from inoperable cancer in at least one-third of patients. A further one-third have considerable but not complete relief of pain, and one-third do not respond. Thus about 65 per cent of patients are helped and 35 per cent are not. Those patients benefiting by this type of treatment may need the pituitary injection repeated after an interval of weeks or months as the relief of pain tends to wear off with time. A subsequent injection usually, but not always, reproduces the benefit obtained by previous treatment.

This method is of great benefit in many patients with inoperable cancer and intractable pain who are not suitable for a percutaneous cervical cordotomy.

Regression of tumours has been seen in a few cases, but no dramatic healing of fungating tumours, or disappearance of lung or bony secondaries, has occurred. However, as the number of patients treated in this way rises such regression should be seen.

Whether regression occurs or not the method should be used for its pain-relieving properties alone.

The method is obviously here to stay, at least until something better takes its place, but the fact that it is accepted as a satisfactory method begs the question as to how destruction of the pituitary gland can relieve pain.

Pain is relieved in most cases gradually but sometimes occurs quickly. It is certain that destruction of the pituitary gland removes the influence of known and unknown hormones and this relieves pain in tumours. It is possible that the removal of growth hormone may on the one hand produce regression of the tumour, and on the other relieve pain as pressure on local tissues from the growing tumour ceases. It could be that metabolites produced by tumour growth have an influence on the production of pain, and on the amount of pain appreciated. The fact that it usually takes a few days for relief of pain to become maximal after a pituitary injection suggests that a humoral element is present. This is the time-scale of relief of pain in tumours with other methods of pituitary ablation.

However, in the pituitary injection of alcohol for destruction of the pituitary gland, and occasionally in other methods, there can be immediate relief of the pain. The author has seen a patient with severe pain in pelvis, lumbo-sacral spines and legs from pelvic spread of a carcinoma of the cervix, have great difficulty lying still on the operating table despite heavy sedation. A pituitary injection of alcohol was performed under local anaesthetic. The patient was in the posture she normally adopted to reduce her pain to a minimum, hips flexed, knees bent, and feet flat on the table top. On completion of the injection it was seen that the patient was slowly allowing her legs to slide down the table, and eventually she stretched them out in normal fashion. This was pointed out to her, her reply being that she was no longer in pain and her legs were now quite comfortable. She had no further pain while she lived.

Relief of pain with this speed is probably due to a nervous pathway. It is not difficult to believe that an injection of alcohol into the pituitary fossa can spread into areas where destruction will interfere with a pain pathway. The hypothalamic region has wide connections with many important regions of the brain, and the hypothalamic region itself is known to be close to centres controlling and appreciating pain. It is more difficult to believe that a surgical ablation of the pituitary fossa carried out under direct vision can do the same thing, yet operators do report some patients who are relieved of their pain from the moment they wake from the general anaesthetic.

Much research needs to be done before these and other interesting problems will be resolved.

REFERENCES

BRITISH MEDICAL JOURNAL (1969) Treatment of Advanced Breast Cancer, 1, 265 (Leading Article).

CORSSEN G., HOLCOMB M.C., MOUSTAPHA ISMAIL, *et al.* (1977) Alcohol-induced adenolysis of the pituitary gland: A new approach to control of intractable cancer pain. *Anes. & Anal. Current Researches,* Vol. 56, 3, May–June.

HAYWARD J.L., ATKINS H.J.R., FALCONER M.A., MACLEAN K.S., SALMON L.F.W., SCHURR P.H. & SHAHEEN C.H. (1970) Clinical trials comparing transfrontal hypophysectomy with adrenalectomy and with trans-ethmoidal hypophysectomy. In *The Clinical Management of Advanced Breast Cancer—Alpha Omega Alpha,* Eds. Joslin, C.A.F. & Gleave, E.N. Cardiff.

KATZ J., LEVIN A.B. & BENSON R.C. (1978) *Treatment of diffuse metastatic Cancer pain by stereotaxic chemical hypophysectomy.* Paper at 2nd World Congress on Pain. Montreal.

LIPTON S. (1978) Current views on the therapy of chronic pain. Percutaneous cervical cordotomy and the injection of the pituitary with alcohol. *Anaesthesia,* 33, 10, 953–957.

LIPTON S., MILES J., WILLIAMS N. & BARK-JONES N. (1978) Pituitary injection of alcohol for widespread cancer pain. *Pain,* 5, 73–82.

MADRID J. (In Press) International Symposium on Pain of Advanced Cancer, Venice 1978. Raven Press, New York.

McEWAN J. Personal communication.

MILES J. & LIPTON S. (1977) The mode of action by which pituitary alcohol injections relieve pain. In *Advances in Pain Research and Therapy,* Vol. 1, pp. 867–869. Ed. J.J. Bonica. New York, Raven Press.

MORICCA G. (1974) Chemical hypophysectomy for cancer pain. In *Advances in Neurology,* Vol. 4, pp. 707–714. Ed. J.J. Bonica. Raven Press, New York.

MORICCA G. (1977) Pituitary neuroadenolysis in the treatment of intractable pain from cancer. In *Persistent Pain,* Vol. 1, pp. 149–173. Ed. S. Lipton. Academic Press, London and New York.

Pituitary Injection needles obtainable from McCarthys, 201 London Road, Liverpool 3, England.

SPINAL INJECTIONS

There are a few important and useful facts that must be considered when using injections round the spinal cord. These are anatomical facts which determine the volume of solution required, the injection site, and the spread of the solution. The dura is fixed above to the edge of the foramen magnum and below usually terminates at the level of the second sacral vertebra. Outside the dura there is a space filled with loose areolar tissue and connected with the paravertebral spaces. This is known as the epidural or extradural space. There is a negative pressure present in this space and use can be made of this to provide a visual indication of entry into it. Various methods are used with the simplest being a drop of fluid hanging on to the end of the spinal needle as it is slowly inserted at the desired spinal level. When the tip of the needle enters the epidural space the hanging drop is sucked into the needle. One of the simplest and most accurate is the one favoured by the author, using a Macintosh balloon. A small rubber balloon is connected to the spinal needle instead of the hanging drop, and a few millilitres of sterile air injected to put the balloon under pressure (sterile air is simply obtained by sucking room air through sterile cotton wool). When the needle tip enters the epidural space the balloon deflates. The balloon will deflate as soon as the smallest part of its lumen enters the epidural space so that it should be carefully advanced a fraction further before threading a catheter through it, if such is to be used.

As mentioned in the section on sacral block through the sacral hiatus, the paravertebral space is continuous below the termination of the dural sac with the space in the caudal canal. As the spinal cord normally terminates at the second lumbar vertebra a needle inserted through the sacral hiatus may perforate the dural sac but is most unlikely to reach the spinal cord. However, there are abnormalities and variations of the bony anatomy of this sacral region and of the lumbar vertebra so care must always be taken.

In addition there are blood vessels in the epidural (and paravertebral) spaces so that after the entry of a spinal needle or catheter in this region haemorrhage may occur. In normal circumstances any haemorrhage is small and speedily stops but the author has heard of paraplegia being produced from this cause. If this happened then it would have to be treated as a surgical emergency and decompressed.

Inside the dura lies the spinal cord suspended by the dentate ligament on each side. The dura is filled with cerebrospinal fluid (CSF) which is continuous with the CSF within the cranium. Thus, if solutions are injected into the spinal CSF they may find their way on to cranial structures. This will particularly apply to substances injected at cervical levels. If the solution injected is a simple local anaesthetic solution producing a respiratory depression which wears off, at the most in five hours, the treatment is simple. Artificial respiration and support of the circulation for some hours will be enough until recovery occurs. If the solution injected is alcohol or phenol then no such simple recovery can occur and prevention is the only cure. The problem is due to the lightness or heaviness of these solutions compared to CSF and in positioning the patient in such a way that these substances enter the cranial cavity. This is discussed later. It is useful to know when a particular nerve root is being affected by the injected solution and this can

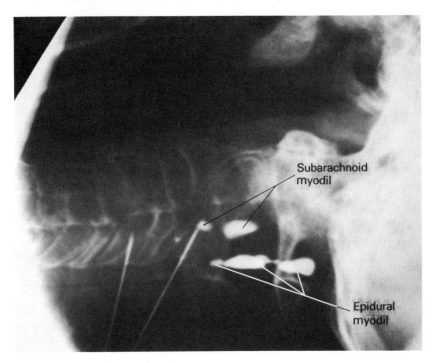

FIGURES 42–46. The use of myodil in subarachnoid block. FIGURE 42. Upper cervical.

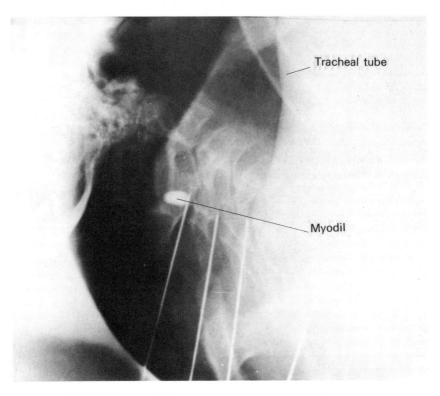

FIGURE 43. Mid and lower cervical.

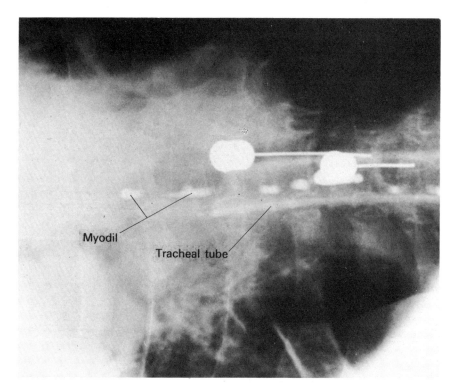

FIGURE 44. High dorsal.

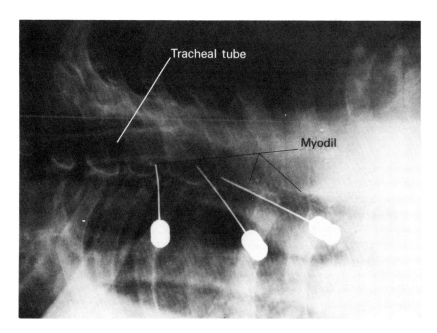

FIGURE 45. Upper–mid dorsal.

be known quite easily by asking the conscious patient of any alteration of sensation. If the patient is anaesthetised the level of the injection can be observed by injecting either air or myodil both of which can be seen on an X-ray film. It is easier to see myodil, which is radio-opaque, than air when an image intensifier is used as the resolution and penetration of this machine is much less than fixed X-ray machines. However, the purpose of the air or myodil is to allow the spinal cord to be levelled or tilted in the correct fashion for the injected solution and definition is not too important (see Figs. 42–46).

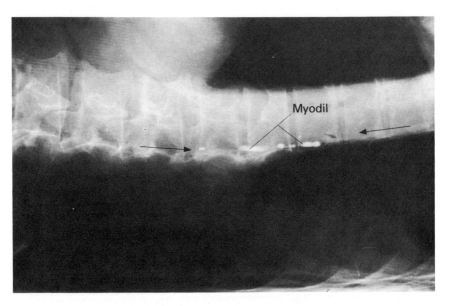

FIGURE 46. Dorso-lumbar. The needles have been removed and the myodil has flowed to the centre of the spinal hollow from both sides (shown by arrows).

There is a difference in the exits of nerve roots through the dura at the upper and lower levels of the spinal cord. Each nerve root as it exits through the dura takes with it a covering of dura. In the cervical region this layer of dura blends with the nerve root after a short distance so that there is only a shallow 'cup' of dura at the exit of each nerve. In the lumbar region this fusion does not occur immediately and the nerve root has a sleeve of dura around its exit. It can be seen that injected solutions can fill these dural cuffs and will remain in contact with the nerves. It is likely that the effect of these injected solutions will be more marked in the lumbar region than higher up.

Subdural injection

There is another type of injection into the coverings surrounding the spinal cord which originally sounds so difficult that it is not worth considering. This is the subdural injection. There is a potential space between the arachnoid and the dura and it is possible to place a spinal needle tip between these layers and inject solutions into them. The technique to carry this out is by one of two methods. In the first the patient is conscious and the spinal needle is slowly inserted until resistance on the dura can be felt. At the same time the patient will usually report a stinging type of pain in the back at the level of the spinal needle. The needle is rotated a few times with a little pressure on it and then a small amount of myodil is injected. An image intensifier is used and a small 'spot' of myodil is seen in relation to the needle tip. If more than a drop or two of myodil is injected then myodil will be seen spreading laterally along the nerve sheaths. The second method is used when the patient is anaesthetised or when the needle has penetrated to the CSF in the first method. In this second method the needle is slowly advanced until it deliberately penetrates the dura and CSF is obtained. The needle is then gradually withdrawn until the CSF flow slows to a trickle and then just stops. From then on the procedure is as in the first method. It is admitted that this is not an easy technique to acquire but all it needs is persistence and a light touch. There are different appearances of the myodil depending where it is in relation to the dura. When it is intrathecal small pools of myodil can be seen on the image intensifier screen which are very mobile. When the myodil is placed subdurally a beaded appearance is produced along the edge of the theca in the antero-posterior view and a thin line in the lateral view. In addition some of the radio-opaque substance will be seen spreading out along the nerves. In the cervical region the spread along the nerves of the brachial plexus can be as far as the edge of the clavicle.

One of the unusual (and valuable) features about this type of injection is that while the injection is being made—the patient being on their side—the injected solution will spread upwards and bilaterally. The solution spreads more on to the dependent side than on to the upper. If it is desired that the solution should move inferiorly this is done by first injecting some air, and the procedure continues using air and myodil solution alternately.

The concentration of phenol in myodil for this subdural block is $7\frac{1}{2}$ per cent phenol in myodil or 5 per cent phenol in glycerine, and the quantity can be up to 3·0 ml. If phenol in glycerine is used then small increments (0·25 ml) of myodil should be injected from time to time and observed on the image intensifier to check that the injection continues in the subdural space. As the patient is head up, any myodil solution which is seen to move upwards and has a beaded or blob-like appearance must be in the subdural space. Any solution which finds its way in to the subarachnoid space will descend rapidly as small blobs or beads. When in the extradural space the appearance is related to the extradural shape when it appears tube-like and somewhat smudged.

Subarachnoid injection

The use of phenol in either glycerine or myodil, and the use of al-cohol within the subarachnoid space, is universal in the treatment of the intractable pain of cancer. It is the one method which can be used through-out the world as it can be carried out using the least sophisticated equipment. A spinal needle, a supply of phenol solution or alcohol, a tilting table are all that is needed. Lest it be thought that the author advocates the use of this mimimum it must be said that he does not, but if an image intensifier is added then standards befitting the last quarter of the twentieth century are available. The use of X-ray equipment removes the element of guesswork in deciding exactly where the needle is inserted, where the highest or lowest point of the spinal cord is, and whether any injected radio-opaque substance

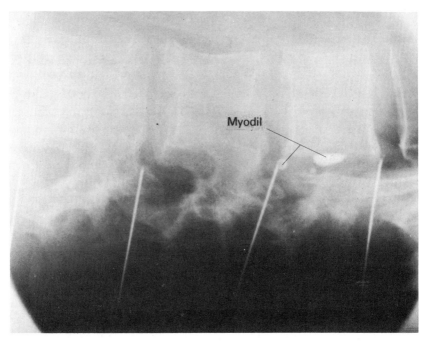

FIGURE 47. Lumbar.

is remaining at the vertebral level it should remain at. Not only that but if radio-opaque materials are used then the patient can be given a general anaesthetic and the operator can be quite certain of the nerve root level that will be affected. This is why the author favours hyperbaric phenol solutions rather than the hypobaric alcohol, as myodil is also hyperbaric.

When using these injections positioning of the patient is extremely important. If hypobaric solutions are used the patient is placed with the painful side uppermost, while if hyperbaric solutions are used the patient is placed on the painful side. Further, as it is the posterior sensory nerve root rather than the anterior motor nerve root that is to be affected, in the case of alcohol, the patient is tilted forwards (anteriorly) to bring the posterior nerve root to the highest position in the spinal theca and thus to the position where the alcohol pools. In the case of hyperbaric solutions the patient is positioned with a posterior tilt to bring the posterior nerve root to the most dependent position where the phenol hyperbaric solution will pool (see Fig. 1c). In addition the patient is tilted so that hyperbaric solutions will affect the nerve root as it lies in the dural cuff, but for hypobaric ones it is the point at which the fasciculi of the sensory nerves enter the spinal cord that is affected. The anterior or posterior tilt necessary is about 45° in each case.

As mentioned in the introduction, phenol in myodil concentration for concentration behaves as a weaker solution than phenol in glycerine. However, phenol in glycerine is a more viscid solution and therefore moves more slowly from the point of injection than myodil solutions and for this reason is more controllable. However, if a mid-thoracic group of nerve roots are to be affected by making a subarachnoid puncture above or below this region and running the phenol solution on to them, phenol in myodil being much more mobile may be the solution of choice. There is one disadvantage of phenol in myodil due to it not being absorbed as is glycerine. It thus remains inside the theca and if a repeat injection of phenol in myodil or glycerine is made at a later date it may not be effective because the dependent nerve roots are protected by the dural sleeve being filled with myodil. This problem occurs particularly in the lumbar region. It can be dealt with fairly simply by lying the patient on the non-painful side and tilting into the trendelenberg position which drains the myodil into the skull. If care is taken when placing the patient into the correct position to keep the head dependent, the myodil will remain in the cranium, long enough for the block to be carried out. This process may be performed more than once and on both sides to drain all the myodil out of the spine. When the block is being carried out care must be taken that the phenol solution does not flow into the cranium. The following doses refer only to inoperable cancer patients.

The quantity of phenol that can be injected varies from level to level of the spinal cord. In the lumbar region phenol in glycerine 1·0 ml at L5 and 1·25 ml at L1 should not be exceeded and spread over three or four nerves will be obtained. A useful method is to insert two or three needles at the level of the nerve roots it is desired to affect and inject a small increment down each one. This is the technique the author uses at all levels of the spinal cord when the patient is anaesthetised. The patient can be levelled off accurately by injecting a small amount of myodil (0·05 ml, literally a drop) and observing its movement in relation to the needle tip. This method has the added advantage that the patient does not 'creep' or gradually alter the position as he does when conscious. At the lower dorsal level phenol in glycerine 1·5 ml rising to 2·0 ml at the upper dorsal nerve roots can be used. The mid-dorsal region needs to be treated with more respect than other levels as the space around the spinal cord is limited and the injected phenol solution seems to come in contact with the cord and I have seen a few patients become mildly ataxic, and with profound loss of sensation at the level of injection. This cleared up to a large extent in a few days and completely within one month.

In the cervical region as much as 2·5 ml of phenol solution can be used. Either 1 in 20 or 1 in 15 phenol in myodil can be used at this level and in the upper dorsal region also this strength (but not this quantity) can be used. If the upper dorsal nerves are affected the sympathetic fibres are also affected. This is shown by a ptosis of the corresponding upper eyelid.

From the above it is seen that very careful positioning of the patient is the key to this technique combined with the correct quantity and concentration of phenol in relation to the vertebral level. Many operators find safety in having the patient conscious and able to answer queries on their sensation to pin prick and scratch and how these change during the procedure. The author would not quarrel with this view though he often uses general anaesthesia for these patients. The doses given are maxima.

One technique where there is an advantage in having the patient conscious is when an intrathecal drop is being carried out for pain in the perineum, usually for a carcinoma of the rectum. The patient is sitting up and a lumbar puncture is performed and the needle withdrawn until the flow of CSF just begins to slow. At this position it is just inside the subarachnoid space. The patient is then tilted posteriorly about 45° so that the lumbar spine is making this angle with the bed or trolley. Enough helpers are required at this stage to support the patient in this position and allow the operator to have both hands free to make the injection. Initially 0·5 ml phenol in glycerine 1 in 20 is slowly injected and trickles down the posterior arachnoid to the lowest sacral nerve roots. The reason for this amount of care is to make as certain as possible that phenol solution does not flow over the S2 nerve roots. These carry most of the nerve fibres from the spinal cord to the bladder and if they are damaged changes in micturition will occur. Often some alteration in bladder control does occur but it will usually recover provided there is no concomitant damage from the primary lesion or consequent surgery. If no pain relief occurs a further 0·25 ml is injected.

If the pain relief is only partial following this injection, then at a later date it can be repeated first using 1·0 ml, or even more in a large man, of phenol in glycerine 1 in 20, and if this only gives temporary relief or wears off in only one week or so, a similar quantity of phenol in glycerine 1 in 15 can be used on a third occasion.

Epidural block

This technique is well described in standard anaesthetic books as it is in world-wide use for midwifery practice. It is not proposed to describe it again here. Some practitioners use phenol epidurally as larger quantities can be used safely.

Chlorocresol

Instead of using phenol 1 in 20, chlorocresol 2 per cent can be used. This substance is said to be longer lasting and more penetrating, but is more difficult to use, as the initial signs that phenol injections produce such as warmth, numbness and tingling, are absent. Mehta uses equal parts of the two agents, while Swerdlow has a large series. The author has no great experience of this substance.

Complications

The various methods of spinal injections produce the type of complications which might be expected. Pain at the site of the needle insertion and injection, motor weakness and alteration in sensation, are directly due to the trauma of the needle and the effect of the injected solution. Headaches, vomiting, meningeal reactions, and alterations in micturition occur following any spinal injection, especially the subarachnoid ones, but there is a higher incidence when foreign substances are injected. The treatment is as for any of these complications occurring during or after a spinal anaesthetic.

REFERENCES

BROMAGE P.R. (1972) Unblocked segments in epidural analgesia for relief of pain in labour. *B.J.A.* **44**, 676.

DAWKINS C.J.M. (1969) An analysis of the complications of extradural and caudal block. *Anaesthesia*, **24**, 554.

GERBERSHAGEN H.U., BAAR H.A. & KREUSCHER H. (1972) Langzeitnervenblockaden zur Behandlung schwerer Schmerzzusände. 1. Die intrathecale Injektion von Neuro-lytica. (trans. Long-term nerve blocks in the treatment of severe pain conditions.) *Der Anaesthesist*, 21. Bd., Heft 3, pp. 112–121.

GREENE M.N. (1961) Complications of spinal analgesia. *Anaesthesiology*, **22**, 682.

MAHER R.M. (1955) Relief of pain in incurable cancer. *Lancet*, **1**, 836.

MAHER R.M. (1957) Neurone selection in relief of pain; further experiences with intrathecal injections. *Lancet*, **1**, 16.

MAHER R.M. (1960) Further experiences with intrathecal and subdural phenol.

MEHTA M. (1971) Extra-dural medication for lumbo-sciatic pain. *Anaesthesia*, **26**, 104.

NATHAN P.W. (1970) Chemical rhizotomy for relief of spasticity in ambulant patients. *B.M.J.* **1**, 1096.

SWERDLOW M. & SAYLE-CREER W. (1970) A study of extradural medication in the relief of the lumbosciatic syndrome. *Anaesthesia*, **25**, 341.

FURTHER READING

MAHER R. & MEHTA M. (1977) Spinal (intrathecal) and extradural analgesia. In *Persistent Pain*. Chapter 4. Ed. S. Lipton. Academic Press, London and New York.

SWERDLOW M. (1974) Intrathecal and extradural block in pain relief. In *Relief of Intractable Pain*. Chapter 7. Ed. M. Swerdlow, Excerpta Medica, Amsterdam.

Chapter 8
Post-Herpetic Neuralgia

It must be stated from the very beginning of this section that there is no treatment that can reliably relieve the pain and discomfort present in the developed condition of post-herpetic neuralgia. Many treatments are advocated for this condition but it is almost fortuitous when a particular case responds satisfactorily. This does not mean that treatment for post-herpetic neuralgia should be abandoned, merely that the expectations of the physician and patient should not be pitched too high.

The treatment that is available needs to be used in the early stages of the disease. In fact, the best results are produced in the most acute stages of the condition. Some information on the infective process of the herpes zoster virus is presented now before discussing the problem of post-herpetic neuralgia which is the problem of the later stages of the disease.

Herpes zoster, or shingles as it is often called, is an acute viral infection which affects the posterior spinal root ganglion of the spinal nerves, or the corresponding ganglia of the cranial nerves. The virus concerned is the same virus that produces varicella (chicken pox) and is of the DNA virus type. The usual form of the disease is varicella in young people and children, and herpes zoster in old age. In occasional cases, zoster occurs in children and varicella in old age. It is thought that the virus lies dormant in the posterior root ganglia after an infection in childhood until the patient's immunity falls in later life when it replicates once again. In the older patient the disease will appear in a local distribution and it tends to be confined in this distribution as immunity rises quickly with the infection.

The segmental level of the distribution of the herpes zoster infection is probably decided by local trauma, infection, muscular activity, or the presence of unsuspected malignancy. It is well known, for instance, that a retroperitoneal sarcoma may first show as a herpes zoster infection in the relevant distribution. This is not to imply that there is a reason for every case of herpes zoster that appears, there is not, as in most cases of post-herpetic neuralgia there is no explanation at all. A similar situation exists in poliomyelitis where the infection tends to present in a nerve distribution where there has been previous vigorous muscular activity. Just as polio-myelitis commonly affects the nerve cells and fibres of the anterior horn, but can on occasion affect other cells in the central nervous system, so does the herpes zoster virus normally affect the posterior spinal nerve root, and to a varying degree the posterior horn, but spreads beyond this in some cases.

Herpes zoster commonly affects the thoracic spinal nerves but can affect other portions of the spinal cord, or the cranial nerves. The most commonly affected of the cranial nerves is the trigeminal, and the most commonly affected branch of the trigeminal nerve is the first division. This may be a reflection of the spinal distribution of the trigeminal nerve, in that the first division has the lowest representation in the spinal cord. The infection is usually unilateral, is most common over the age of 50, and is more common in males than females. As implied in the previous paragraph, the infection can be symptomatic and is common in debility. Occasionally the virus invades the spinal cord or the brain producing a myelitis or an encephalitis.

The acute disease usually presents with severe continuous pain in the distribution of the affected nerve. The general effect on the patient can be trivial, or the pain can present with pyrexia and malaise. The diagnosis can be in doubt and is often not resolved until the skin eruption appears. This usually occurs on the third or fourth day when the skin appears reddened and the vesicles appear. During the early stages before the rash, the patient suffers paraesthesiae and shooting pain, which may develop into the con-tinuous type of pain mentioned previously.

At first there is exudation of fluid into the skin forming blebs and vesicles, which are clear at first, but soon become infected, and eventually scabs form. The vesicles dry up in five or six days leaving small scars behind, but sometimes the resulting scarring can be most marked. When the areas of vesicular eruption spread until they become confluent, a widespread and continuous scar results. However large or small, the scars produced are anaesthetic. There is some controversy as to the cause of the skin eruption, some believing that a ganglionitis in the posterior root ganglion produces an autonomic imbalance. Certainly sympathetic blockade is a useful and often successful method of treatment in the acute phase as will be seen later. Others believe that the skin eruption is the result of the virus passing along the nerves, reaching the skin, and initiating an inflammatory reaction. This latter explanation seems the most likely.

In some cases of herpes zoster, the skin eruption is minimal, with only a few vesicles in the acute phase, and thus very few scars to see in the chronic condition of pain, if this develops. It is postulated that some cases of post-herpetic neuralgia can occur without any scars being present. In other words, the original infection produced damage in the central nervous system, resulting in a neuralgia, without producing any vesicles or scars in the skin. Certainly most physicians have seen a patient suffering from what appears to be a post-herpetic neuralgia without there being any trace of scarring in the corresponding dermatomes. Practically speaking, it does not matter what the causative virus is, as if damage of the zoster type in the central nervous system is produced, then pain will result. In the acute stage of the infection a rising zoster antibody titre will confirm that the infection is produced by a zoster virus and this would be the only way to confirm that the disease had occurred in the absence of skin scars.

When the disease occurs in the ophthalmic division of the trigeminal nerve, vesicles may appear on the cornea, and if corneal ulceration occurs, the danger of scarring and impairment of vision will be a real one.

Usually the pain of herpes zoster presents in the acute phase, subsides as the eruption fades, but especially in old people this may not happen and the pain continues. The patient may then suffer from a persistent and intractable post-herpetic neuralgia that lasts for months or years. When the acute inflammatory viral process is not confined to the posterior root ganglion and the posterior horn, but also affects the anterior horn, motor disabilities will be present. Again these tend to be confined to a segmental distribution, thus if the brachial plexus is involved there may be sensory changes in the lower two or three roots of this plexus, and in addition motor weakness or paresis in the same distribution. Usually these motor defects are reversible and in that case the time scale for recovery may be over several years. In other, occasional and more severe infections, there may be no recovery, or only limited recovery.

There are even rarer residual effects which follow on from bulbar and encephalitic zoster but they are common to any widespread viral infection and are not specific to zoster.

Intractable pain arises in many cases of zoster in the older patient. The acute phase settles but the pain, dysaesthesia, and hyperaesthesia remain. The usual story is that the pain first begins as a discomfort of the skin which is increased by any stimulus to the skin. This discomfort increases in severity and there are occasional sharp stabbing pains as well. The discomfort has an element of burning or heat, and hyperaesthesia and hyperalgesia can be intense. In most cases the disease terminates in the third week and the pain, dysaesthesia, and hyperalgesia, begin to disappear. After about five weeks or so the scabs formed on the dried-up vesicles separate, leaving pink scars which are usually anaesthetic. The hyperaesthesia and hyperalgesia may persist for a month or two but will gradually subside. The scars become pale, and retract, forming the typical 'pocks', but they remain insensitive and this does not alter even after long periods of time.

In some patients, and the proportion increases with their age, the pain, burning dysaesthesia, and hyperalgesia, persist for very long periods of time. There is a tendency for the condition to improve slowly, but once the condition has been present for six months the prospect of a complete cure is remote. Often the patient maintains that the pain slowly increases, but this is probably due to slow reduction in the patient's pain threshold similar to that which occurs in any long-standing painful state.

It has to be realised that there are two elements to the discomfort produced by post-herpetic neuralgia. One is pain, which is constant, never varying, and often has a feeling of heat about it. The patient is always conscious of this pain only getting relief in sleep. Most patients will say that when they wake in the morning the pain does not appear as long as they remain perfectly still but as soon as they move the slightest amount the pain appears in its normal severity. In the chronic stage of post-herpetic neuralgia the patient usually suffers from hyperpathia. In this condition the patient has a higher threshold to the pain which has a peculiarly unpleasant and radiating character. This is the type of pain which is often associated with damage to a peripheral nerve, the spinothalamic tract, or the thalamus and is thought to be due to a reduction in the number and proportion of conducting nerve fibres. In the acute phase of the condition there is a hyperalgesia where pain is produced at a lower threshold than normally.

The second element in the discomfort is not really a pain though the patient will often interpret it as pain, it is the presence of dysaesthesiae. These are uncomfortable sensations which have an element of unpleasantness about them. The patient may be unable to bear even the lightest of clothes to touch the skin. This can be present to the extent that patients will cut out portions of their clothes so that on removing their outer coat the affected portion of the skin can be viewed without them undressing further.

This dislike of touch on the affected part can be so sensitive that even a slight draught or breath of wind is sufficient to initiate an additional paroxysm of pain. Not only is the patient sensitive to touch and the uncomfortable feeling it gives, but the actual touch itself stimulates the production of pain. It is interesting that most patients say that they can stand firm pressure on the painful part but not light pressure. So much so does this apply that they will often spend much of their time pressing a hand over the painful region, or they wear an extra specially tight garment.

Sometimes the patient has a feeling of formication and describes it as a feeling of worms under the skin or ants crawling over the skin. Some of the descriptions used by the patients are highly pictorial and fantastic.

Gate control theory and its dual input theory of pain would seem to explain some, at any rate, of the features involved in the production and persistence of pain in post-herpetic neuralgia. This theory postulates that pain is carried by small unmyelinated or small myelinated nerve fibres to the central nervous system. There the input provided through these channels is modified by that through pathways in larger myelinated nerve fibres. Both types of fibres are stimulated by any severe stimulation which produces pain. The transmission of nerve impulses is faster in large myelinated nerve fibres than in small unmyelinated ones, and this has a bearing on the pain modulation (see Chapter 3).

In the acute herpetic process destruction occurs of nerve cells and nerve fibres in a rather selective fashion. There is a tendency, proportionately, for far more large fibres to be damaged and destroyed than small fibres. Regeneration of large fibres is slower than that of the small fibres and also many large fibres after regeneration do not have as large a diameter as previously. Thus the range of nerve fibres changes, tending towards an increase in the smaller fibres. According to the Gate Control theory this would be exactly the situation where minimal small fibre stimulation might produce the sensation of pain as the normal modulation of larger nerve fibre stimulation is no longer present. In addition, whenever there is damage to nerve fibres peripherally or centrally then so-called 'protopathic' pain arises, i.e. pain with unpleasant characteristics. There is one final possibility in that continuous stimulation of central neuron pools may result in perseverating pain arising and then continuing, and this could well occur after the loss of modulation following the zoster infection. One of the features of an abnormal central nervous system of this type is that relatively slight stimulations in the affected dermatomes, or in neighbouring ones, will trigger off paroxysms of pain, and the pain has an unpleasant quality about it.

There are added features in post-herpetic neuralgia in that there is an increasing incidence with age. This may be related to the fact that the proportion of large fibres to small nerve fibres falls steadily throughout life. It is obvious that this will increase the factors tending towards a post-herpetic neuralgia.

Treatment of post-herpetic neuralgia is unrewarding. As stated in the opening few words of this section there is nothing that the author has tried which can reliably relieve the developed condition. This means that there are two methods of approach to the question of treating post-herpetic neuralgia. One is quite obvious, and is to prevent the condition from developing in the first place. The second is to carry out those measures which might improve, but will not cure it.

Prevention can be developed on three different lines of treatment. The most logical of these is to prevent the disease from developing at all. The DNA virus, of which zoster is one, can be inhibited by idoxuridine. There are other substances which have a similar effect but this is the simplest to use (*B.M.J.* editorial). The herpetiform rash usually clinches the diagnosis of zoster, and until that stage it would be unwise to use potentially dangerous agents in its treatment. Thus treatment with idoxuridine is begun when the rash appears and consists of covering the affected area with idoxuridine 40 per cent in dimethylsulphoxide (DMSO). This is painted on, or pads of lint moistened with the idoxuridine solution are used for about four days. There can be problems with toxic effects, and the idoxuridine is somewhat expensive in this form due to the quantity used. It is commonly used in viral corneal ulcers, when the quantities used are small and the cost can be kept reasonable. It is most effective for this condition, and is said to be equally effective in zoster eruptions where it rapidly reduces the pain and heals the vesicles. It can abort the infection and thus reduce the chance of a post-herpetic neuralgia developing. The evidence suggests that its effect is variable. It does not remove the possibility of a post-herpetic neuralgia developing, as this depends on the stage of the disease when the idoxuridine is used, the virulence of the infection, the resistance of the patient, and the amount of damage to nerve fibres produced before the infection resolves.

It would seem reasonable to use this form of treatment in the early stages when the rash has just appeared, and in the older group of patients, say over 50 years of age, who are the group particularly at risk from post-herpetic neuralgia. Unfortunately at the present time treatment of zoster with an average area of rash to cover requires idoxuridine costing about £30, and many patients who would benefit from its use do not receive it because of this high cost. A second reason is that the potential value of idoxuridine in the prevention of post-herpetic neuralgia is not widely realised.

There is one other problem in the use of idoxuridine in relation to the DMSO used as a vehicle for the active ingredient. DMSO is an irritant and has an unpleasant smell, and may produce a maceration of the skin. It has one benefit in that it has a bacteriostatic effect. Cytarabine can be systematically in place of the idoxuridine but it is not a drug to be used lightly as there is a real risk of producing a dissemination of the zoster infection.

The second method, which has widespread use in the treatment of zoster infection, is the use of steroids, though the author thinks that this is a dangerous method of treatment. The steroids are used topically on the rash when it appears, or in massive doses started within the first ten days, and continued for up to three weeks. Prednisone is the usual cortico-steriod used in dose of up to 60 mg daily for one week, then 30 mg daily for one week, and finally 15 mg daily for another week. With the topical cortico-steroids there is the danger of wide dissemination of the rash locally. With systemic cortico-steroids there is the danger of spreading a neurotropic virus infection, and this has been reported as happening on occasion. The benefit of the cortico-steroid treatment is said to be a reduction of pain and scarring, and a prevention of post-herpetic neuralgia developing. These claims do not seem to be borne out in practice.

The third method of treatment of the active stage of zoster infections is by sympathetic and systemic nerve blocks (Colding 1969). There is no doubt that a block of the sympathetic ganglia can relieve pain and vesiculation in herpes zoster in dramatic fashion in the acute stage in some patients. Whether it is reasonable to claim subsequent post-infection freedom from pain as due to this is doubtful, as most post-herpetic patients do not develop post-herpetic neuralgia.

There is some logic in treating the acute herpetic condition with sympathetic nerve blocks. The primary lesion in herpes zoster is an acute inflammatory state of the posterior root ganglion, and this may cause increased sympathetic vasoconstriction segmentally. Blocking this ganglion may interrupt sensory afferent impulses through the sympathetic fibres and ganglia proceeding to the dorsal roots, as well as producing a vasodilatation. If this method is to be adopted then either a long-acting local anaesthetic solution should be used, or the sympathetic blocks must be repeated daily. The rationale of this treatment depends on a fairly constant interruption of the sympathetic impulses to the affected segment of the skin. This means that the block must extend at least one segment above and below, and as the thoracic region of the body is the most commonly affected it may mean that a considerable number of paravertebral blocks are required. A more satisfactory method for continuously blocking the required region would be to place an epidural catheter and leave it in position for several days. This would be a much kinder method as far as the patient is concerned.

These three methods are designed to avoid the problem of a post-herpetic neuralgia in the future, by taking precautions during the acute phase of the infection. As far as the pain clinic is concerned this is academic as the patient will present with the developed condition of a post-herpetic neuralgia. The complaint is one of continuous and intolerable pain which has a most unpleasant element to it. In addition there will be hypersensitivity of the affected skin but there may be a raised threshold of stimulation, i.e. a hyperpathia rather than a hyperalgesia.

On examination there will be scarring of a more or less obvious degree, and this will be in a dermatomal distribution. The scars are present in those areas where a peripheral nerve transmits impulses from skin, and thus the scars tend to be arranged in groups where particular peripheral branches penetrate from the deeper structures. This is seen most easily in the distribution of the upper intercostal nerves where there are three groups of scars. One group is usually found posteriorly where a branch of the posterior primary ramus supplies the skin over and near the vertebrae. Another group is lateral, being the lateral branches of the anterior primary ramus, and thirdly the terminations of the intercostal nerves penetrate the overlying tissues to be distributed to the skin of the anterior chest wall and there form a group. If the infection has been widespread and severe then the scarring can be more or less continuous. It is usually accepted that the herpetic infection is confined to one side of the body and this is usually so. However, in many cases the scars in the thoracic region do spread over the mid-line, and this happens more frequently in the posterior chest wall than in the anterior. Under these circumstances no possible treatment on one side only of the body is going to relieve the pain completely. Fortunately, when this happens there is usually only a small area of overlap. There is no doubt that when this occurs the nerve supply is from the opposite side, and why the process should be confined to a very small area rather than spread throughout the whole of the peripheral nerve distribution is difficult to understand. Presumably the infection does not spread from the central nervous system to the periphery, but is due to a local spread along small nerve fibres in the skin. This process probably occurs during an overwhelming local infection at the time of skin vesiculation, when the antibody titre has risen so that retrograde spread along the whole of the peripheral nerve is impossible.

It is not certain that if an individual intercostal nerve is affected that all its branches will be affected. Often, if the scarred area is observed, it will be seen that one intercostal nerve has posterior scars, while the ones below or above have them laterally or anteriorly, or in both of these places, or in all three.

The scars themselves are completely anaesthetic whereas it is the skin between the scars that is sensitive. Often it will be a particular area of skin which is especially sensitive, the remainder of that dermatome being, if not normal, then not unduly painful. This means that treatment can be confined to a relatively small area of the body.

The author believes that the best time to relieve the pain of post-herpetic neuralgia is within the first three months, after that period the pain may be improved but not usually cured completely. As some of the patients who have post-herpetic neuralgia at three months obtain spontaneous cures, it is not always possible to decide which patients obtain relief spontaneously and which by treatment. If the therapist adopts an expectant policy of a nil result (as the author does) he may be pleasantly surprised from time to time. This is not to suggest for one moment that it is not worthwhile treating the post-herpetic neuralgia patients as vigorously as is possible—it is. In many cases the condition can be improved, the pain partially relieved, and the patient's quality of life improved. Unfortunately this is a condition caused by an imbalance of nervous activity and a consequent central nervous system misinterpretation of an abnormal input. This defect cannot be altered but it may be affected in such a way that the patient's well-being is improved.

Treatment can be of many varieties but there does not appear to be any way of distinguishing beforehand which particular treatment will be successful. The method adopted at the Centre for Pain Relief is to have a series of treatments which are tried successively. Before treatment begins the patient is given a simplified explanation of the cause of pain in post-herpetic neuralgia on the lines of 'the original shingles infection which produces scabs on the skin also damages the nerves inside the body. Just as the scars cannot be removed afterwards so the nerve damage cannot be removed, and it is this damage to the nerves which causes the pain. The pain tends to improve gradually with time, but this can take a very long time, sometimes years. It is often possible to help the pain, but once it has lasted over three months the best thing to expect is that it will improve. The treatment you will get is designed to improve your pain but you may be lucky and have it disappear completely.' This will prepare the patient for a prolonged and probably varied programme of attempts at pain relief.

It is now completely outmoded to use vitamin B12 in the treatment of nervous disorders unless these are of the pernicious anaemia, sub-acute combined degeneration type, but very occasionally a patient suffering from post-herpetic neuralgia obtains some benefit from this. In most cases this treatment is used in patients in the early stage of the post-herpetic state, say in the first three months, and as mentioned before there will be a number of spontaneous cures in this period. It is always difficult to assess results under these circumstances but as injections of Cyanocobalamin 1000 μg. given weekly for six weeks are innocuous, and may help, there is no reason to withhold them. In the very early stages of the condition, in the first four weeks after the scabs separate, they may be combined usefully with analgesic tablets, and sympathetic blocks. The arrangement of treatments can be altered in the early stages if it is thought that one particular method of treatment has more prospect of success than another. At a later stage there is no point in varying the order of the methods used.

Non-addictive drug therapy has not been discussed so far and there is no need to go into it in detail here. The problem is that there is no known combination of drugs that will relieve the patient of their pain for any length of time. It is the belief of the author that this class of patient should be kept on non-addictive drugs and on no account be prescribed addictive ones. The usual history with these patients is that they go on to a particular analgesic drug regime and for a time their pain, while not entirely relieved, is improved. After an interval, usually shorter rather than longer, this particular dose no longer relieves them. The dose is increased and they obtain benefit for a shorter period this time. The process continues with another drug, and the patient returns, each time asking for more or stronger drugs. If these patients are given narcotics they will become drug addicts. These patients 'suffer' in the real sense of the word. It is not only pain which makes them wretched but the dysaesthesiae and hyperpathia, and there is no prospect that drug therapy will be able to relieve these sensations. It is important to tell the patient when informing them of the cause of the pain, that there are two types of sensation present. Once the patient is told that there is pain on the one hand and uncomfortable feelings on the other, they usually say that that is exactly the sensations they feel. At this stage they should be told that while it is possible to improve the pain, it is very difficult to alter the sensations of discomfort that they feel. It is possible, in fact, for the pain to be entirely relieved without affecting the discomfort at all.

It is obvious that there is a 'psychic' element to the pain and it might be thought that drugs of the psychotropic type would be of benefit. The combination of substituted phenothiozines and tricyclic anti-depressants has been tried vigorously (Taub and Collins). Fluphenazine not more than 4 mg daily is used, and as depression may develop, or is already a feature, amitriptyline 75 mg at night is added as an anti-depressant. This regime is continued for at least a month as relief of pain, when it occurs, is progressive up to this time. In the Centre this regime has not been of help.

One feature of patients who suffer from post-herpetic neuralgia exists which has not been mentioned so far. This is a function of the age of the patients, who in the English-speaking countries find that they, having outlived most of their contemporaries and their immediate family, have to live on their own. A lonely existence of this kind, with time hanging heavily on their hands potentiates the problem. The patient has too much time to think about his own problems and misery. The best that a patient with a post-herpetic neuralgia can do is to 'get out and about', but it is realised that this is not always possible, even if the patient can be stirred out of the mental misery and sloth which envelopes them.

The series of treatments continues with a trial of the *cold spray*. There are a number of these in use, which in its simplest form makes use of an ethyl chloride spray. As there are problems with this when used in a confined space, the modern version uses a mixture of trichlorofluoromethane 85 per cent in dichlorodifluoromethane 15 per cent in a spray can (P.R. spray Boots). The technique is to use the can to jet fluid over the whole of the painful area, beginning at the upper level and working down. If the painful region is on the face or is near mucous membrane, care must be taken as it will sting. The method is to 'wash' the cold fluid over the whole of the painful region and then let it evaporate, cooling the area. The 'wash' is repeated twice more at one-minute intervals until the skin is thoroughly cooled, this being one 'treatment'. When of value a treatment will relieve the pain for a varying time. As soon as the pain returns to near its former intensity the spray is repeated. This means that when the treatment by this method begins the patient will be spraying very frequently indeed, at least every hour. If the patient is working it is best to start this method at the weekend when the patient can rely on two clear days for treatment. Before initiating such a course of treatment the patient should be tested for suitability. This is done very simply by using a test of one set of three sprays and unless the patient obtains some obvious and immediate benefit there is no point in trying the method further.

If the patient responds satisfactorily the period during which pain relief occurs gradually becomes longer. Eventually the patient's pain is relieved by two or three sets of sprays per day. It must be made very clear to the patient that they are meant to spray frequently in the initial period of the treatment. If this is not carried out the trial is not a fair one, and the already small prospect of benefit from this method will reduce to zero. Often patients find some benefit even if it does not relieve their pain completely. It can be used in combination with say, analgesic drugs, or to help the patient over a period when their pain or dysaesthesiae is particularly troublesome. Some patients find that this method is useful just before they settle themselves for sleep at night.

It must be carefully explained to the patient that spraying must not be continuous, as this might cause a frost-bite. Some patients when they are being tested for suitability of the spray technique will complain that the spray exacerbates their pain. There is no point at all in bothering further with the spray in these patients, even as an adjunct.

A subcutaneous injection below the scarred area is the next method to be used in the scheme of treatment for post-herpetic neuralgia. This injection can be with or without cortico-steroids. As a first measure a simple anaesthetic agent such as $\frac{1}{2}$ per cent Marcaine plain (Bupivacaine B.P.) can be injected under the most painful scars. The quantity used depends on the anaesthetic agent used and its toxicity, but about 30 ml will be necessary in the thoracic region when two out of the three main areas usually affected can be treated by this quantity in the average case. When the patient has a number of painful areas, as occurs in most post-herpetic neuralgia in the thoracic region, it is possible to leave one area untreated to act as a control. If treatment is effective in the injected areas the untreated portion is dealt with at the follow-up visit. The frequency of injection depends on the response. In all cases there will be relief of pain while the local anaesthetic has its primary effect. In most cases this will be the only effect, but in some the pain relief will last much longer than the expected period, perhaps forty-eight hours or more, and then return gradually over a variable period of a few days to a week. In addition to this some patients obtain benefit in regard to the hyperpathia that troubles them. This also lasts for a variable time. The use of the control area is a valuable adjunct to treatment because it often allows the patient to see that there is some difference produced by the treatment.

It is also valuable to the physician to confirm that the treatment is helpful, and that he is not just wasting his time. The question 'do you want me to inject the area which we did not inject last time?' soon informs the physician of the value the patient puts on the method.

If this simple injection does not produce enough benefit or fails completely, then a similar injection with the addition of a long-acting cortico-steroid is made. The long-acting steroids are usually the acetate compounds, such as Methylprednisolone acetate B.P. (Depo-Medrone), and this one is given in 40 or 80 mg doses mixed with local anaesthetic. The method of action of the local anaesthetic agent and of the cortico-steroid acetate is unknown, but it is most likely that the local anaesthetic blocks stimulation to overactive neuron pools in the spinal cord reducing their activity. When the peripheral nerves become active again they may have their input into normal or near-normal neuron pools. This reduction in activity may gradually increase again, the patient returning to his previous sensitivity but the hope is that they do not quite return to their previous state and if the injections are repeated his condition gradually improves. The use of cortico-steroids seems to be indicated in those patients where there is a marked element of hyperpathia, or where there has been no response to previous treatment.

If there is no response from injections after the combination of local and long-acting cortico-steroids have been used on two occasions, this particular method is useless in that patient.

The next method is to carry out those nerve blocks which can be done without having an effect on motor power. This type of block is particularly valuable in the thoracic region where the intercostal nerves are accessible. It is best first to carry out a test block with simple local solutions, such as Marcaine $\frac{1}{2}$ per cent plain, to see if this will remove the pain. If it does a long-acting local anaesthetic such as 2 per cent Benzocaine in Arachis Oil, followed by twice the quantity of 6 per cent Urethane, injected down the same needle without moving the position of the needle can be used. This combination of solutions produces a long period of analgesia as it only tends to block small fibres. The period of block varies from three or four weeks, to a more usual three months. On one occasion the author has seen such a block last over one year for relief of pain in a secondary carcinoma in rib.

Once a long period of pain relief has been obtained there is the prospect that when the block wears off the relief may be permanent. The block may need to be repeated on more than one occasion.

Another type of injection but using a similar method is to produce a temporary neurolysis of the small afferent fibres, whilst leaving the large fibres untouched. This is performed with a solution of 5 per cent ammonium sulphate (Dam and Larson). This solution is painful so bupivocaine is added to it. The injection may have to be repeated if the patient is not kept pain-free for two months by the initial block.

Paravertebral blocks are the next type of injection to try if the previous blocks have not given acceptable pain relief. These have the advantage that they block the sympathetic fibres centrally and this is an acknowledged method of treatment in the acute phase of the disease. It is also well worth trying in the chronic stage. There appears to be an advantage in combining nerve blocks with sympathetic blocks and this is most easily carried out by the paravertebral injection.

Sympathetic blocks can be made at the stellate ganglion for the upper quadrant of the body, while a lumbar sympathetic block performed at the lumbar sympathetic chain at L.2 level will deal with the lower limb. It is well worthwhile carrying out these blocks at any stage of the post-herpetic process but they are most likely to respond in the acute phase.

Intrathecal injections of alcohol or phenol can be used when all else has failed. Intrathecal phenol 5 per cent in glycerine in small quantities of 1·0 to 2·0 ml have sometimes produced benefit in the author's experience in the past. This is no longer used by him as, although this method does tend to relieve the painful part of the condition, it does not usually relieve the dysaesthesia and hyperpathia, or if it does alter these, it is either only for a short time, or to a minor degree. There is the normal problem present which follows the use of phenol for any painful condition of the pain relief not lasting for more than two to three months. There is the added factor that as a large proportion of post-herpetic neuralgias occur in the thoracic region then the phenol injection will need to be placed in the thoracic theca. An intrathecal placement of a spinal needle in the mid-thoracic region is the most difficult of all the intraspinal injections due to the imbrication of the mid-thoracic spines. It is not an injection to be made lightly in a patient who otherwise has a normal expectation of life. It is important with intra-thecal phenol in glycerine injections that the spinal tap must be clear. There should be no blood in the cerebro-spinal fluid (CSF). Blood will show that the spinal needle may have damaged the surface of the spinal cord, and if that has happened then the phenol may fix to this region of the cord and penetrate into the tissues. In addition to this, the rather narrow space between the cord and theca at this level means that the phenol may rest against the cord surface, usually posteriorly. The phenol may then be absorbed on to the surface of the cord and penetrate it. There may well be a period of alteration of position sense and unsteadiness of gait following the procedure. Fortunately on the few occasions when this has happened at the Centre for Pain Relief these complications have only lasted from a few days to a few weeks.

Instead of phenol in glycerine the intrathecal injection can consist of 100 per cent alcohol. The benefit of this substance is that the spinal tap can be made well away from the level to be blocked. Theoretically phenol in glycerine can also be deposited well away from the painful dermatomes, but technically this is more difficult as phenol in glycerine spreads slowly being viscous, and will affect the spinal nerves that it flows over. Alcohol also travels over the intermediate spinal nerves but tends to do this much more quickly than phenol in glycerine. There are, of course, the usual differences between intrathecal injections of alcohol and phenol. Phenol in glycerine is hyperbaric, therefore the patient must lie on the painful side and be tilted posteriorly to bring the posterior roots to the most dependent position. Alcohol is hypobaric and therefore the painful side must be placed upper-most, and the patient is tilted anteriorly to position the posterior rootlets uppermost. There is one final difference, the phenol in glycerine is aimed at the exit of the nerve at dural level, while for alcohol the aim is to deposit it around nerve rootlets as they come off the spinal cord and before they unite to form a root. Alcohol is less controllable than phenol, and very occasionally produces strange effects at unexpected spinal cord levels.

For the above reasons the author has given up using intrathecal injections of long-acting chemicals in the relief of the intractable pain from post-herpetic neuralgia as it is unsatisfactory. However, in the case of patients threatening suicide it can be used as it may well give some relief and help to tide the patient over a critical period.

Finally, there is the question of neurosurgical operations for the relief of this type of intractable pain. This problem must be decided on the same criteria that are used to prevent the patient becoming a drug addict. It is known that there is no non-addictive narcotic which can reduce the level of the patient's appreciation of pain over a prolonged period, it is also known that there is no neurosurgical operation which will irrevocably remove, or destroy, pain pathways so that the patient will be unable to transmit the sensation of pain permanently. It is possible to alter the patient's appreciation of pain by altering its effect. Such methods as frontal leucotomy will change the patient's appreciation of pain such that although he still has pain, and knows it is there, he is no longer worried by it. In other words, it has altered his ability to suffer. The whole question of alteration of the patient by such operations is constantly exercising the minds of physicians and lay public because of its overtones of brain-washing. They are rarely used.

The percutaneous cervical cordotomy is often requested for patients with intractable pain due to post-herpetic infection. This request comes from either patient or physician and in the author's opinion there are only two circumstances when it is reasonable to do this. The first is if it is believed the patient is truly suicidal, and all other methods of pain control have failed. The second is when it will make the difference between a breadwinner being able to support the family through a critical year.

The patient and physician must understand the limitations, and possible complications, of the cordotomy, before the operation is performed. It is as well if the patient's relatives also understand these. The patient has to realise that the original herpetic infection may have spread throughout the nervous system, and if it has spread beyond the spinal cord level where the cordotomy will be carried out, the pain cannot be relieved, and it will be impossible to relieve it. It should be mentioned, so as not to paint an incorrect picture, that in most cases of herpes this does not happen, but it most definitely occurs in some patients and there is no way of picking out those that will get no pain relief. The next point to emphasise is that this operation is best performed for patients who have their intractable pain from cancer, and who will die before any of the possible complications appear. There are also difficulties, first that it proves impossible to perform the operation, next that having performed the operation properly pain relief does not appear, or if it appears it wears off quickly in a few days. Thus, the patient may go through the ordeal of the operation and either have no relief because it does not develop, or may get analgesia of their body without relief of their post-herpetic pain. When the operation is performed properly and the expected relief of pain results there is always a tendency for the pain relief to wear off after a more or less prolonged period of time. This length of time may be no more than eighteen months, though it is usually longer. There are a number of side-effects produced by the operative process, such as weakness on the normal side of the body, and after six months or so the patient may begin to feel dysaesthesiae, and these get worse as time goes on. In patients with inoperable cancer these uncomfortable feelings are not a factor in the recommendation for the operation as the patient does not live long enough for these to develop to any extent.

It must be emphasised to the patient that under the worst possible combination of circumstances their body might be completely analgesic but without any relief of pain at all. If, then, dysaesthesiae develop the patient will have a complete set of disadvantages without any benefit at all. There is one final complication to warn the male patient about, especially the younger patient, and that is that even in the unilateral cordotomy there is a small possibility of impotence resulting, and this can occur whether the result is satisfactory or not.

There are very good reasons for avoiding this operation in non-malignant conditions but if, after all these explanations to the patient and their relatives have been made, they still desire the operation then the author for one would be prepared to carry it out.

Having said that the author would also reinforce a point made in another chapter that a large part of the problems that have followed percutaneous cordotomy operations have occurred in patients who had this done for a non-malignant condition. When dysaesthesiae develop they tend to increase steadily until the analgesia produced by the operation has worn off. In a few unfortunate patients they do not disappear even then.

There is another non-destructive method which can be tried in post-herpetic neuralgia. This is the application of external electrical stimulation to the affected dermatomes.

External electrical stimulation

The use of this technique in the relief of the intractable pain of post-herpetic neuralgia has been very thoroughly recorded (Nathan and Wall). The technique is based on the gate control theory where it is postulated that stimulation of the skin at non-painful levels of stimulation will increase activity along the larger myelinated nerve fibres. This will increase the modulation at spinal cord level of painful impulses which travel along the smaller myelinated and unmyelinated fibres. The total effect of this system is to decrease the pain appreciated by the patient. It will be obvious that those patients who had total, or near total, destruction of their large myelinated fibres during the original zoster infection cannot benefit from this method. They have no, or too few, large fibres to transmit enough modulating stimulation, and therefore there must be a number of patients who cannot obtain satisfactory results from this method.

There is no doubt that some patients respond very well to external electrical stimulation, and as the apparatus involved can be made quite small and electrodes can be left in position on the skin for long periods, the patient can carry on normal activity at work or home with the apparatus in use. The stimulator itself can be tucked away in a pocket, or hung on the belt, while the connecting wires can be hidden easily. Thus, the patient may be receiving treatment without anyone else being the wiser.

The results obtained at this Centre are by no means as satisfactory as those reported by Nathan and Wall, but are still satisfactory enough to be worth trying in these most intractable of cases. It is most interesting indeed that they report two patients, who after using the apparatus for long periods of time had total relief of their pain, abandoning the machine. These patients had had their original zoster infection many years previously. This has never happened in our series.

The great advantage of this method over any of the others mentioned is that it is eminently suited to patients with a prolonged period of life ahead of them. It is, therefore, recommended that this method should be tried before any of the destructive methods. It may also happen that even when the pain relief obtained by electrical stimulation is insufficient, it may in combination with simple analgesics give an improvement in the quality of life.

REFERENCES

CHEMOTHERAPY FOR VARICELLA-ZOSTER INFECTIONS. (1976) Editorial, *B.M.J.* **2**, 1466-1467.

COLDING A. (1967) Regional block in acute herpes zoster. *Der Anaesthesist*, **16** (6), 172.

COLDING A. (1969) Effect of regional sympathetic blocks in the treatment of herpes zoster. *Acta. Anaesth. Scandinav.* **13**, 133-141.

COLDING A. (1973) Treatment of acute herpes zoster. *Proc. roy. Soc. Med.* **66**, 541-543.

DAM W. & LARSON J.J.V. (1974) Peripheral nerve blocks in relief of intractable pain. In *Relief of Intractable Pain.* (ed.) M. Swerdlow, pp. 134. Excerpta Medica, Amsterdam.

JUEL-JENSEN B.E. (1973) A new look at infectious diseases. Herpes simplex and zoster. *B.M.J.* **1**, 406.

NATHAN P.W. & WALL P.D. (1974) Treatment of post-herpetic neuralgia by prolonged electric stimulation. *B.M.J.* **3**, 645-647.

TAUB A. & COLLINS W.F. (1974) Observations on the treatment of denervation dysaesthesia with psychotropic drugs: Post-herpetic neuralgia. Anaesthesia dolorosa, Peripheral neuropathy. In *Advances in Neurology*, Vol. **4**, pp. 309-315. Raven Press, New York.

Chapter 9
Electrical Stimulation in the Control of Pain

The modern use of electrical stimulation to control the sensation of pain is based on the Gate Control theory of pain (Melzack and Wall). It must be understood from the beginning that stimulation of peripheral receptors in the skin is interpreted at cerebral levels as touch, pin prick, hot and cold. If the stimulation damages the tissues then it may be interpreted, and usually is interpreted, as pain. The nervous stimulation and transmission from the peripheral receptor through peripheral nerves to the spinal cord through the brain stem and on up to the cerebrum is not pain stimulation. It is a transmission of nerve impulses which under the correct circumstances may arrive at consciousness as the sensation of pain.

The Gate Control theory is concerned with the way this transmission of nerve impulses from periphery to centre is modified. The theory tries to explain why an identical stimulation on one occasion does not even reach consciousness, while on another it may be interpreted as a pin prick, and on another as pain.

The theory states that at spinal cord level there is an input of nerve impulses which is the resultant of inputs from small C fibres and delta fibres on the one hand and the larger myelinated fibres on the other. The mechanism is said to be that of a pre-synaptic inhibition though it is specifically mentioned in the original paper that the authors had no doubt that this could take place at any level of the spinal cord and that they had no doubt that post-synaptic inhibition could take place as well.

The Gate Control theory is based on previous work which was designed to evaluate two phenomena. One is known as the dorsal root reflex and the other is called the dorsal root potential. The dorsal root reflex is a discharge of nervous activity which originates in the posterior horn cells and is conducted antidromically to the periphery in peripheral cutaneous and muscular nerves. Wall (1959) showed that if depolarisation of the afferent fibre terminals was great enough, spontaneous impulses would develop and they would travel in both directions along the nerve fibre. Impulses running peripherally in the posterior nerve roots would constitute the dorsal root reflex.

Barron and Matthews, as well as Wall (1958), showed that the dorsal root potential is due to depolarisation of afferent fibre terminals in the grey matter. While they are depolarised, transmission cannot take place ortho-dromically and thus there is a type of blocking of the afferent nerve which can be partial or intermittent. This effect is still present when the relevant nerve root is divided. The nerve input into near-by nerve fibres continues the activity. Wall (1964) concluded that afferent fibre terminals can be held in a partially depolarised state and act as a trigger mechanism on which other incoming impulses act. Eccles called this phenomenon pre-synaptic inhibition.

There is no point in going into great detail on the experimental work which has been carried out to evaluate the Gate Control theory of pain. The value of any theory is to advance knowledge and to provide tests of its viability. By these criteria the Gate Control theory has been most productive. The various methods of external and internal electrical stimulation can, and do relieve pain in many patients. Nevertheless, there are some deficiencies in the Gate Control theory of pain and these with a huge bibliography are most adequately dealt with by Nathan (1976).

ELECTRICAL METHODS

The basic concept of the Gate Control theory that the gate is closed by stimulation travelling along the larger nerve fibres immediately suggested that there might be a method of relieving pain by increasing this stimulation. This type of stimulation can be 'injected' into the central nervous system from the periphery by stimulating the skin, or by the implanting of electrodes near the spinal cord, or directly into the brain (see Figs. 48 and 49).

Originally, stimulation was carried out at either the periphery or over the posterior columns of the spinal cord. Stimulation travelling from the periphery along peripheral nerves to the spinal cord was believed to have an effect on the gate reducing transmission of stimuli which could at cerebral levels be interpreted as pain. By surgically implanting electrodes over the posterior columns which mainly consist of the larger fibres, it was believed that a similar inhibition could be provided by antidromic activity travelling from the posterior columns downwards to the gate.

However, it soon became apparent that it was not necessary to stimulate the posterior column, similar results could be obtained by stimulating the anterior quadrant of the spinal cord. Further, when stimulation of the

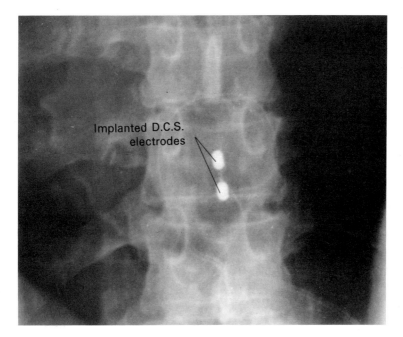

FIGURE 48. A–P view. Dorsal column stimulator (DCS) implant.

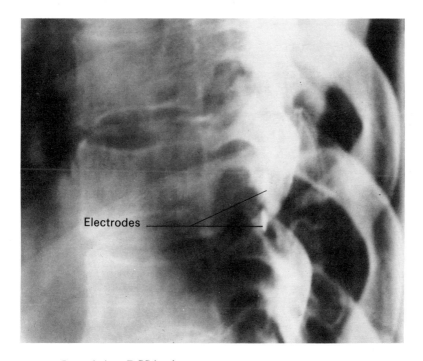

FIGURE 49. Lateral view. DCS implant.

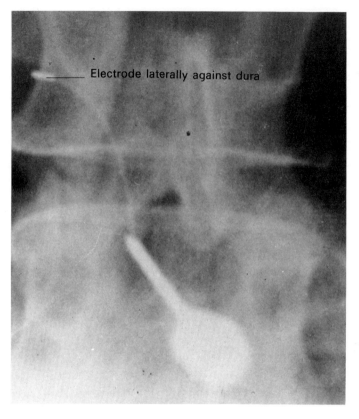

FIGURE 50. Lateral electrode.

FIGURES 50–54. Electrodes usually track fairly easily but not always.

posterior columns occurs the patient appreciates that stimulation is present by a buzzing or tingling sensation below the dermatomal level of the stimulation. When the anterior columns are stimulated the patient has no such sensation at all. At a later stage electrodes were implanted into the posterior limb of the internal capsule and near the peri-aqueductal grey matter and near-by regions of the brain stem with excellent effects.

When used at the periphery carbon rubber flexible electrodes are usually used and the electrical stimulation has a pulse frequency which varies between 15 to 200 pulses per second, the pulse duration varies between 50 and 500 micro-seconds, and the output is adjustable between 0 and 50 milli-amps. Usually a constant current is used into an electrode impedance of 0 to 1,000 ohms. The pulse shape used is a modified rectangular pulse and the power density and current density at the electrode are kept to levels which do not produce skin damage.

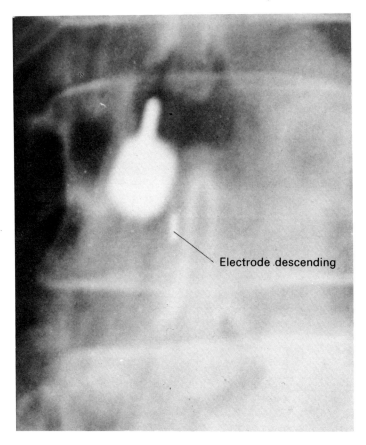

FIGURE 51. Electrode descends.

For implantation on to the spinal cord or into brain tissue the parameters are very similar. The electrode naturally tends to be much smaller under these circumstances and some thought has to be taken to keep the electrode surface area as large as possible so that the power and current densities are kept as low as possible.

There are many varieties of peripheral and dorsal column stimulators produced and at the Centre for Pain Relief the stimulators used are those of Stimtech, Medtronic, Shackman, and Avery. For diagnostic testing using epidural temporary electrodes Avery electrodes are used (see Figs. 50-54), while the brain electrodes are provided by Medtronic (see Fig. 55). The Avery electrodes are also used for long-term temporary implants in disseminated sclerosis patients.

Peripheral stimulation is useful in many mildly painful conditions. There

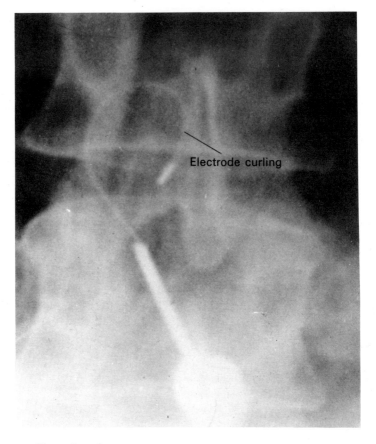

Electrode curling

FIGURE 52. Electrode curls.

is a huge bibliography and treatment ranges from post-herpetic neuralgia to sciatica. It has also been used post-operatively to relieve the pain of post-operative abdominal and pulmonary operations. Sterile flexible electrodes are placed on the wound post-operatively and gently stimulated. It is said that healing rate is also increased under these circumstances. The author has no experience of its use for this purpose.

Many thousands of dorsal column stimulators have been implanted in the U.S.A. but the long-term success rate is not good. This is believed at the Centre for Pain Relief to be a fault of selection and a series of twenty-five patients suffering from phantom limb pain have been treated with a high success rate (Miles 1977).

Logically, if implanting electrodes at spinal cord level does not relieve pain then stimulation at higher levels of the central nervous system might produce benefit. This has been done in the posterior limb of the internal capsule (Hosobuchi 1973). A few cases have been treated by this method at the Centre for Pain Relief with encouraging results and one incidental find-

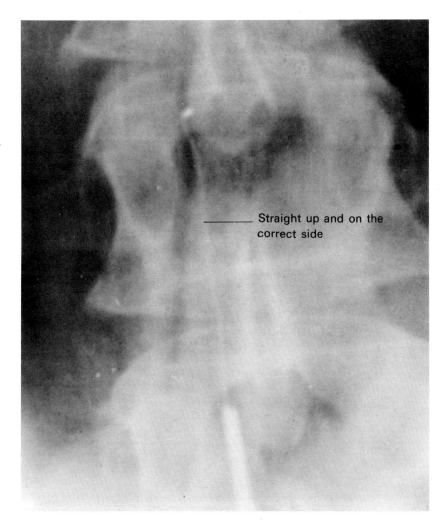

Straight up and on the correct side

FIGURE 53. Good position in A-P view.

ing (unpublished so far) as that during stimulation high levels of encephalin can be obtained from the lumbar cerebro-spinal fluid.

There is a growing belief that acupuncture, stimulation of musculo-fascial trigger points, and peripheral nerve stimulation by electrical means, all act in similar fashion and therefore when using the external electrical method to relieve pain it is wise to seek out any trigger areas first and try the stimulation on these initially.

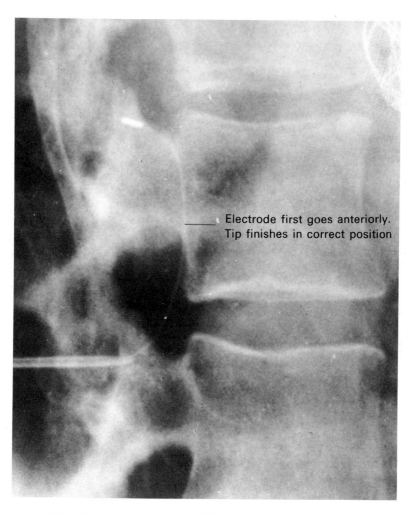

Electrode first goes anteriorly.
Tip finishes in correct position

FIGURE 54. Lateral view shows electrode in Fig. 53, curves anteriorly then posteriorly (but a useful result).

It would appear that there is a fruitful field for research and treatment using these methods, but as success cannot be predicted, it has to be tried on those patients where it may be suitable.

MULTIPLE SCLEROSIS

There have been numerous reports that passing small electric currents through the spinal cord of patients suffering from multiple sclerosis will improve their condition. In particular it is said to improve the spasticity of muscles which may be present.

At the Centre for Pain Relief fourteen patients have been treated in this fashion. Two of them obtained no benefit whatsoever, but there was objective improvement in some of the others. However, this condition is

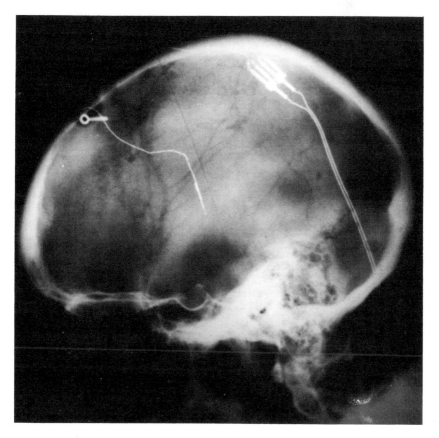

FIGURE 55. Brain electrode (thalamus).

notorious for producing remissions of longer or shorter degree and there-fore improvement in some patients is of no great significance. In due course further patients will be treated in this fashion to see if there is any statistical basis for continuing with the method.

In the X-ray shown, two temporary Avery electrodes were implanted in

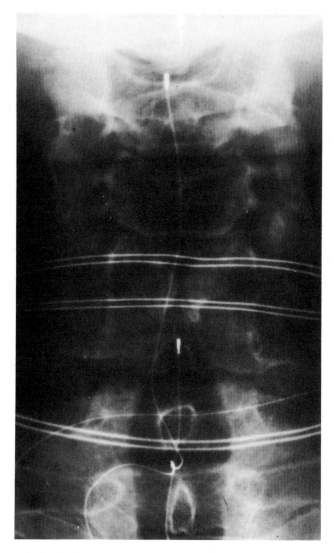

FIGURE 56. Twin electrodes for M.S.

the epidural space through a Tuohy spinal needle under local anaesthesia and using an image intensifier X-ray control (Fig. 56). The particular patient whose X-rays are shown in the figure had the electrodes in position for ten weeks. The common method of dealing with this type of patient is to place the electrodes as mentioned and then if any benefit occurs within a relatively short period of not more than twenty-four hours the electrodes can be immediately implanted subcutaneously.

REFERENCES

BARRON D.H. & MATTHEWS B.H.C. (1938) The interpretation of potential changes in the spinal cord. *J. Physiol. (Lond.)* **92**, 276–321.

ECCLES J.C., SCHMIDT R.F. & WILLIS W.D. (1963) Depolarisation of the central terminals of cutaneous afferent fibres. *J. Neurophysiol.* **26**, 646–661.

FIELDS H.L. & ADAMS J.E. (1974) Pain after cortical injury relieved by electrical stimulation of the internal capsule. *Brain*, **97**, 169–178.

HOSOBUCHI Y., ADAMS J.E. & RITKIN B. (1973) Chronic thalamic stimulation for control of facial anaesthesia dolorosa. *Archs. Neurol.* **29**, 158–161.

MELZACK R. & WALL P.D. (1965) Pain mechanisms: a new theory. *Science, New York*, **150**, 971–979.

MILES J.B. (1977) Stimulation for the relief of pain. In *Persistent Pain*, pp. 140–146, Ed. S. Lipton, Academic Press, London and New York.

MILES J., LIPTON S., HAYWARD M., BOWSHER D., MUMFORD J. & MOLONY V. (1974) Pain relief by implanted electrical stimulators. *Lancet*, **1**, 777–779.

NATHAN P.W. (1976) The gate-control theory of pain: a critical review. *Brain*, **99**, 123–158.

OLIVERAS J.L., BESSON J.M., GUILBAUD G. & LIEBESKIND J.C. (1974) Behavioural and electrophysiological evidence of pain inhibition from midbrain stimulation in the cat. *Exp. Brain Res.* **20**, 32–44.

SHEALY C.N. (1974) Six years experience with electrical stimulation for the control of pain. In *Advances in Neurology*, Vol. **4**, pp. 775–782. Ed. J.J. Bonica, Raven Press, New York.

WALL P.D. (1958) Excitability changes in afferent fibre terminals and their relation to slow potentials. *J. Physiol.* **142**, 1–21.

WALL P.D. (1959) Repetitive discharge of neurons. *J. Neurophysiol.* **22**, 305–320.

WALL P.D. (1964) Presynaptic control of impulses at the first central synapse in the cutaneous pathway. *Progress in Brain Research*, **12**, 92–115.

FURTHER READING

CAMPBELL J.N. & LONG D.M. (1976) Peripheral nerve stimulation in the treatment of intractable pain. *J. Neurosurg.* **45**, 6, 692–699.

ILLIS L.S., OGYAR A.E., SEDGWICK E.M. & SABBAHI AWADALLA M.A. (1976) Dorsal column stimulation in the rehabilitation of patients with multiple sclerosis. *Lancet*, **2**, 1383–1386.

RICHARDSON D.E. & AKIL H. (1977) Pain reduction by electrical brain stimulation in man. Part 1. Acute administration in periaqueductal and periventricular sites. *J. Neurosurg.* **47**, 2, 178–183.

RICHARDSON D.E. & AKIL H. (1977) Pain reduction by electrical stimulation in man. Part 2. Chronic self-administration in the periventricular grey matter. *J. Neurosurg.* **47**, 2, 184–195.

Chapter 10
Acupuncture

It is said that the Yellow Emperor talking to his physician said 'My people are dear to me, look after them, keep them fit and well, prevent their illnesses. Let them earn and I will tax their earnings.' The Yellow Emperor in this light is one of the great innovators, not only ordering the systematising of acupuncture knowledge, but also introducing income tax. As is mentioned later it is unlikely that any one man produced the first book on acupuncture (or that the above conversation ever took place).

Acupuncture is the ancient Chinese system of medicine in which a needle pierces the skin to a greater or lesser depth, is left there for a variable time, and may be rotated, pushed in and out, or stimulated in some other fashion. It must be emphasised that it is a complete system of medicine, put together in a highly sophisticated fashion, in which the patient is observed and examined, a diagnosis made, and therapy instituted.

Acupuncture was not discovered 'de novo' but apparently knowledge of it gradually accumulated over a period of time. There are records of acupuncture on bone etchings dating about 1600 B.C. In the period 200–300 B.C. the book now known as the Yellow Emperor's Book of Internal Disease was written.* It is really two books, one being concerned (in part) with acupuncture therapy, while the other is more concerned with particular aspects of internal medicine and often takes the form of a dialogue between the Yellow Emperor and Chi-Po, a skilled physician.

It is generally agreed that this book was produced by a group of writers rather than being the work of one man. It is, of course, written in the Chinese language of the day and translation of it is not a simple matter. In addition to this one has to take into account the oblique approach and hyperbole that is present in Chinese writing and it is obvious that there will be difficulties in understanding what was meant so many years ago.

* References for Chapters 10–13 appear on pages 304–5.

The author has one additional suggestion to add to this complexity. Most likely, whether or not the book was written by one, or more than one physician, it would have been prepared for publication by the civil service of the day. It is also unlikely that any civil servant could refrain from 'improving' the book, correcting the English (or rather the Chinese), the phrasing, the punctuation, and so forth. It seems to be a universal fact that few civil servants will use one word when two will suffice, and there is no reason to believe that the Chinese civil service of two thousand years ago, behaved in any different fashion. Thus we can expect wordiness, repetition, obliquity, and great systematisation. Such does appear to be the case, and this is corrected or converted into modern language to a greater or lesser extent, by the skill of the translator. The western-trained person must rely on translations but the reliance should be of the same order that would be given to any translation of material 2,000 years old.

It is thought that the 'Yellow Emperor's Book' was not compiled at one time but was a collection of oral teachings some of which date from between the third and seventh century B.C. It was completed in the first half of the first century A.D.; the Yellow Emperor probably lived around 2,500 B.C.

A book describing the meridians and the connection between them and the organs was published in the eleventh century A.D., and in 1027, according to the Chinese, bronze figures were cast showing the meridians and acupuncture points. Copies of these in different sizes are used today for teaching purposes.

Apparently it was Jesuit priests who first mentioned the strange form of medicine they had witnessed in the Far East, and there are books published by others, all of this occurring in the seventeenth century. The method did not become popular although many books have been written about it.

In 1822 the Chinese government tried to discontinue the practice of acupuncture by decree but obviously without much success, and in 1929 there was another attempt to ban acupuncture but this failed because the opposition was too strong. It was in this period that Soulie de Morant translated the basic medical texts of acupuncture into French and with the spread of this knowledge the use of acupuncture increased and to some extent became popular.

Only fairly recently, as news of acupuncture anaesthesia came out of China, did the western world become really interested in it. A number of medical study groups from various countries have been to China over the past few years, but the most recent information suggests that acupuncture anaesthesia (really analgesia) is not used as frequently as was first believed. This will be expanded upon later.

There are differences in style between classical and modern acupuncture, but for the present an appreciation of the classical style will be given in fair detail.

Part of the problem for the western mind in understanding the Chinese approach to acupuncture is due to the fact that there is no distinction between physical facts and metaphysical concepts. They were not alone in this as most early religions had the concept of a life force or 'something' which penetrated the heavens and the earth. The early European idea of the ether which pervaded everything is one such. Some of the concepts used in acupuncture are also to be found in the western world. For instance, classical Chinese acupuncture uses the concept of the world being divided into five elements, wood, fire, earth, metal, and water. Everything on earth belongs to one of these, or to a combination of them. Our bodies also and in particular the various major parts of them, come in to one of these categories, which must, of course, be taken into account before the correct acupuncture points can be arrived at.

This idea is reminiscent of the four elements of earth, water, air, and fire, which formed the basis of the European idea of the components of the world until quite recent times. Thus it would appear that acupuncture is a form of folk medicine having features common to folk medicine in other countries. If this view is a correct one, then most acupuncture theory can be dismissed immediately. There is, however, the undoubted fact that acupuncture treatment on occasion obtains benefit for the patient that has been unavailable from conventional medicine. This should not be taken to mean that all the ideas of acupuncture have to be accepted. There is no discrepancy in believing that acupunture is based on false premises and also accepting that on occasion it works. It merely means that the reason for the effective action is obscure and has to be worked out. It also means that that part of acupuncture which works can be accepted into conventional western medicine. In fact, it would be very remiss of the modern physician if he failed to do so under these conditions. This is the attitude adopted at the Centre for Pain Relief in the treatment of chronic painful non-malignant conditions which have not responded to the usual standard treatment.

There is one further idea which has to be considered. There is no country in the world, however primitive, or however advanced, which does not have the knowledge that if properly applied a small pain will relieve a larger pain. In one form or another the use of counter irritation is practised everywhere. The ancient English custom of cupping and blistering is well known. In cupping, the 'cup', which is variable in size but often about the size of a wine glass and made of metal, is heated and placed on the skin of the part to be counter irritated. The air inside the cup cools, a vacuum forms and the skin is sucked up into the cup with great force. Damage occurs under the skin with rupture of small vessels and a blister or haematoma results. It is excruciatingly painful. A less-damaging method is the well-tried mustard plaster. In more primitive countries more vigorous forms of counter irritation are used such as the use of red hot nails to blister the skin. Melzack at the International Symposium on Pain in Seattle (1973), and at the Fourth European Congress of Anaesthesiology in Madrid (1974), showed a film of an African being treated for headache by a local native doctor. This consisted of making a cruciate incision over the scalp, which was then reflected with somewhat crude but effective instruments. The bone of the vault was then scraped away by means of a rasp and some bone was removed. Penetration to the dura did not occur and the scraping went on until the patient (who was sitting on the ground), the relatives (one of whom was holding the bowl into which the blood was freely running) and the doctor agreed that enough had been done to relieve the patient's headache. No stitches were inserted. The wound healed perfectly and the headache was relieved. A most successful procedure for all concerned. It is interesting to note here that not only did the patient not feel pain during the operation but the pain was relieved afterwards. Everybody concerned expected that the operation would be painless and the patient was not expected, and did not expect, to have any problems. Also they all knew that this operation relieved this type of pain and he was expected to be cured. The patient really had a lot to look forward to. The western explanation would be either that the patient had produced a state of self hypnosis, or that the enormous peripheral nerve stimulation that was present produced a central inhibition. Some rather interesting concepts are raised by either of these ideas when one comes to consider how acupuncture anaesthesia works.

Acupuncture has a relationship with the ancient Chinese religion known as Tao, which to describe it briefly is a way of maintaining harmony in this world as well as the next. It is postulated that there is an invisible force existing throughout the world and in all things, animals and people. In acupuncture this is called Ch'i (sometimes called Qi) the life force. It is the force which converts ice to water, produces a storm, or the change from day to night. It produces the growth of plants and gives life to the body. It is convenient to the western mind to understand Ch'i as a life force but a more definitive description would be to call it a change of energy. If this is done it is easier to understand another feature of Ch'i in that it is formed of two complementary parts, which are antagonistic to each other, being at opposite

ends of two extremes in the perfect and ideal state. These are known as the
Yin and the Yang. These can never be regarded as being in a perfect and
ideal state as they are always in transition and therefore there is always part
of one in the other. They cannot exist in an absolutely static condition.
There is always some Yin in Yang, and Yang in Yin.

Yin and Yang

The Chinese have formulated this idea into a universal law. One of these
dualities, the Yang, is regarded as the positive active state, while the Yin,
is regarded as the opposite where these positive things do not exist. The yin
is not so much an inactive state as a zero state due to the absence of yang.
Nevertheless, there is some of each in the other and there is a constant
blending and changing from one to the other. Thus yang things are the day,
spring or summer, hot, the sun, as opposed to yin things which are their
opposites such as the night, autumn or winter, cold, the moon. The same
applies to the human being where the body surface, or a male, is yang, while
the interior of the body, or the female, is yin. Similar differences exist for
the different components of disease processes.

The Meridian

Acupuncture is based on the idea that there is a flow of the life force round
the body. This occurs in what, for want of a better term, is called a Meridian.
This is a channel so fine that it has not been demonstrated to exist as far as
any anatomical or physiological preparation is concerned. In 1964 Kim
Bon Han published a monograph on the 'Kyungrak System', which was
a new anatomico-histological system distinct from the vascular and nervous
systems. He described the Bonghan ducts which were extravascular and
intravascular and linked the internal organs to Bonghan corpuscles on the
surface. Insertion of a small needle into a superficial Bonghan corpuscle
caused a 'unique movement' (that) 'well coincides with the practice of
acupuncture treatment of a long tradition'. There is no supporting evidence
of this system to date and as far as can be gathered the meridians are to be
regarded as hypothetical lines and are so regarded in modern China. They
are certainly regarded as such at the Centre for Pain Relief.

Each meridian consists of a series of points on the skin and is in direct
relationship with one of the internal organs of the body. In the system of
Chinese acupuncture there are twelve such organs divided into two groups
of six. One group is yang, concerned it is thought with nutrition and excretion, and are the hollow organs. They are the gall-bladder, the small intestine,
the stomach, the large intestine, the bladder, and the organ usually translated

as the triple warmer or tri-heater. This latter is a new organ to western doctors, it is said to have a function which concerns the absorption of energy. The other group is yin and consists of the solid organs which are concerned with the circulation of the blood. They are the liver, the heart, the spleen, the lung, the kidney, and the pericardium, or heart constrictor. Here again the pericardium would not normally be regarded as an organ in western medicine. In Chinese medicine it has more of a function than just being an organ; it is concerned with those diseases affecting the pulse and in depression.

As there are twelve organs it follows that there must be twelve meridians. In actual fact there are many more than this but there are twelve main or principal meridians. The course of the main meridians is symmetrical as they are bilateral, but there are two exceptions to this due to the presence of two extra meridians which run along the posterior and the anterior median line of the body. The posterior one, called the Governing Vessel, is a yang meridian, while the anterior one known as the Conception Meridian is yin. These two form part of eight meridians, which are in addition to the twelve main meridians, and are classically described as being outside the main meridians. There are also the conjunctive meridians which connect the main meridians to each other. All these additional meridians, except the two median ones already mentioned are bilateral.

The life force circulates around the main meridians in a definite order, and when they lie on the same limb a yang meridian is coupled with a yin one. The circulation of the Ch'i follows these pairs of meridians as follows: from lung to large intestine (which are coupled), to stomach and then spleen (coupled), to heart to small intestine (also coupled), then bladder to kidney (coupled), followed by the pericardium to the triple heater (coupled), and finally to the gall bladder and then the liver (coupled). The circuit is completed by a link between the liver and lungs (see Fig. 57). There are relationships of many kinds established by the relationships of the meridians to each other. The simplest kind are when two meridians lie close together on a limb, or are connected to the same organ in the circulation of Ch'i.

The life force in normal health fills the meridians with a certain volume and force. In disease states the quantity or quality of the life force may be at fault. If it can be discovered which meridian or meridians are abnormal, the flow of Ch'i can be corrected by inserting a needle in the correct place on the meridian. This place is known as an acupuncture point. The whole basis of acupuncture is knowing which is the correct position. This is not to say that inserting the needle or needles in a different position to the correct one will not get a result. It may well be so, but first it will not do so as quickly or effectively as the correct one, and secondly it may do harm.

Choice of acupuncture point

Naturally there are rules and regulations in working out which is the correct
point. Not only must the correct point be used but when the needle is
inserted in this correct point, it is inserted for a specific time to a specific
depth. The Qu'i moves through the twelve meridians in a twenty-four hour
cycle beginning at 3 a.m., and those meridians which are twelve hours apart
in this cycle are related in that if the one is mildly stimulated the effect is

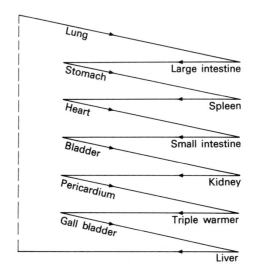

FIGURE 57. The circulation round the meridians.

obtained on that meridian and organ alone, but if it is strongly stimulated
the connected meridian and organ is stimulated in the opposite fashion. For
instance, if the liver is strongly stimulated the effect on the corresponding
small intestine will be sedative. Further this principle is more effective if
a yin organ is stimulated at a yin time, which is midday to midnight, and
a yang organ is stimulated at a yang time, which is midnight to midday.
There is an effect if the yang organ, for instance, is stimulated at a yin time
but it will not be as great as if it were stimulated at a yang time. The organs
are arranged through the twenty-four hours in the same order as previously
given and it is therefore simple to work out which organs are twelve hours
apart (see Fig. 58). As long as it is remembered that the cycle starts with the
lung at 3 a.m. those organs coming in the yin time can be distinguished from
those in the yang.

The Elements

The Chinese concept that the world is composed of the five elements wood, fire, earth, metal, and water, mentioned previously, can now be expanded. Everything on earth is considered to belong to one or several of these categories. If these elements are arranged round a pentagon in clockwise fashion, then each element has a similar effect on the next in line, to that which is produced on itself (see Fig. 59). Each element is allocated two

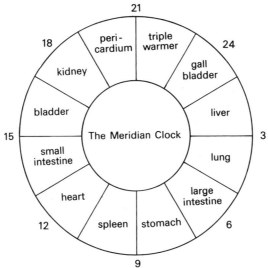

FIGURE 58. The meridian clock.

organs, one yin, one yang. Thus, wood is liver and gall bladder, fire is heart and small intestine, earth is spleen and stomach, metal is lung and large intestine, water is kidney and bladder, and pericardium and triple heater are also fire. Stimulation of an organ is known as tonification and the reduction in activity is called sedation. Thus tonification of the wood elements on the liver and gall bladder will also produce some tonification on the next along on the fire element which is the heart and small intestine. Which particular fire organ is tonified is decided according to the meridian stimulated by the acupuncture needle. If liver is the one over-stimulated then it is the heart and not small intestine, as both liver and heart are yin, whereas the small intestine is yang.

There is another feature of this pentagonal arrangement which has to be taken into account as although one element will affect the next one along in the same fashion as it itself is affected, the next but one along is affected in the opposite way. Thus in the example given above, tonification of wood produces tonification of fire but sedation of earth. In Chinese acupuncture the first element tonified or sedated is known as the mother and the second point is known as the son. In the phraseology of China 'the mother nourishes the son'. On each meridian there are acupuncture points which correspond to each of the elements, and if, for instance, the stomach meridian is found to have a deficiency of energy, this can be supplied from the 'mother' organ,

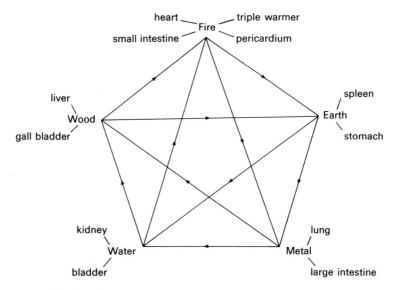

FIGURE 59. The five elements.

in this case the small intestine which is a fire element. The method of treatment is to use the stomach meridian and to insert the acupuncture needle at the fire point. This point can be read off from charts. If the stomach meridian had an excess of energy this would have to be transferred to the son organ, in this case into the large intestine. The large intestine meridian is a metal element and therefore the large intestine meridian would be used at the point of metal to disperse the excess energy.

There is not usually an excess or deficiency of Ch'i in a global sense because an excess in one part of the body is balanced by a deficiency in another. Illness is due to an imbalance which is set to rights by the acupuncture treatment. As might be expected the diagnosis as to which meridian to treat and which point or points to use is not a simple one. If there is a great deficiency in one element and the 'son' draws on the 'mother', this might not be enough and other elements are drawn on. In fact it is possible that there may be a reversing of the flow in the pentagon. As far as an excess of energy is concerned the points of dispersion are forbidden points unless it is possible to act on the affected meridian because the son is deficient. This is to follow one of the cardinal precepts of acupuncture that energy must be conserved. Excess energy is only drawn on to fill a deficiency. It is better to acupuncture a meridian with a deficiency than one with an excess.

The combination of yin and yang organs with the elements is of value in diagnosis as all parts of the body, its secretions, behaviour, the natural forces of the weather, the available drugs and foods can be classified as one of the elements. These will correspond to the deficiency or excess of Ch'i, the meridian in which this occurs and the selected acupuncture point.

Apart from points of tonification and sedation already mentioned there are what are called the source points. Stimulation of a source point can produce either tonification or sedation. This depends on whether a gold or silver needle is used, whether the needle is rotated clockwise or anti-clockwise, whether it is inserted in the direction of flow of the energy or against the flow and whether the patient is inhaling or exhaling at the time this is being performed. Mann maintains that whichever way the source is stimulated the effect is to correct the imbalance whether this is a deficiency or an excess.

There are also alarm points, associated points, connecting points, accumulating points, and many others. They each have their special functions and the reader is referred to one of the textbooks mentioned in the bibliography.

The pulse diagnosis

This is the key to acupuncture as the detailed examination of the radial pulse and its interpretation provides the only method by which any imbalance between the various meridians can be detected. In other words it is the method used to decide which meridian is selected for attention. The Chinese distinguish three pulses on the right wrist and three on the left, and also between the superficially felt pulses and those palpated with a deep pressure. Thus there are twelve different pulses palpated at the wrist and each one corresponds to one of the meridians.

The three pulses at each wrist are not randomly selected. The styloid process is taken as the mid-position, above and below this and separated by the width of a finger tip are the other two positions. Each wrist is palpated in these three positions, first, with a very light superficial pressure, this provides six pulses. Next, the same six positions are palpated but this time with a deep, heavy pressure. This will provide another six pulses, in all a total of twelve. Those on the left wrist with superficial pressure correspond to the small intestine, gall bladder, and bladder, in that order, from the periphery proximally (see Fig. 60). The corresponding meridians on the right hand are the large intestine, stomach, and triple heater. The pulses on deep pressure are for the left wrist, the heart, liver, and kidney, and for the right, the lung, spleen, and pericardium. In early classical Chinese acupuncture mention is made of using pulses other than the radial. For instance,

PULSE DIAGNOSIS

Left Pulse		Position	Right Pulse	
Superficial	Deep		Superficial	Deep
small intestine	heart	1	large intestine	lung
gall bladder	liver	2	stomach	spleen
bladder	kidney	3	triple warmer	pericardium

FIGURE 60. Pulse diagnosis.

in the Yellow Emperor's Book of Acupuncture, the pulse at the elbow is specifically mentioned. In the modern Chinese usage attention appears to be confined to the wrist.

It is difficult for western-oriented people to understand that the liver meridian, for instance, is not solely concerned with the liver as an organ but with the whole concept of 'liverishness'. This implies much more. Perhaps it is just possible for the westerner to understand this overall view as far as the liver is concerned as it is well understood what 'being hungover', or feeling 'yellow', or 'being off colour' means. It is even accepted that in the main this combination of symptoms (and signs) is due to dysfunction of the liver. The Chinese physician would normally accept that this combination could be amended by correcting a faulty flow of energy in the liver meridian, and would expect to feel this in the pulse diagnosis. It is, however, more difficult if not impossible for a westerner to understand that the bladder meridian is concerned with 'bladderishness' and what this implies. He might well understand that it has to do with all those diseases related to alteration of water metabolism, transport, and excretion. From this it follows that there must be some special relation with the kidney meridian for obvious reasons.

Classically the pulse diagnosis should be taken early on in the day when the patient is fasting and the stomach empty, and ideally each suspected meridian pulse should be felt at another time for confirmation. Early in the morning the meridians are said to be quiescent and the conjunctive vessels are empty. At this time if the pulse feels normal then the patient is healthy. A normal pulse has a tone or tension to it, but is nevertheless compressible and elastic. These characteristics are unaltered throughout its length. Although health is normally reflected in the pulse it is not 100 per cent so. Mann records feeling a normal pulse in someone who was ill and mentions that the method of pulse diagnosis is not foolproof. If the pulse felt at a particular meridian pulse point is full and hard the organ is hypertonic, i.e. the energy in the organ is in excess. When the pulse is feeble and soft, the organ is empty and deficient. It does not necessarily follow that only one particular pulse will be abnormal, as it is possible for all three pulses on one wrist to be affected in the same way.

A western-trained physician finds it difficult to believe that three different portions of the radial pulse over a very short interval can show much difference between the portions. This being quite apart from his accepting the whole concept of the pulse diagnosis. In fact, it is quite easy to postulate that as the radial artery at the wrist lies at varying depths, and sometimes against bone, it is logical that different portions of it might feel different to palpation, and that this is due to purely anatomical considerations. At various times attempts have been made to demonstrate that there are differences in the pulses, i.e. at the three places by means of experimental methods using pressure transducers. No such differences have been demonstrated. The author on a few occasions believes that he has felt such differences. Chinese experts in this method are said not only to detect the present illness the patient has but former ones. In addition as a disease process begins a variable time before the overt disease manifests itself and this is reflected in the pulse, the expert can forecast future illness and treat it. This is done by correcting the imbalance in the pulse through acupuncture to the involved meridians. In this way the circulating life energy is brought back into equilibrium.

Purpose of acupuncture

The use of acupuncture is in two stages. If disease is already present then the pulse diagnosis is unreliable as it is affected by the secondary effects of the illness. In this case the disease is treated by acupuncture using points laid down in tables for treating symptomatically. Once the disease is brought under control the pulse will reflect the underlying cause of the illness and this will then be treated by using the meridians and acupuncture points indicated by the pulse diagnosis. In this way the life energy circulation is brought back into equilibrium, and prevents the patient having a relapse. Thus the most important reason for using acupuncture treatment is to maintain a patient in good health rather than to treat him once illness develops. In other words, acupuncture is concerned with prevention rather than with cure, though it does both.

Acupuncture is said to help or cure any disease that can be corrected by normal physiological processes. It is unable to reverse something which has become irreversible such as an arthritic joint, though the effects can be mitigated and possibly the disease process arrested.

Cauterisation

Treatment by acupuncture traditionally involves the use of the cautery, or moxibustion as it is commonly called. The dried leaves of Artemesia are formed into a small cone and placed on the skin at the point selected. The tip is ignited and the patient feels an increasing degree of heat and pain as it burns down towards the skin. This will produce a small blister from a burn and a considerable stimulation at the acupuncture point. It may well produce a scar and for this reason an acupuncture needle is usually inserted at the point selected and a small ball of moxa is stuck on to the head of the needle and ignited. Heat is thus transmitted down the metal of the needle to the skin. There are other ways of modifying the amount of heat the patient obtains. Cauterisation always produces a stimulation never a sedation. There are certain points on the body where the use of moxa is forbidden and conversely, there are other points which are forbidden to the needle but moxa can be used. There are also a very few points where both are forbidden.

Insertion and use of the acupuncture needle

Traditionally there are many ways of inserting the needle. In the main they can be divided into those that are placed superficially, those placed at a medium depth and those placed very deeply indeed. In addition the needle can be inserted rapidly or slowly, can be left in place or stimulated in one of many different ways. It can be inserted once only or several times and can be withdrawn from the skin and reinserted, or brought superficially and replaced deep. In some diseases points distant from the affected part are used and in others near points are chosen. There are different lengths and thicknesses of needle, and the tips can be rounded, can have short points or long points. The needle can be rotated clockwise or anticlockwise and fast or slow. When either inserted or removed this can be done during inspiration or expiration.

Take

When the acupuncture needle is inserted to the correct depth, the sensation called 'Take' is experienced by the patient. This is derived from the Chinese word Te-Ch'i and implies a numb sensation which occurs in a few seconds and spreads from the site of acupuncture. The description of this feeling varies from patient to patient being described by some as sore and heavy, and by others as tingling. All agree that it spreads outwards from the acupuncture site. There is a general agreement that the sensation of take is important as if it occurs promptly the results are likely to be good, and if not present then results tend to be poor. Associated with these sensations is warmth of the skin, and in fact, some patients say the skin is not merely warm but is burning.

Frequency of treatment

There is a complete diversity of ideas in this respect, presumably corresponding to the usual agreement to differ over their own treatment that occurs in western medicine between western physicians. In some Chinese clinics the patient will be seen and treated daily for a week or two, or even longer if it is considered necessary. Kaada mentions treatment for psychiatric conditions involving three treatments per day, for thirty minutes each time of electrical stimulation of about 100 hertz. This was given into both pre-auricular regions. At the same time the patient received other treatment, including drug therapy, group activity, practical activity, and so on. How long this treatment continues was not mentioned. In lists of diseases which can be treated by acupuncture and which give a prescription of the points to be used—one point, two, three or more, there is often an indication as to how frequently the treatment is to be given. Usually this is daily. There is also an indication as to how gently or severely the acupuncture point should be stimulated, and to what depth the needle should be inserted. Mann considers that there is a difference in treating a patient in the acute phase of a disease when frequent treatments may be necessary and in the chronic or recovering phase, when preventive medicine is practised. He considers that the average patient who has a number of mild chronic complaints, in addition to the one which brought him to the acupuncturist in the first place, will need about seven treatments. There is a variable period between treatments depending on the response, which may take place immediately, or occur gradually over a few days or even weeks. Improvement can occur up to two weeks after an acupuncture treatment and therefore he tends not to treat at shorter intervals than this, once the acute phase is over. Once a patient has been cured and the pulse is normal a twice-yearly check-up by means of the pulse diagnosis is all that is required. There is general agreement that twice-yearly check-ups by means of the pulse diagnosis are a necessity and that if there is any abnormality of the pulse this should be corrected, and that if this is done the patient will remain healthy.

Contra-indications for acupuncture treatment. In the main these are fairly obvious and self-evident, as acupuncture is not to be performed on a patient who is drunk, has had a fit, is in a rage, or has just had sexual intercourse. There is also a ban on using acupuncture at certain times, and in certain places, such as after a meal acupuncture is not used on the epigastrium and during pregnancy no puncture is to be made below the umbilicus. After five months of pregnancy, needling is forbidden anywhere on the abdomen. There are also special points which are never used in the case of pregnant women, for instance, the small intestine 4 point. There are also certain areas which are never needled under any circumstances in any person.

It is fairly obvious that certain areas must be particularly dangerous to needling such as the chest wall where there is the ever-present danger of penetration of the chest wall and production of a pneumothorax. In children, points on the head, i.e. near the open fontanelles are forbidden, and in women points on the breast should be avoided.

Acupuncture should not be used on patients who are especially nervous, or over tumours. If a patient has fainted during the needling the needle should be removed and no further acupuncture performed that day.

Precautions during acupuncture therapy. Proper sterilisation of acupuncture needles is important if infective hepatitis is to be avoided. Again for hygienic reasons the skin should be cleaned and sterilised before puncture and the needles examined for hooked ends and bends and that the shaft and needle are firmly attached.

After the acupuncture therapy has been completed, the needle is removed but sometimes it is gripped by the deeper tissues and will not slide out easily. In this case the needle should never be dragged out as if it is left alone for a little while it will be released. If there is a haematoma or a little bleeding produced after removal of the needle (both rare with the finer needles) local pressure with a finger for a few minutes will keep the amount to a minimum. In general, it is a good idea to put a little pressure on the site of acupuncture for a brief period after withdrawing the needle whether or not there is any abnormality.

To avoid the danger of syncope it is best to perform acupuncture with the patient lying down though this is by no means essential.

Some patients are hypersensitive to any form of stimulation and acupuncture is no different. It is as well to grade the amount of stimulation to the reaction of the patient. For instance, if the needle is to be rotated the amount of rotation and its vigour can be reduced.

Response to acupuncture

Usually a patient will notice benefit during or shortly after the treatment and as mentioned this will last for a variable time when a further treatment will be needed to reinforce it. The benefit obtained may develop its maximum effect immediately or this may take time to develop (from a few days to a week or two).

Sometimes there are other reactions. On occasion the acupuncture therapy can make the patient's condition worse and in that case the next session should have the vigour of the treatment reduced. This being done after re-evaluating the patient's condition by examination, observation, and pulse diagnosis to ensure that a mistake has not been made. If there has been no mistake then further treatment should be most effective as a hyper-reaction does show that the patient is responsive to acupuncture therapy.

Another type of reaction that sometimes occurs, and is not confined to the reactive type of patient, is extreme tiredness and lethargy after the acupuncture. Sometimes this occurs so rapidly that the patient will say that the treatment is making him feel very sleepy while the needles are in position. Others will mention at the next session that they went home, went to bed, and slept for fifteen or more hours. Very occasionally they mention that this lethargy lasted more than one day. It is a good idea before the first acupuncture treatment to mention the possibility of a feeling of tiredness after it. If it does occur then the vigour of subsequent treatments is reduced, in addition the patients do seem to become accustomed to the treatment and after a time the somnolent effect becomes less marked, although it never entirely disappears. Development of lethargy is a positive indication that the chosen acupuncture is on the correct lines and a good response can be expected. Once the lethargy wears off it is replaced by a feeling of alertness and well being, which is the normal feeling after a successful acupuncture treatment.

Localisation of points

The acupuncture positions are in very constant situations provided allowance is made for the normal differences of size between people and between the sexes. Initially they are located by very precise anatomical coordinates, for instance, the second lung point is two inches lateral to the nipple and six and a half inches above it in the hollow below the clavicle. The acupuncture points are invariably located in small hollows or depressions in the body, and this fact helps in finding them (see Figs. 61–66). However, there are precise methods of location by using measurements but the measurements are of a special kind called 'osteological' inches by some, and 'pouce' by others. This unit is divided into smaller distances, for instance, the pouce is divided into tenths called 'fen'. Mostly there is correlation between different authors as to the way they assess the distance of the osteological inch but sometimes there are discrepancies. In two recent publications the distance between the xiphisternum and the umbilicus is given as seven units in the one and eight units in the other. It must be admitted that there is room for variation in these measurements depending on whether the position used as the anatomical landmark has the measurement taken from its upper or lower border. Classically it is believed that the acupuncture points are small areas and therefore have to be very precisely located and thus the instructions for finding these places are carefully and meticulously given. For example, to return to the second lung point used above, the full instructions would read 'this point is located 2 osteological inches lateral to the nipple and 6·5 osteological inches above it in the hollow under the medial end of the clavicle'. It also has to be borne in mind that there are different ways of numbering the acupuncture points of the meridians and what is lung 2 in one nomenclature may be 3 or 4 in another. In general terms, the numbering of these points is surprisingly constant but it is as well to choose one author's method and to stick to it. It is of course essential to have some method of

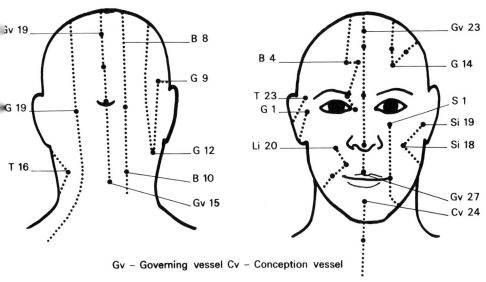

Gv – Governing vessel   Cv – Conception vessel

FIGURE 61. Face.

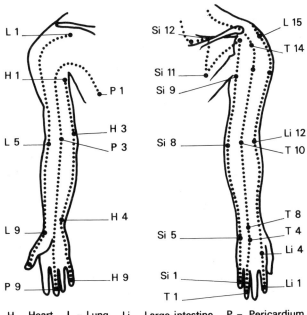

H – Heart   L – Lung   Li – Large intestine   P – Pericardium
Si – Small intestine   T – Triple warmer

FIGURE 62. Arm.

FIGURES 61–66. The meridians with some acupuncture points marked.

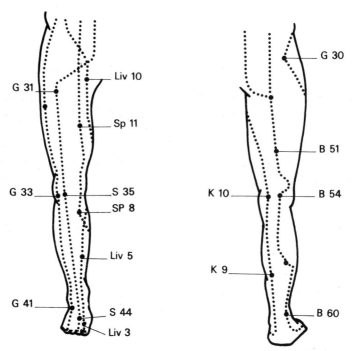

B – Bladder G – Gall bladder K – Kidney Liv – Liver
S – Stomach Sp – Spleen

FIGURE 63. Leg.

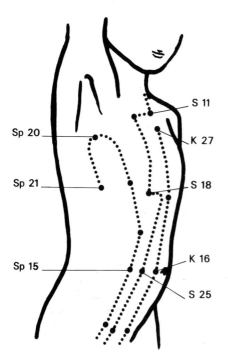

FIGURE 64. Lateral torso.

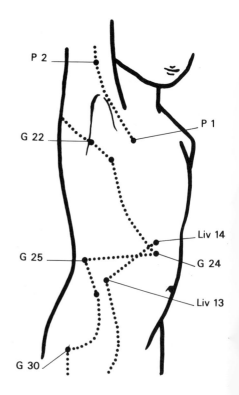

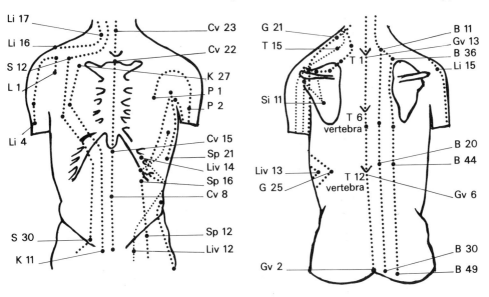

FIGURE 65. A–P and posterior torso.

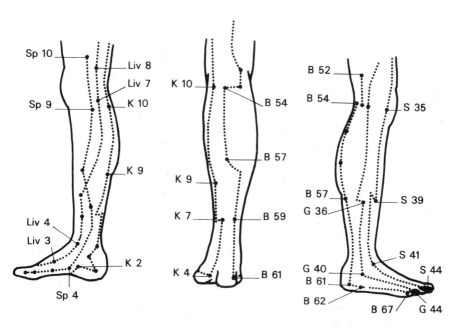

FIGURE 66. Leg.

making notes in a case sheet so that the points used on one occasion can be recalled in the future. The atlas used by the author is that of Mann.

The osteological inch that has been mentioned is not a constant measurement but varies with the size of the patient, thus, in a small woman there would be an appreciable difference between her osteological inch and that of a large man. Another method of estimating one unit of distance is to take the length of the second phalanx of the second finger when it is bent to touch the thumb, that is between the creases made by the first and second phalanges and the second and third phalanges. Here again there is room for error as this measurement can be taken towards the dorsal or towards the ventral surface of the finger. When taking this measurement the left hand is used for a man and the right hand for a woman.

Tender points

Very often acupuncture points which are of particular importance in treating the disease of a given patient will prove to be tender or painful on pressure. Treatment at these sites is of particular importance provided it is remembered that it is possible to stimulate too vigorously at these sensitive areas. There is one school of thought which believes that imbalance in the Ch'i is always reflected by some of the acupuncture points becoming tender and their treatment will consist of carefully searching throughout the whole body for such places and treating them by acupuncture at these places. Needling is performed at the tender positions even if these do not lie on meridians at known acupuncture points. Results by this method are said to be as good as by any other, and its protagonists use the pulse diagnosis to indicate where the initial search for tender areas should be carried out, and when they are found and needled, the needles are left in position until the pulse becomes normal or as normal as it can be expected to become at the treatment. The process is continued over a period of time.

REFERENCES (*see* pp. 304–5).

Chapter 11
Auriculotherapy

The use of acupuncture points on and around the ear has been known from the earliest records of the method, but over recent years the method of auriculotherapy originated in France and has now spread throughout the acupuncture world, including back to China. The basic idea is that anything that can be accomplished by the classical acupuncture using limb and body points can be equally satisfactorily dealt with by using corresponding points on the ear.

Around 1953 Dr. Paul F. M. Nogier had the concept that if an embryo was superimposed curled up, but inverted over the ear then the various portions of the foetal limbs, body and head, would correspond to the portions of the ear with which they coincided. In this concept the whole antihelix represents the spinal column and the head has correspondence in the antitragus. From this beginning he developed his ideas, expanding on them in major written works (see Fig. 67).

The basic idea of this variety of acupuncture is shown in the first two diagrams. As might be expected considering the small area in which points affecting the whole body have to be fitted in, there has to be a detailed knowledge of the shape of the ear, how it varies from person to person in age, health, and disease (see Fig. 68).

Fig. 68 shows the various portions of the external ear from the lateral approach but this amount of knowledge of the shape of the external ear is only a beginning. In addition it has to be remembered that there is a medial surface to the external ear, and also a portion where the ear is attached to the head.

Examination of the ears for auriculo-acupuncture therapy starts as in any other variety of medicine by observation of the parts, in this case the ears. It becomes immediately obvious that rarely are the two ears exactly the same shape. How then should the two ears be used; for instance, is one of them more important than the other? Differences between the two ears are found in the examination of the patient which takes place whatever form

of acupuncture is to be used. However, in auriculotherapy the examination
is more specific and precise than the classical variety of acupuncture, except
perhaps when searching out painful or tender acupuncture points.

The examiner usually positioned behind the patient first of all palpates
the ears. This is said to give information on the general well-being of the
patient according to the presence or absence of tonicity and resilience of the
tissues of the ear. Palpation of the two ears takes place simultaneously and
symmetrically, starting at the power portion and working upwards, i.e.
from the lobule upwards. Particular attention is paid to any obvious alteration of sensation of any part of the ear, either to lack of sensation or to
hypersensitivity.

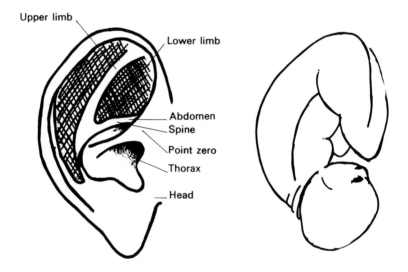

FIGURE 67. Ear and embryo.

After this rather simple examination a more detailed observation of the
sensitivity of the external ear is made using any rigid instrument to apply
pressure to the surface. The instrument will therefore have to have a tip of
fairly small surface area, and recommended ones often have cork tips which
avoid producing sensations of hot or cold. Alterations in touch can be found
in this way either by pressure directed at right angles to the skin or by means
of stroking the area quite gently. This type of stimulation will distinguish
areas of normal, hypo- and hyper-sensitivity, and these reactions are believed
to correspond to major peripheral disease. In addition these areas are explored
by both fine-tipped points and blunted feelers. In this way small points can

be distinguished which are sensitive when the surrounding area is insensitive, or conversely insensitive when the surrounding area is sensitive.

Two further tests are made, one for points in the ear sensitive to cold, the other sensitive to heat. Tests for cold are performed when the ear is at normal temperature, when a metal rod is dipped in ice-cold water and used dry as the probe. Whether the test is for cold or hot the probe is only touched to the ear for a very brief period. In this way points which are hypoaesthetic to cold can be distinguished. In a similar fashion the ear is tested for its

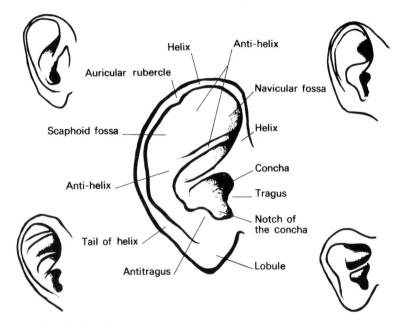

FIGURE 68. Variations of shape.

response to heat. This is done by means of a probe heated to a temperature of between 38–40 °C. In this case there are points which are both hypo- and hyper-sensitive to heat.

Auriculotherapy originated with the belief, or flash of inspiration, that the spinal column is represented by the antihelix of the ear. The edge of the helix crosses the antihelix at the lumbo-sacral hinge. The vertebrae are spaced out along the antihelix quite regularly and so the homologous vertebrae can be picked out on the antihelix in this fashion.

There is another most important relationship to be made and that is the one known as point zero or the fulcrum. This is situated in the concha at the root of the helix and is regarded as the centre of the antihelix. Once the positions of the vertebrae are known on the antihelix, lines can be drawn from the fulcrum to each vertebral homologue and other important relationships worked out according to where these lines cut the various portions of the external ear.

Instead of using mechanical probes to detect places where there is tenderness or increased sensitivity to hot or cold an electrical detector can be used. These are of many types but all work on the principle of either detecting points of low resistance compared to the surrounding area of higher resistance, or detecting areas of higher electrical resistance compared to surrounding areas of lower resistance. Electrical apparatus of similar types can be used for treatment either by applying stimulation direct to the ear or by inserting ear acupuncture needles and then connecting them to the electrical apparatus. These machines are essentially producing small alternating currents of a square wave type that are not dangerous to the bodily functions.

Auriculo-Cardiac reflex

Nogier mentions his recent discovery which he calls the Auriculo-Cardiac reflex. When certain portions of the external ear are touched the pulse alters. There may be an acceleration or decrease in its speed, or there may be an increase or a decrease in amplitude. The ear is explored gently with a cork-tipped probe as mentioned previously while at the same time palpating the pulse. Any alteration is noted and the same procedure is used while stimulating the pulse with cold and hot probes, again as in the fashion previously described. The responses to hot and cold may not be of the same kind nor in the same direction as the touch probe.

Gold and silver needles

These are believed to have different actions and are used according to the following scheme. If the auriculo-cardiac reflex is increased by the cork stimulation and also by the hot stimulation, but reduced by the cold stimulation, then further stimulation of the kind produced by the cold stimulation is most likely to correct the imbalance present if applied to the correct acupuncture point. The correct point is where the alterations in the auriculo-cardiac reflex occurred. The stimulation either hot or cold which corrects the effect of touch on the auriculo-cardiac reflex is the one to use for therapeutic purposes.

It is believed that as the cold cannot provide a practical method of treatment it is replaced by a silver needle or a negative current. Similarly if heat corrects the auriculo-cardiac reflex then a gold needle or a positive current should be used. If when the cork probe alters the auriculo-cardiac reflex in one direction and both hot and cold probes alter it in the opposite direction then a steel needle is used. There is no suggestion as to which electrical current is suitable in this case.

Indications for Auriculotherapy

These will be very briefly mentioned here and then only in slight detail. Nogier divides the conditions for treatment into major and minor depending on the statistical prospect of success, pointing out that auriculotherapy is of major value in any pain which is a result of trauma and can rapidly and lastingly relieve such conditions. Traumas are divided into those pains which result following surgery of any type, and those produced by stiffness or pain due to immobility either during the operation or in the post-operative period. Along with these go the general conditions of sleeplessness and worry.

The functional rehabilitation of the patient after fractures can be improved by the relief of pain. This is done by adding in the stimulation of the required ear points to the normal medical treatment of the patient with consequent saving of convalescent time.

Much benefit can be obtained in pains from trauma but of the type in which surgical intervention is not necessary. In this group of conditions are twists and strains, muscle or ligamentous tears, and abnormal positions of bones, especially those of the vertebrae, all of which may produce pain of a greater or lesser degree but of some chronicity.

Pain due to one or other of the various neuralgias can be treated by auriculotherapy but the efficacy is not the same in all of these conditions. While sciatic neuralgia is effectively treated by auriculotherapy that of the cervico-brachial axis is not so easily obtained. Probably the most difficult of all the neuralgias to treat under normal circumstances in western medicine is that known as post-herpetic neuralgia, and the longer the condition has been present the more difficult it is to treat. It is said that many of the facial neuralgias have reflex connections with the cervical region and that good results can be obtained by auricular treatment. The same is said to hold for post-herpetic neuralgia provided it is not of long standing.

Phantom limb pain can be relieved by acupuncturing the external ear not at the point corresponding to the stump, but at the place corresponding to the phantom.

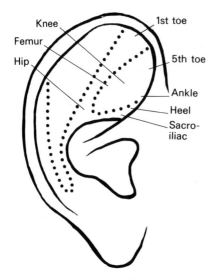

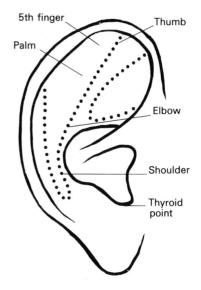

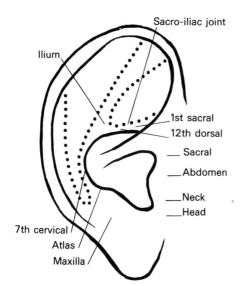

FIGURES 69-71. Position of some body points on the ear.

Minor conditions for auriculotherapy include most of those conditions not mentioned above, bearing in mind that the above list is not meant to be comprehensive. Further information can be obtained from the original authority. The term minor condition merely means that the statistical probability of obtaining a good result is not as certain as those in the first group, it does not mean in any particular case that the method should not be tried out. It is quite possible that a good or very good result will be obtained but the prognosis is less certain and this should be taken into account when discussing the possibilities with the patient and the relatives.

Contra-indications

An absolute contra-indication is if there is any local infection on, or in, the tissues of, or near, the ear. If acupuncture causes spread of infection to the cartilage of the ear then this may be destroyed and all shape lost to the concha. Auriculotherapy is not used, as in classical acupuncture, when the condition is irreversible and there is no hope of a cure or of improvement. It is also not advocated when there is a standard well-proven method of treatment of orthodox western medical style, which should be used instead. As with classical acupuncture, needling of certain areas of the ear is forbidden during pregnancy, such as the notch and the hypothalamic point. On the other hand, the complaints of the first month or so of pregnancy can be treated by stimulating the lobule. Acupuncture is not advisable on the ear after vigorous exercise, a heavy meal, and during early menstruation. Nor is it used during a chronic illness of long duration or in anaemia. It will be seen that there is a correlation between the contra-indications in auriculotherapy and those for the classical acupuncture. There is the added feature that as auriculotherapy arose under conditions associated with western medicine there is a readiness to use some features of this medicine which are not present in classical acupuncture.

The positions of some points for auriculotherapy are shown in Figures 69–71.

REFERENCES (*see* pp. 304–5).

Chapter 12
Acupuncture Analgesia

From general knowledge of the conditions in which acupuncture is effective there is no doubt that on occasion pain of quite severe degree can be controlled by this method of treatment. It was used for some time in the relief of post-operative pain before an attempt was made to use it for pain relief during operations. It would appear that acupuncture produces a rise in the pain threshold but leaves the other sensory modalities unchanged. Thus as far as its use in operative surgery is concerned there is no anaesthesia but a variety of analgesia.

Acupuncture analgesia for operative surgery was first used in 1958 in China for an appendicectomy. Since that time it has been used in many types of operations with a proportion of successful results in all the types, some being more successful than in others. The technique used has changed considerably over the short period of time in which it has been used, for instance, in a major operation such as pneumonectomy a large number of acupuncture points were initially used to produce enough analgesia for operative purposes. Nowadays only a few points are needed to produce perfectly adequate conditions.

It is claimed that in China about 90 per cent of cases in which acupuncture analgesia is used are successful, the remainder requiring supplements of local or general anaesthetics. It is probable that this is a fair assessment though it has also to be admitted that this percentage will cover those cases where the patient is completely comfortable throughout the whole of the operation and requires no supplement of any sort, and is perfectly at ease mentally and physically; and those cases where, although the operation is completed under acupuncture analgesia, there are periods when the patient wriggles around on the operation table, phonates, and the operation has to be slowed or stopped for a short period, and/or a supplement of pethidine or a local anaesthetic agent has to be injected. It has to be understood that even under the latter circumstances the operation is performed under acupuncture analgesia because the supplements used in combination with fairly heavy premedication are still not sufficient to allow that particular operation to take place without some form of anaesthesia as that is understood in western medicine. Thus it has to be said that acupuncture analgesia does add something extra to the operative technique since without it no operation could take place.

Various medical study groups from different countries have visited China over the past five years or so to study and investigate the phenomenon of acupuncture analgesia. There was a British study group, but before this there were study groups from Norway, Canada, and the U.S.A. Initially it appeared that about 80 to 90 per cent of all operations performed in China were done under acupuncture analgesia. This does not now appear to be the case, even if it ever was so. Nowadays 80 to 90 per cent of operations performed under acupuncture analgesia appear to be successful on the lines mentioned above but the total number of operations performed under this method is no more than 10 per cent. It is most likely that the correct figure is around the 6 per cent level.

Perhaps it should be emphasised that acupuncture analgesia is most important because a method which is safe with no danger from general or local anaesthetic drugs must be examined for use in the western hospitals. Think, for instance, of the boon this would be in childbirth in having a method for relieving the pain without affecting the mother or the child. This would only hold good if it proved to be a reliable and a repeatable method. Unfortunately this does not appear to be the case. However, from the research and interest point of view it does not matter at all that the method is unreliable for routine use, it is enough that it works only now and again for it is essential to find out the mechanism of action for the light it may throw on our knowledge of pain conduction and the appreciation of pain. It looks as though the major value of acupuncture analgesia will be as a research tool.

Choice of patient

From reports by members of the British study group it would appear that only those patients who were particularly interested in having their operation performed under acupuncture analgesia were assessed for it. Most often the operative sessions were carried out under general or local anaesthesia and acupuncture was not the method of choice. Those patients who expressed a desire for acupuncture analgesia were given full instructions in the method and what would happen to them on the operating day, and also what would be expected of them. There was much discussion about all this, in which other patients who had had acupuncture analgesia performed successfully took part. The patient tended to come into hospital rather earlier than is normal in the West and when not taking part in meetings extolling Chairman Mao and the virtues of the little red book, and provided they were fit enough, acted as ward orderlies according to their capabilities. How much of the subsequent results were due to suggestion or self-hypnosis is impossible to say but there may be some element of this. Also, there is the factor that it is not in human nature to be pleased at the idea of making a fool of oneself after opting specially for acupuncture, and there may be some self-induced pressure on the patient from this angle, though it has to be admitted that if this were the only factor involved it would be surprising if the patient could lie still on the table during say abdominal surgery. Again it is possible to believe that an occasional patient might be sufficiently motivated to keep still but to believe that 6 per cent or more of the population would do so is unlikely.

All the patients were carefully selected for acupuncture analgesia and those who wavered in the slightest were withdrawn from this type of analgesia, in other words, only those patients who were quite solid in their desire to have acupuncture and who showed no signs of having second thoughts right up to the moment of the operation were allowed to go on to have this type of pain relief for surgery.

Premedication

This was fairly heavy involving a barbiturate in the ward followed by 50 mg pethidine. The pethidine might be repeated in the same dose after about thirty minutes. The patients often walked to the operating table but needed some support, as the premedication was heavy enough to produce a certain amount of unsteadiness. Again it should be emphasised that this amount of premedication would not be enough on its own to allow surgery to be performed.

Acupuncture analgesia

In most cases this takes up to half an hour to develop. Stimulation of the acupuncture needles was done either manually or by an electrical method. In this electrical method the needle twitches from each electrical pulse due to direct stimulation by the electrical current of the muscles in that region of the body. It was these twitches that caused movement of the needles and thus the stimulation. In general terms an electrical method was used when more than a few acupuncture needles were inserted. If the needles were stimulated manually then they were not manipulated continuously but in bursts with intervals of a few minutes between each series of stimulations. During the operation stimulation continued but again in an intermittent fashion.

Because of the time taken to develop acupuncture analgesia it is not the method of choice if an emergency operation is required. In addition, there is insufficient time to prepare the patient mentally for the method as it does seem that a tranquil mind is a very helpful factor in the production of effective analgesia.

In some cases the acupuncture analgesia developed over fairly narrow areas, in others over a widespread area. It might be taken that in an emergency where one type of operation might need extending into another, or where one operative field might be combined with another in an entirely different area, acupuncture analgesia might not allow a sufficiently flexible approach to surgical anaesthesia. It would, therefore, be contra-indicated in these circumstances.

Acupuncture points

Naturally there are two schools of thought as to which acupuncture points to use for the production of analgesia. The first are the traditional point users, as opposed to those who believe that ear points provide all that is necessary. Apparently those using the ear tend to use similar points for similar operations, though one unkind thought could be that as the ear is such a relatively small organ its limited area cannot provide all that many different positions for analgesia. The users of traditional points, i.e. those on the body and limbs showed great individual variation in their choices. It might be thought that an operation such as a thyroidectomy (or thyroid lobectomy) with a fairly standardised incision, would have a fairly standardised type of acupuncture analgesia with standard acupuncture points used. This was not apparently so, further, the area of analgesia produced varied with the different methods but seemed to bear no great relation to the number of acupuncture needles inserted. On occasion an operation was performed under a technique using but one needle, while another analgesist at the same or a different hospital on the same day might use eight or more. There did not seem to be much logic in the choice of the acupuncture needle sites. There was a tendency to insert the needles in a dermatomal distribution, and this idea was quite deliberately followed by some of the more modern acupuncturists. This in fact is not only followed in acupuncture analgesia but also in treating non-surgical medical conditions, particularly those where pain is a feature.

Types of operation

It appears that acupuncture analgesia is not used in children very much—
'as they cry'. If questioned if it was used in children the answer invariably
was 'yes, in the hospital down the road but not here'. The method is not used
for abdominal surgery, or rather it is not the method of choice for abdominal
surgery, as the relaxation produced by acupuncture analgesia is poor. There
is also a great deal of stimulation when the parietal peritoneum is penetrated
and for this reason when acupuncture analgesia is used it is combined with
a little local anaesthetic solution into the parietal peritoneum if the patient
shows anything more than a mild reaction at that stage. Even if the patient
responded to parietal stimulation of the peritoneum once the surgeon was
past that hurdle the patient usually settled down without difficulty.

Cranial surgery was not uncommonly performed under acupuncture
analgesia as was thoracotomy. Patients having thoracotomy performed had
a period of training in breathing beforehand designed to minimise respiratory problems associated with an open chest and absence of control over the
airway by means of a cuffed intratracheal tube or similar type of technique.
The Chinese method involved teaching the patient to breathe very shallowly
to minimise mediastinal shift in an open chest, and also to breathe out against
a resistance formed by the pursed lips which will tend to keep the lungs
inflated and prevent shunting. It has to be admitted that the best of these
operations showed patients in apparently fine condition—not distressed in
any way. On the other hand, there were patients who were by no means
happy and seemed in very poor shape indeed. If required the open chest
operation patients were given oxygen through a mask, not continuously
but from time to time. As this oxygen was given under pressure and through
a tight face-mask it appeared that a form of inflation of the lungs was being
performed.

The operation which is most favoured for acupuncture analgesia is the
partial thyroidectomy, as about 50 per cent of all the operations for which
acupuncture analgesia is used is for this condition. The operation performed
tends to be more of a lobectomy than the corresponding operation in the
western world and is performed through a much smaller incision. In fact,
a small incision is a feature of Chinese surgery under acupuncture analgesia.
Chinese surgeons have adopted their surgery for these operative conditions, by means of slow, careful movements, injection of small quantities of
local anaesthetic solutions into sensitive areas, and small incisions. Incidentally, the quality and the results of the surgery were good.

The surgical technique used was designed to avoid traction reflexes as much as possible as these result in pain and increased muscle tone. In addition, pain will produce anxiety and there is no doubt that it is easier to obtain satisfactory acupuncture analgesia in a quiet relaxed patient. Many patients who undergo satisfactory operations under acupuncture analgesia, and stay quiet and fairly still during the procedure, do not in fact have complete freedom from pain. As was mentioned before, the patients can be divided into three types in this respect. First are those patients who are completely pain free and relaxed, these are the perfect demonstration cases. At the other extreme are those patients whose analgesia is insufficient to cover the operation performed and who must then have their analgesia supplemented by local or general anaesthesia. In between are a group of patients who at the one end are almost perfect and except for perhaps a moment or two of mild discomfort have no unwanted sensations at all, and who at the other extreme have so much pain as opposed to discomfort that supplemental anaesthesia is absolutely necessary. At this extreme it is only by encouragement of a high order that the operation can be finished under the original acupuncture analgesia. It is difficult to be sure of the relative percentages of each of these groups but not more than a third can be considered to be satisfactory or very satisfactory, and it must be remembered that this is in a group of patients selected carefully by the Chinese themselves as being most suitable for acupuncture analgesia.

Advantages

Acupuncture analgesia is said to be a very safe method of operative pain relief. Kaada reports no death or serious complication had been reported at the time of the Norwegian visit. However, as it is not used or tends to be useless in children, and in old people; and is not used in patients with severe blood loss, hypovolaemic shock or in coma, or in operations which last more than two hours or so, a large number of the potential difficulties are removed long before the operative theatre is reached.

Other advantages lie in the fact that the patient is awake and can co-operate with the surgeon, which can be useful in some circumstances.

There is said to be little disturbance in many bodily functions such as in the circulation, respiration, fluid, or electrolytic balance. Post-operative nausea and vomiting is infrequent, as are post-operative complications such as urinary retention, or respiratory tract infection. Abdominal distention or ilius are uncommon. The method therefore is of particular benefit in the poor-risk patient, who is debilitated or suffering from liver, renal, or hepatic complications.

One of the most useful benefits of acupuncture analgesia is due to the fact that the analgesic effect does not disappear immediately after the stimulation is removed but continues into the post-operative period and provides a very useful measure of post-operative analgesia. The analgesia lasts for two to three hours post-operatively and sometimes for much longer than this (up to twenty-four hours) so that post-operative medication is reduced.

REFERENCES (*see* pp. 304–5).

Chapter 13
Modern Acupuncture

It has been previously mentioned that it has long been known that a small pain could relieve a much larger severe pain by the use of the technique known as counter irritation. This does not mean that a great deal is known of the method by which counter irritation produces its results but some details are known from observation and empirical use. Counter irritation is used in the area of referred pain, though on rarer occasions it is used on distant apparently unaffected regions with good results. Thus in the main, if counter irritation is to be used, it is used in a dermatomal distribution.

In the myofacial syndromes it is common knowledge that there may be tender areas in muscles or tendons with pain referred to distant areas of the body. These areas may be in dermatomal or scleratomal distributions or may have no apparent relationship to the precipitating tender area or nodule. Often there is a history of mild or very minor trauma to the tender region which may have been in the very distant past.

Treatment of the myofacial syndromes is directed to the tender areas when these are demonstrated and usually benefits or cures the condition. Sometimes a single injection into a painful nodule is all that is necessary for a cure to result but usually, if the condition has been present for any length of time, a series of such treatments is required. The use of physiotherapy, heat, massage, and manipulation are other methods which are well tried and are of known beneficial effect. All these methods act, in one way or another by improving the circulation, relieving pain and spasm, and restoring or allowing normal function.

It is not necessary to understand why and how these methods work to make use of them. It is sufficient for practical purposes that a particular method does produce a useful result. It can then be used in the confident knowledge that it will not harm the patient and in most cases will help the condition.

There are similarities between the use of counter irritation and the treatment of the myofacial syndromes on the one hand, and the use of acupuncture in the treatment of pain and disease on the other. There is no doubt that acupuncture produces useful results in a way that are not understood. This avoids the question as to whether the results are better, as good as, or worse than the corresponding ones obtained by other methods. What is known is that the method of action of acupuncture is not understood at the present time. Much research work is being conducted into acupuncture and no doubt in due course some answers will come out. Already there does appear to be a correlation between the length of time it takes to develop acupuncture analgesia, and the depression of post-synaptic evoked responses following suitable stimulation. Acupuncture analgesia is normally said to require about twenty to thirty minutes stimulation by acupuncture needle before it appears in any degree, and the depression of the evoked response takes about twenty minutes to reach its maximum. Further the degree of depression is correlated with the duration and intensity of the acupuncture stimulation, and wears off after the stimulation ceases.

When it comes to deciding which point on the limb or body is to be the acupuncture point there is great room for controversy. Traditionally there is only one position allowed for each of the known (and named) acupuncture points, but this is disputed by those of the modern school who believe that acupuncture points are at best only an approximation, and that any position within a centimetre or so is equally effective. Also there are other schools of thought who believe that acupuncture points correspond to areas of 'high nerve density' and that most of the important acupuncture points are situated near nerve trunks or where there are arbourising branches coming through from the deeper structures. Another school believes that acupuncture is merely a form of strong peripheral nerve stimulation and that it does not matter particularly where the stimulation occurs but that it is most effective in the dermatomal distribution of the area which it is desired to influence.

There is some recent work on animals suggestive that the acupuncture points correspond to the motor points of muscles. These motor points are defined as the skin locations where maximum muscular contraction is elicited with electrical stimulation. It must be realised that this research continues to progress and although most encouraging too much should not be read into the preliminary results. In similar fashion it is believed that the position of the acupuncture points can be picked out by the use of various electrical methods. These involve measuring the resistance of the skin over small areas by the use of suitable electrodes and there are a number of commercially available units to do this. Whether they do in fact accurately place the acupuncture point is still not decided and there is no doubt that one of the difficulties is that if a small electrical current is passed through the skin the resistance of the skin is altered anyway. Many of these methods of picking up the acupuncture points in the skin do so by the measurement of the small electric currents generated by the effect of the body salts on bimetallic junctions, or by passing small currents through the skin and measuring the resistance. In either case there are electrical currents developed which pass through the skin and may affect it.

From assessment of the previous ideas it is possible to arrive at the following tentative conclusions:

(A) It is admitted that acupuncture stimulation has an effect on painful conditions.

(B) It is not admitted that there is any proof that acupuncture treatment has, by itself, cured any medical or surgical condition. There are trials in progress in the western world which suggest that in some cases this has happened, but until these trials are completed it is impossible to know whether these known and occasional results are statistically significant.

(C) There is no acceptable proof that acupuncture points exist. It does appear that there are certain areas in the body where stimulation by an acupuncture needle has widespread effects at a distance from the area of stimulation. Stimulation by any other means would have the same effect, and the area over which the stimulation is effective is about 2 cm in diameter.

(D) The most effective region to stimulate is one in the dermatomal dis-tribution of the part to be affected. The effects obtained are not confined to the dermatomal or local distribution. They may be at widespread areas either on the same or the other side of the body.

(E) The greater the stimulation the more effective and prolonged the result except in the case of those patients who are hyper–reactors. Hyper–reactors have low pain thresholds and over-stimulation will result in adverse responses.

(F) As the most effective areas to stimulate seem to be areas either of high nerve density in the skin, or sensitive areas in muscles, the best depth for the acupuncture needle will be about 1 cm deep. In areas where there is no muscle deep to the superficial tissues penetration beyond the subcutaneous tissues is not warranted.

It is then possible to make some further assumptions and the main one is that if the previous six tentative conclusions have any relation to reality it should be possible to obtain the benefits of acupuncture, or some of them without having to spend three years or so learning the basic points and techniques of traditional acupuncture. It is quite possible to do this, but

if any accurate conclusion is to be made as to whether the results obtained
are as good as those which could be obtained by the traditional method of
acupuncture then a properly trained traditional acupuncturist must be used
as a control. In other words a proper research technique is necessary. One
of the problems in assessing acupuncture treatments effectively is in obtaining properly trained acupuncturists to conduct the control side of the
trial.

SIMPLIFIED TECHNIQUE OF ACUPUNCTURE

Nomenclature

It is convenient to use the traditional acupuncture maps of the human body
to record the places where acupuncture stimulation of the skin is performed.
There are various types of 'atlas' produced and any which aids the
physician concerned is suitable, provided it is easily obtainable and is
clearly marked. The author uses the one published by Mann.

Stimulation

Many varieties of this are used in traditional acupuncture but for convenience and for their ready availability the traditional acupuncture needle
might as well be used. For the average purpose a two-inch needle will cover
all normal needs. This should be made of stainless steel and have a one-inch
handle and a one-inch needle portion. The handle is traditionally wound
round with fine wire which provides a very good and non-slip grip. It is
important that the needle and hub are properly connected as some poorly-
made acupuncture needles can come apart at this place leaving the needle
in the tissues.

Sterilisation

The acupuncture needle of the type just described is not very expensive
and could be used as a disposable item. However, it is made of stainless steel
and unless the point is allowed to hit bone and become blunt, it will last for
a dozen or more occasions. There is no danger in this provided effective
sterility is observed. The principal disease to avoid is infective hepatitis
spread from unsterile needles, and autoclaving or chemical sterilisation is
effective when adequate safeguards are used. Before puncturing the skin

the same precautions of sterilising the surface should be taken that would be used in any other type of injection therapy. Again the particular technique does not matter as long as it is effective.

Pulse diagnosis

A decision will have to be taken as to whether the physician concerned is going to bother with the traditional pulse diagnosis. If the decision is not to bother then the method of carrying on follows after this section. However, most physicians would be interested in deciding for themselves whether it is possible to appreciate any differences and the following simple method of pulse diagnosis is suggested. This idea is not the author's own but was suggested to him and others by Dr. Mann.

The basic idea in this method is that as the meridians are paired structures and as one of these pairs, if stimulated, has an effect on the other, all one needs to know is which pair of meridians is involved. Thus it is not necessary to know which of twelve pulses is abnormal by assessing both superficial and deep pulses, merely which of six pairs. Thus in this modified form of the pulse diagnosis three fingers are placed on each radial pulse in the fashion described before, and the various pulses are then compared. The pulses at the right and left first position are compared, either at deep pressure or light pressure or at any intermediate pressure that suits the physician. This is followed by similar study at the second and then the third position. It is useful to have had some help initially from somebody skilled in the pulse diagnosis to explain the types of pulses that can be felt and the nuances that are looked for, but with the simple method described above all that needs to be looked for is a difference, any difference, on the two sides. Thus this method can be used when the physician concerned has never palpated a Chinese pulse diagnosis before. If some idea of the traditional Chinese descriptions of the pulse can be obtained beforehand from a traditional acupuncturist (e.g. what is meant by a 'wiry' pulse) then feeling the three positions may become more interesting and more information for research purposes may be obtained.

If no difference can be palpated in the pulse diagnosis then carry on with the scheme below. If there is a difference in the pulse diagnosis then the two meridians concerned are noted and may be used in deciding the acupuncture points to select. If there is a difference in more than one of the six pulses then some assessment should be made of the relative abnormality between them and most notice taken of the pair of meridians corresponding to the most abnormal pulse.

Combinations

Traditional Chinese medicine does not list its diseases in systems but in symptoms, and this is why quite diverse diseases may have the same, or share many of, the acupuncture points used. One of the essentials for the practice of acupuncture is to have a library of 'good points'. The bibliography at the end of this chapter provides a good start and very soon experience will suggest that some are more useful than others. The basic idea of traditional acupuncture is to overcome the acute phase of any disease by making use of the body of knowledge represented by the so-called combinations of acupuncture points which are available in the literature or handed down by word of mouth (see end of this chapter for examples). Once the acute phase is over then treatment is continued by means of the pulse diagnosis. Thus for chronic or long-lasting conditions the combination points may be used for a prolonged period, in addition to others added in from the pulse diagnosis.

Frequency of treatment

This will depend on the reaction of the patient but in the acute stage a treatment every day, or even twice per day is not unrealistic. It is rather time-consuming and therefore a more realistic frequency of every other day could be used. After the initial period the treatment is extended to once per week and then once every two weeks. When the pulse diagnosis method is being used to keep the patient in health by means of corrective acupuncture a frequency of two to four visits per year is necessary.

Meridian points

The affected meridians are diagnosed by the simple method given previously. A careful search is made over the patient in the dermatomes of the affected area to pick up any tender or painful places or nodules. Any such places are treated by acupuncture needling at the painful point, especially those which are in the distribution of one of the meridians already chosen by the simplified method. If there are no painful or tender areas the acupuncture atlas is consulted to see if any of the meridians which traverse the affected part, includes those which have been abnormal on the pulse diagnosis. If it does then this is the meridian to use and one of the acupuncture points shown on the atlas on this meridian is needled. If there is any doubt as to which acupuncture point on this meridian to use consult the list of combination points for the condition to be treated. There will be a list of the usually effective combinations, then a list of other less effective or less commonly used combinations. There will probably be, in addition, a note that certain points are most efficacious in the particular condition and if one or other of these specially mentioned points is on the selected meridian then this is the point to use.

If there is no mention of special points in the list of combinations or there are no such points on the selected meridians there are two methods of approach. A textbook of acupuncture is consulted and the individual points on the selected meridian studied, if one of these points mentions the condition of which the patient suffers then this is the acupuncture point to use. The second method is to ignore the selected meridian or meridians and to choose the one from the atlas which traverses the centre of the affected region. If more than one region is affected then more than one meridian is chosen. Once a meridian has been chosen in this way, then the process outlined previously can be carried through.

If all these methods do not produce a satisfactory acupuncture site then ignore all methods of choosing the point and use those on the liver or bladder meridian at their distal and peripheral portions to the affected part.

Non-acupuncture stimulation

From what has been previously stated there are many acupuncturists who believe that there is no merit in the traditional method of selecting a meridian and the acupuncture point and that either dermatomal stimulation is as effective and should be used, or knowledge of neuroanatomy should be used to choose places of high nerve density. These two methods are particularly apposite for western-trained physicians to adopt and they can be used as a fall-back system when the methods mentioned previously fail to be effective. Alternatively the simplified methods can be ignored or kept in reserve and the two methods of non-acupuncture stimulation used from the beginning of treatment. It will be found that despite the method chosen to select the acupuncture needle site that stimulation for painful conditions will be of benefit. Further that the sensation of 'take' can be obtained at these stimulation sites. As this is one of the ways of distinguishing that a needling has occurred at the correct position of an acupuncture point it can be concluded that either there are many more acupuncture points than have been described, or the methods mentioned are satisfactory in picking out the acupuncture points, or the acupuncture points are not points but areas and relatively crude methods are sufficiently accurate to obtain the position of these areas.

An alternative explanation is that the whole basis of acupuncture is built on false premisses.

Once again the author suggests that it would be sensible to see acupuncture performed on at least one occasion before trying it out oneself for the first time. If it is impossible to do this then there is no reason why the beginner should not use the technique.

Stimulation technique

If an electrical apparatus is used then there will be instructions on the parameters to use for pulse width, power, and frequency. By the use of one of these instruments a period of continuous stimulation can be carried out at a stimulation level acceptable to the patient.

Under some conditions, and these are mentioned in the combinations or in the instructions on individual acupuncture points, a needle is inserted and just left *in situ*. It is not stimulated in any way. The time it is to be left in position is often mentioned but not always. The traditional method in deciding how long to leave the needle in place is to perform the pulse diagnosis and remove the needle when the pulses return to normal or approximately so.

If the acupuncture needle is to be stimulated by hand this is done by rotating the needle between the first and second fingers. The vigour with which this is done determines the amount of stimulation the patient receives. It has to be recognised that acupuncture performed in this way is very painful indeed or can be very painful if the needle is twirled vigorously. It is best to stimulate under these circumstances in short bursts with a rest interval between each period of stimulation. Each period of stimulation is about three to five seconds long and about three such stimulations can be done in one minute. But the stimulation given and the intervals between depend on the patient's reaction. It is not the purpose of the acupuncturist to produce agony, the amount of stimulation used must depend on the patient's ability to accept it.

EXAMPLES OF COMBINATION POINTS

Condition	*Acupuncture Points*
Angina Pectoris	G 20, G 21, Si 15, B 15. B 18, L 4, L 5, P 6.
Aphthous Stomatitis	S 4, Gv 26, Gv 24.

Dysmenorrhoea	L 3, L 8.
	Cv 4, Sp 6, L 5.
Frozen Shoulder	L 1, Si 16, Si 9, Si 11.
	Li 15, L 5, G 34.
Headache	Liv 3, B 2, Li 4.
	Li 8, Li 14, B 18 or B 19.
	K 5, L 6.
	B 62, Li 4.
Hot Flushes	L 9, H 7.
Insomnia	H 7, L 9, S 36, Sp 6.
Metatarsalgia	Sp 3, B 65, K 1.
	G 42, Liv 3, B 60.
Migraine	Bilateral Liv 2.
	G 5, Li 4, Liv 3.
Nasal Cold	Li 4, G 20, B 12.
Painful Breast	L 9, H 7, S 18, S 15.
Pain and Swelling in Arm	Si 16, H 1, H 7, L 9.
	H 8, T 4, T 8, T 9, L 3.
Pain in Neck (with Headache)	Si 16, G 20.
Premenstrual Tension	Sp 9, Sp 10, Liv 1, Liv 3, Liv 6.
Pruritis	L 5, L 9, Li 4, Li 11.
Tennis Elbow	Si 16, Gv 14 or Li 4, G 34.
Tranquillise. (Sedation)	H 7, Li 4, P 6, Gv 15, Gv 26.
	B 13, B 15, Cv 14, Cv 12.
Toothache. (Upper Jaw)	Li 5, S 8, T 20.
(Lower Jaw)	Li 4, S 6, K 4.

Meridians

B...Bladder. Cv...Conception Vessel. G...Gall Bladder. Gv...Governing Vessel.
H...Heart. K...Kidney. L...Lung. Li...Large Intestine. Liv...Liver.
P...Pericardium. S...Stomach. Si...Small Intestine. Sp...Spleen. T...
Triple Warmer.

Depth of insertion of acupuncture needle for the combination points (in inches).

Bladder. 2, 12, 15, 18, 19, 60, 62, 65.
$\frac{1}{4}$ $\frac{1}{4}$ $\frac{1}{4}$ $\frac{1}{4}$ $\frac{1}{4}$ $\frac{3}{4}$ $\frac{1}{2}$ $\frac{1}{4}$

Conception. 4.
$\frac{1}{2}$

Gall Bladder. 5, 20, 21, 34, 42.
$\frac{1}{4}$ 1 $\frac{1}{2}$ 1 $\frac{1}{2}$

Governing Vessel. 14, 24, 26.
1 $\frac{1}{2}$ $\frac{1}{4}$

Heart. 1, 7, 8.
$\frac{1}{2}$ $\frac{1}{2}$ $\frac{1}{4}$

Kidney. 1, 4, 5.
$\frac{1}{2}$ $\frac{1}{4}$ $\frac{1}{2}$

Lung. 1, 3, 4, 5, 6, 8, 9.
$\frac{1}{2}$ $\frac{3}{4}$ 1 $\frac{1}{2}$ $\frac{3}{4}$ $\frac{1}{2}$ $\frac{1}{4}$
Large Intestine.   4, 8, 11, 14, 15.
1 $\frac{1}{2}$ 1 1 1

Liver. 1, 3, 6.
$\frac{1}{2}$ $\frac{3}{4}$ $\frac{1}{2}$
Pericardium.   6.
$\frac{3}{4}$
Stomach.   4, 6, 8, 15, 18, 36.
$\frac{1}{2}$ $\frac{1}{4}$ $\frac{1}{2}$ $\frac{1}{2}$ $\frac{1}{2}$ 1
Small Intestine.   9, 11, 15, 16.
1 $\frac{3}{4}$ $\frac{3}{4}$ $\frac{1}{2}$
Spleen.   3, 6, 9, 10.
$\frac{1}{4}$ 1 1 1
Triple Warmer.   4, 8, 9, 20.
1 $\frac{3}{4}$ $\frac{3}{4}$ $\frac{1}{4}$

REFERENCES

BONICA J.J. (1974) Therapeutic acupuncture in the People's Republic of China. *J.A.M.A.* **228**, 12, 1544–1551.

BONICA J.J. (1974) Acupuncture anaesthesia in the People's Republic of China. *J.A.M.A.* **229**, 10, 1317–1325.

KAADA B., HOEL E., LESETH K., *et al.* (1974) Acupuncture analgesia in the People's Republic of China. *T. norske Laegeforen*, **94**, 417–442.

KIM BONG HAN (1964) *On the Kyungrak System.* Foreign Language Publishing House, Pyongyang, D.P.R. Korea.

LIPTON S. (1974) Acupuncture—A problem for the Anaesthetist? *Proc. roy. Soc. Med.* **67**, 8, 731–732.

MANN F., BOWSHER D., MUMFORD J., LIPTON S. & MILES J. (1973) Treatment of intractable pain by acupuncture. *Lancet*, **2**, 57–60.

MELZACK R. (1973) How acupuncture can block pain. *Impact of Science on Society*, **23**, 1, 65–75.

National Health and Medical Research Council of Australia. (1974) Report on Acupuncture. Canberra, Australian Government Publishing Service.

STEWART D., THOMPSON J. & OSWALD I. (1977) Acupuncture analgesia: an experimental investigation. *B.M.J.* **1**, 67–70.

WALL P.D. (1972) An eye on the needle. *New Scientist, July*, **20**, 129–131.

ADDITIONAL READING

Acupuncture, The Ancient Chinese Art of Healing (1971) Ed. Felix Mann. Heinemann, London.

Chinese Acupuncture (1962) Ed. Wu Wei-P'ing, Translated and adapted by J. Lavier and P.M. Chancellor. Health Science Press, Northamptonshire, Great Britain.

An atlas of acupuncture; points and meridians (1972) Ed. F. Mann. Heinemann, London.

The Acupuncture Treatment of Pain (1976) Ed. L. Chaitow. University Press, Oxford.

The Yellow Emperor's Book of Acupuncture (1962) Ed. Zhang Jin-an. The Shanghi Scientific and Technical Publishing House, Peking.

The Yellow Emperor's Book of Acupuncture (1973) Translated by Henry C. Lu. The Academy of Oriental Heritage, Vancouver, Canada.

Treatise of Auriculotherapy (1972) Ed. P. F. Nogier. Maisonneuve, Moulins-les-Metz, France. (English translation available.)

Chapter 14
Useful Nerve Blocks

The technique of nerve blocking has been revolutionised by the use of the semi-portable image intensifier. This can be swung through 90° to give lateral or antero-posterior X-ray views quickly.

It is perfectly possible to carry out blocks without the use of the image intensifier and this was normal in the past. At the most a few check X-rays were taken, and with practice great expertise was developed. The reason for carrying out a block is to deposit anaesthetic solution near a particular nerve or nerve plexus and the use of the image intensifier introduces more accuracy. In the techniques described later it is taken for granted that an image intensifier, having a television screen with good definition, is available and is used.

Various local anaesthetic solutions are available, and commonly used ones are Benzocaine (Americaine), Procaine (Novocain), and Chloro-procaine (Nesacaine). Chloroprocaine is the least toxic of these, which are all esters of para-aminobenzoic acid. They diffuse much less than the other large group of local anaesthetic agents which are amines. These consist of such well-known local anaesthetics as Lignocaine (Xylocaine), Prilocaine (Citanest), Etidocaine (Duranest), and Bupivacaine (Marcaine). The latter two have the longest effect and in general terms are less toxic.

As in regional anaesthesia, toxic effects, and duration of the block depend on the total dose of the local anaesthetic agent used. When a large amount of dilute solution is used, as in the 'flooding' technique where an area is bathed in the solution, there are as many toxic effects as when a similar dose in concentrated solution is used. Toxic effects depend on dosage, the pharmaco-logical structure of the drug used, and the technique of injection. The quantity of drugs actually injected in the techniques to be described do not usually cause toxic symptoms, though there is always the possibility of a patient being sensitive to the agent used.

One difference between the esters and amide group of drugs is that the former are hydrolysed by pseudocholinesterase. In patients with a deficiency of this substance the local anaesthetic agent cannot be hydrolysed at the normal rate and thus there is also a reduced tolerance. When a general anaesthetic is given to cover the block and suxamethonium chloride (Anectine) forms part of the anaesthetic regime, prolonged neuromuscular blockage may occur and an increase in toxicity, if ester local anaesthetics are used. In this circumstance it is preferable to use an amide local anaesthetic agent, since this is metabolised mainly in the liver by microsomal enzymes.

If the patient has liver disease the amide drugs can be reduced in quantity, or using esters may be preferable.

The local anaesthetic agents commonly used at the Centre for Pain Relief are Lignocaine 1 per cent and 2 per cent for the short-acting blocks, and Marcaine $\frac{1}{2}$ per cent plain for long-acting ones. Rarely are solutions with added Adrenaline used.

When long-lasting blocks are required 6 per cent Phenol in saline or 100 per cent Alcohol (dehydrated alcohol) are the agents used. Alcohol tends to produce neuritis and is only used for the Trigeminal nerve blocks and intrathecally. There is no particular reason why it should be used in this way on the trigeminal nerve except long usage has given consistently good and reliable results. The newer and better method of destruction of this nerve by means of a radio-frequency electric current (RFC) producing a heat coagulation is now used at this centre and is mentioned in detail elsewhere.

Another long-acting block can be produced by the combination of 2 per cent Benzocaine in Arachis Oil followed by twice the quantity of 6 per cent Urethane injected down the same needle without any movement of the needle so that mixing occurs in the tissues. This is extremely useful for subcostal blocks for a secondary tumour of a rib.

All the blocks that are mentioned here are in regular use at the Centre for Pain Relief. They are only included if they have worked satisfactorily and reliably in our own and our trainees' hands. Sometimes to elucidate a difficult chronic pain problem other blocks than those mentioned are used, and in fact are sometimes 'manufactured' by reference to the anatomy books, or to our Anatomical Associates. It is felt that rare blocks have no place in a practical book such as this.

Apart from somatic nerve blocks there are three common autonomic nervous system blocks which are in constant use. These are those of the Stellate Ganglion, the Lumbar Sympathetic Chain, and the Coeliac Plexus, and these will be described first.

STELLATE GANGLION BLOCK

The Stellate Ganglion is formed by the fusion of the inferior cervical ganglion and the first thoracic ganglion. When these two ganglia are separate structures the inferior cervical ganglion lies in front of the transverse process of the seventh cervical vertebra, and the first thoracic ganglia lies anterior to the neck of the first rib. The stellate ganglion can have various shapes and may be formed by a number of closely linked small ganglia, but in its common position it forms a single structure which lies along the neck of the first rib extending upwards into the space above. Thus anaesthetic solutions deposited anterior to the neck of the first rib, or anterior and below the transverse process of the seventh cervical vertebra must block the stellate ganglion or the ganglia forming its constituent parts.

The cervical portion of the sympathetic trunk, of which the stellate ganglion is a portion, lies directly behind the carotid sheath on the fascia covering the longus capitis and longus cervicis muscles. Further posterior are the transverse processes of the cervical vertebra, and anteriorly is the subclavian artery and its branch, the vertebral artery. Below and anteriorly is the pleura (see Figs. 72 and 73).

There are three basic methods of carrying out the stellate ganglion block. These may be called the lower cervical chain block, the anterior stellate ganglion block and the posterior stellate ganglion block.

The lower cervical chain block makes use of the anatomical relationship of the cervical chain being anterior to the fascia covering the paravertebral muscles. Any anaesthetic solution deposited anterior to this fascia will diffuse along this fascial plane and if the patient is sitting up, or the head is raised, the solution must spread downwards under the influence of gravity. It will reach and bathe the stellate ganglion as well as those portions of the cervical sympathetic chain over which it passes.

The technique is straightforward. The patient lies flat with one pillow under the head (and not the shoulders). The head is slightly extended as this stretches the major vessels in the neck, and also the oesophagus tends to lie in the mid-line behind the trachea. Standing (or sitting) by the side of the patient to be injected, the fingers of the most convenient hand are pushed into the tissues of the neck and the carotid artery felt and pulled laterally out of the way. At the same time these fingers feel one or other of the cervical transverse processes and a 10 ml syringe with a 21-gauge 4 cm needle is inserted through the skin down to the selected transverse process, without preliminary injection into the skin. The needle is withdrawn about 0·25 cm after touching bone to place the point anterior to the paravertebral fascia, and the solution is then injected after an aspiration test has proved negative. An almost immediate Horner's syndrome should result, and in any case the patient's head and shoulders are raised a little. The Horner's syndrome does not indicate that a stellate ganglion block has been carried out but merely that the upper sympathetic nerves to the head have been interrupted. The Horner's syndrome consists of anhydrosis, enophthalmos, ptosis, and miosis. Additional signs with a complete stellate block are vaso-dilatation of the area affected which is the whole of the upper limb and half of the face. This tends to be seen as a flushed face with injected con-junctival vessels, and a blocked nose.

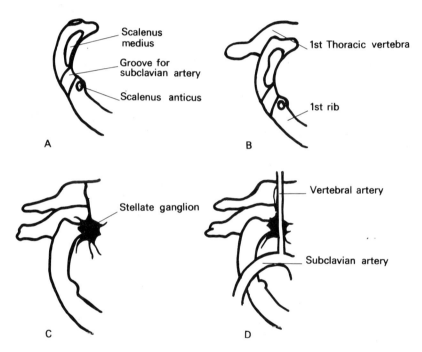

FIGURE 72. Relations of stellate ganglion (A–D).

The volume of fluid used is 10 ml of 1 per cent or 2 per cent Lignocaine. Longer-acting solutions can be used if prolonged effects are required.

Complications are few with this approach. A hoarse or weak voice due to recurrent laryngeal nerve paresis may occur but will disappear when the block wears off. Similarly there can be a spread on to the brachial plexus with varying degrees of weakness of the arm. The patient is reassured that both of these will wear off in time. Formation of a haematoma is a possi-bility, and there is the danger of an intravascular injection of local anaesthetic

Chapter 14

solution. If the needle misses the transverse process it can hit the vertebral artery, or can penetrate a dural sleeve accompanying the somatic nerve producing a spinal blockade. Pleural puncture and pneumothorax is very unlikely in this approach unless there is a considerable bulge in the dome of the pleura, but it is a complication which has to be borne in mind in the other two methods, and particularly the next.

The anterior stellate ganglion block is designed to place solution directly on to the stellate ganglion, or very close to it. This (or the posterior approach) would be used if a very long-lasting block were required for, say, a status anginosus and absolute alcohol was to be used.

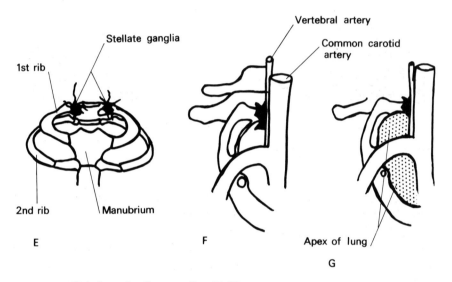

FIGURE 73. Relations of stellate ganglion (E–G).

In this method the injection is made at the level of the transverse process of the seventh cervical vertebra and this is at the level of the spinous process of the sixth cervical vertebra posteriorly and about 3 cm above the sterno-clavicular joint anteriorly. The patient is placed in the same position as for the lower cervical block and a subcutaneous wheal raised 1·5 cm lateral to the mid-line and 3 cm above the sternoclavicular joint. An 8 cm 20-gauge needle is then directed through the wheal in the direction of the transverse process. When in the correct place the needle will contact the base of the transverse process and it is then withdrawn 0·5 cm and the aspiration test carried out as in the previous method. Problems begin when the transverse process is not contacted by the needle on the first insertion and repeated insertions are necessary to find it, or when the first contact is too lateral and

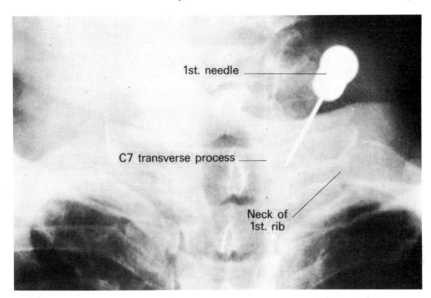

FIGURE 74. First needle too medial on seventh transverse process.

FIGURES 74–76. Injection at neck of first rib (stellate ganglion).

more medial reinsertion is necessary. X-rays can be taken after the first insertion (see Figs. 74–76), but the method advocated is to use an image intensifier from the beginning of this approach. In fact, if this is the case then the approach can be modified by inserting the needle higher in the neck, further away from the sternoclavicular joint and adopting a more oblique angle. The position of the needle tip can be followed by frequent observations on the television monitor. This is a much safer approach than the 'low' one as there is much less chance of producing a pneumothorax.

The third method can be used when permanent or semi-permanent block of the stellate ganglion is required and is a safe method when the image intensifier is used.

Posterior stellate ganglion block is carried out in the sitting position with the image intensifier at an angle to the horizontal, being almost in the line of the upper ribs. This provides X-ray views with less overlapping of the upper ribs than the usual antero-posterior ones. The seventh cervical transverse process is identified by using the image intensifier and a skin wheal is raised 4 cm lateral to the mid-line (usually lateral to the spinous process of the sixth cervical vertebra). An 8 cm 20-gauge needle is inserted through the skin wheal and directed downwards and medially to make

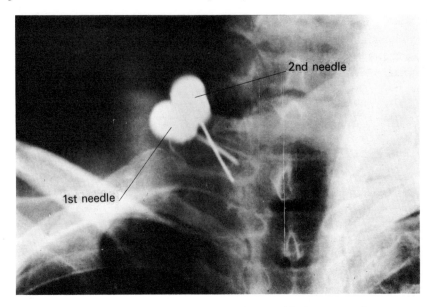

FIGURE 75. Second needle inserted lower. First left as a guide then removed.

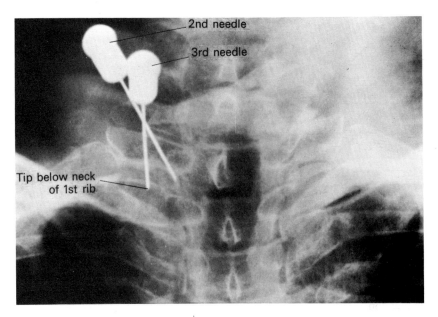

FIGURE 76. Third needle placed on lower edge of neck of first rib. (It tends to slip off but can be held on for the injection.)

contact with the upper border of the transverse process of the first thoracic vertebra and the neck of the first rib. This can be observed on the television screen and the progress of the needle point can be observed intermittently. Contact should be made and kept with these upper borders and when it is lost the needle is advanced a further 0·5 cm to place the tip anterior to the paravertebral fascia. If destruction of the stellate ganglion is not desired then the position of the needle tip is not critical (as long as it is anterior to the paravertebral fascia), and the anaesthetic solution can be injected in either a medial or lateral position along the transverse process, after carrying out the aspiration test for blood, cerebrospinal fluid, or air.

When destruction of the ganglion is required a test dose of 1–2 ml of 2 per cent Lignocaine is injected and only if an immediate Horner's syndrome develops is it followed up with not more than 3 ml dehydrated alcohol injected in divided doses. Alcohol produces a long-lasting block but 6 per cent Phenol in saline or water can be used without the same danger of neuritis developing. Repeated blocks with marcaine can be carried out on a daily basis for a week or so.

This particular block is useful where there is circulatory insufficiency in the arm and hand, producing pain and damage, and where there is pain carried over the sympathetic nerves as in sympathetic dystrophies. It is extremely useful in cases of long-standing angina after a preliminary diagnostic block has demonstrated that it is effective. Surprisingly it is also effective in early cases of coronary thrombosis when a left-sided diagnostic block may relieve the pain for a week or more. In fact in many cases recovery of cardiac function takes place in this time and pain does not recur. Blocks must not be carried out when a patient is on anti-coagulants.

Simultaneous bilateral stellate ganglion block is avoided in case bilateral recurrent laryngeal nerve palsy develops producing problems with respiration.

LUMBAR SYMPATHETIC CHAIN BLOCK

The lumbar sympathetic chain lies on the antero-lateral surface of the lumbar vertebrae. Theoretically there should be five ganglia but as the twelfth thoracic and first lumbar are usually joined, and as some of the remaining ones may join, three or four is the common number. Further, these ganglia do not have constant positions, and it is unlikely that the lumbar chains on either side are mirror images. The most constant ganglia is found in relation to the body of the second lumbar vertebra.

They lie medial to the origin of the psoas muscle, and anteriorly on the right side is the inferior vena cava. On the left side anteriorly is the aorta but this lies more medially so that it rarely actually covers the lumbar sympathetic chain. The sympathetic chains are covered by the retro-peritoneal fascia and thus there is a fascial compartment containing the lumbar sympathetic chain which is limited by the vertebral column, the psoas sheath, and the retro-peritoneal fascia. Anaesthetic solutions deposited in the compartment will travel up and down the chain having a wide effect (see Fig. 77). Two techniques for carrying out the lumbar sympathetic block are available.

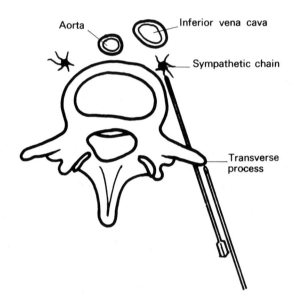

FIGURE 77. Lumbar sympathetic chain.

The first is when a single injection of anaesthetic solution is made. The patient lies in the lateral position with a pillow under the waist. This straightens out the spine and makes it easier to carry out the injection. A wheal is made lateral to the spinous process of L2 vertebra. The distance of this wheal from the mid-line is variable being from 5–8 cm, and depends on the personal preference of the operator and whether the transverse process is to be used as a landmark. At a distance of about 8 cm from the mid-line the distance to the transverse process is about 5 cm, and the distance to the lumbar chain is about twice this, i.e. a further 5 cm. In the method using the transverse process a skin wheal is made level with the upper border of the spinous process of the vertebra to be injected. This is usually level with the middle of the transverse process of the same side. First the needle is introduced and impinges on the transverse process. The depth marker is placed the same distance from the skin that the needle has already penetrated and is then inserted towards the antero-lateral border of the vertebra avoiding the transverse process until the marker is flush with the skin. If the needle hits the lateral border of the vertebra it is withdrawn and reinserted further laterally until it is felt to scrape past the vertebral body. In fact as the measurement is only approximate, the only certain way of placing the needle tip correctly is to feel the lateral border of the vertebral body and advance a little beyond that point.

The use of the image intensifier simplifies this block. The patient is placed in the position mentioned above, and also 'curled up'. The skin wheal is made between the upper borders of two adjacent spinous processes and a 20-gauge 12 cm, or longer, needle is inserted and directed to the desired position under intermittent X-ray vision. The transverse process can be avoided by this method or can be deliberately used to get some idea of the depth required. The antero-posterior X-ray view is used in the initial stage and gives a direction to the lateral surface of the vertebral body, later the lateral X-ray view is used to place the tip of the needle about 1 cm posterior to the observed anterior edge of the vertebral body (see Figs. 78 and 79). A test injection is made and there should be no resistance to the anaesthetic solution being injected. 15 ml of 2 per cent Lignocaine or $\frac{1}{2}$ per cent Marcaine will be sufficient to produce a complete block of the sympathetic chain. Some authorities advocate a much larger volume of solution to fill up the fascial compartment using 25-30 ml but for ordinary purposes 15 ml is sufficient.

However, when the block is being used to decide whether a surgical lumbar sympathectomy would be effective in relieving a deficient circulation this simple injection is not enough. In these circumstances electrical skin thermometers are placed on each leg at corresponding positions on thigh, calf, and foot. Both legs must be exposed to the air and not covered for fifteen or twenty minutes to allow for equilibrium to take place. The patient is in the lateral position ready for the block while the skin thermometers are reaching equilibrium. Three needles are inserted along the lumbar sympathetic chain at approximately the upper border of L2, the middle of L3, and the lower border of L4. These positions are not critical as long as they are spaced out. 5 ml of 2 per cent Lignocaine is injected into the upper one and the temperatures noted over a period of about five minutes, then 5 ml are injected into the middle one and the results noted, after a further five minutes the third one is injected. The first injection will produce a marked effect in the thigh, probably in the calf also, but if there is vascular

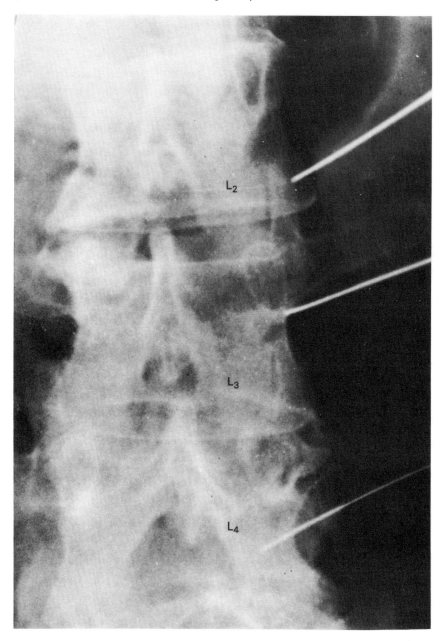

FIGURE 78. A–P X-ray view.

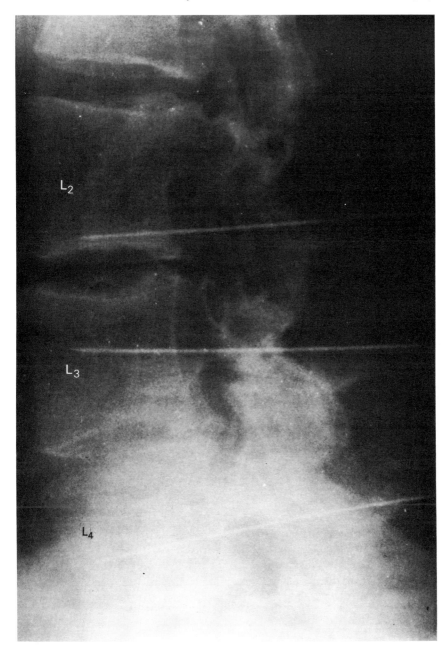

FIGURE 79. Lateral X-ray view.

disease there will be little, if any, temperature change in the foot. After the second injection there will be a further increase in the thigh or calf with a little more in the foot, but after the third there will be little added effect in the thigh and calf but there may well be an added increase of temperature in the foot. This increase will only be slight but it may make the difference between an amputation and retention of the limb. It is an indication for the surgeon to make an extremely thorough removal of the lumbar sympathetic chain.

If it is desired to have a prolonged test of lumbar sympathetic blockade then either a large bore needle is used and an epidural or other catheter threaded down it and used for intermittent injections to prolong the block, or after an initial small test injection to check that there is a temperature rise and that no somatic block is developing, an injection of 15 ml of 6 per cent Phenol in saline or water is made in divided doses. If necessary, this can be done on both sides but it must be remembered that 30 ml of 6 per cent Phenol is a large dose and can produce a methaemoglobinaemia.

Complications of this technique are rare and involve hypotension, intravascular injection, and haematoma. Painful sensations may be produced during insertion of the needle from stimulation of somatic nerves and these are more likely to be avoided if the insertion through the skin is made well laterally. Subarachnoid injection could occur through a fault in technique.

This block is most useful in peripheral vascular disease and in painful conditions of the lower limb. Its use in intermittent claudication is unlikely to help for any long period of time as the underlying vascular condition is progressive. If there is an operable narrowing in the vascular tree of the lower limb then this can be corrected, otherwise the lumbo-sacral block advocated by Feldman, mentioned later, should be used for the pain alone.

It should be remembered that there are somatic nerves running in the psoas sheath which may be affected by neurolytic agents and may develop a neuritis.

COELIAC PLEXUS BLOCK

The coeliac plexus is a large prevertebral plexus which is not a homogeneous structure but a number of loosely connected subsidiary ganglia. These are bilateral structures which interconnect to form the coeliac plexus which itself splits up into smaller distributive ganglia. In area it is quite large, about 4 cm by 3 cm, lying between the two adrenal glands in front of the body of L1 vertebra and extending upwards over part of T12. Behind the coeliac plexus lies the aorta centrally between the crura of the diaphragm and the coeliac ganglia; and anteriorly and to the right is the inferior vena cava and the right renal vessels (see Fig. 80). On the left is the pancreas and the left renal vessels. The plexus is surrounded by loose arealar tissue in which the local anaesthetic solution diffuses and spreads easily. Thus any injection made to affect this plexus must be made about 1 cm in front of the anterior border of the L1 vertebra, where it is dangerously close to large vessels. Anaesthesia of this plexus produces vasodilatation of the whole of the lower half of the body and the lower limbs and thus hypotension of a marked degree will result. It will also interrupt those afferent fibres from the upper

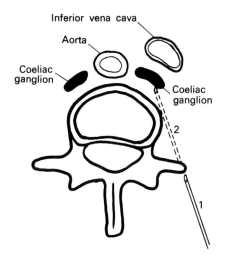

FIGURE 80. Coeliac ganglia.

abdominal viscera in particular which convey pain. It is commonly believed that a block of this plexus will not affect the afferent nerves from the pelvic organs but in practice it is worth carrying out a diagnostic block as it often helps.

The coeliac plexus block is particularly useful in the pain of chronic pancreatitis and for relieving pain in inoperable cancer of the upper abdominal organs, such as the liver, stomach, and spleen.

The technique of Bridenbough is the one most commonly used but there is no necessity for complicated methods when an image intensifier is available. The problem of carrying out a coeliac plexus block is related to the position of the twelfth rib (see Fig. 81). An injection made above this structure will penetrate the pleura, thus the position of the skin puncture depends on whether the twelfth ribs are set at narrow or wide angles to the vertebral column. In the former case, the insertion point is relatively close to the spinous processes (say 5 cm), while in the latter it can be perhaps twice this. There is an advantage in being as far lateral as possible as the needle tip can be placed more medially.

The position of the patient can be lateral or prone. The author prefers the prone position as a more effective block is produced if an injection is made from each side, and technically the prone position is easier for this. If possible the dorso–lumbar region should be flexed to open out the spinous processes. The position of the spine of the first lumbar vertebra is marked, as is that of both twelfth ribs. A 12 cm, 20-gauge needle is used or longer for large patients. A 22-gauge needle can be used for this block (and for that

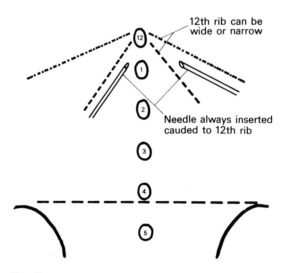

FIGURE 81. Twelfth rib.

of others mentioned) but the pressure required for the injection increases the longer and finer the needle used. At the length suggested a 20-gauge needle is reasonable and is also not as flexible as the 22-gauge one.

The skin wheal is raised 5 or 6 cm lateral to the upper border of the spinous process and the needle inserted through this. The direction is obtained by using the image intensifier and the tip is directed to the anterior border of the first lumbar vertebral body. There should be no difficulty in avoiding the transverse process of the first lumbar vertebra, but if there is the point of insertion should be altered. A preliminary view of the antero-posterior X-ray will also indicate how far from the mid-line the point of insertion should be to avoid penetration of the pleura. In most cases, this will mean that the plane of insertion will be below and parallel to the twelfth rib. The transverse process, depending on the angle of approach, is between 3 cm and 4 cm from the skin, and the antero-lateral portion of the vertebral body is about 5 cm beyond this. The coeliac plexus is about 1 cm further on, thus the needle will need to be inserted to a depth of about 10 cm. However, when using the image intensifier there is no need to guess the situation of the plexus as the lumbar vertebral body can be seen in the lateral view and after this direction is correct the antero-lateral view will show how far to direct the needle tip medially to slide past the lateral vertebral body wall. When the needle tip is advanced 1 cm anterior to the first lumbar vertebral body as shown in the lateral X-ray view, it will appear medial to the lateral vertebral body wall in the antero-lateral view (see Figs. 82 and 83).

This process is repeated on the other side and should be easier as the line of the second needle can be copied from the direction of the first.

If a diagnostic block is required then 10–15 ml of local anaesthetic solution is injected on each side, and if a prolonged block for some hours is required then 0·5 per cent Marcaine plain is the drug of choice. If the diagnostic block is to be followed by a semi-permanent block then small quantities, such as 5 ml of 2 per cent Lignocaine, are used and a wait of half an hour allows the local anaesthetic solution to be absorbed so that there will be little dilution. The solution used for the long-acting block is 25 ml of 50 per cent alcohol on each side injected in divided doses. This alcohol may cause pain not only in the abdomen but also in the shoulders due to diffusion on to the diaphragm. It may be necessary to cover the injection with intra-venous Diazepam (Valium) or a short-acting local anaesthetic. A minority of patients have little or no pain during the injection.

It is most important to carry out the aspiration test before injecting any solutions. The large vessels can be easily penetrated if the needle is inserted too far and apart from the danger of intravascular injection there is the danger of haematoma formation. Unless the needle is inserted far too deeply (which should not be done when the image intensifier is used) there should be no peritoneal injection. Local anaesthetic intraperitoneally is not painful but 50 per cent alcohol would produce severe and widespread pain. The other danger is of intradural injection and this also should be impossible using the image intensifier.

The principal complication in the coeliac plexus block is a prolonged hypotension. The vasoconstrictor fibres are blocked and postural hypo-tension results. The patient may have a profound fall in blood pressure on standing and is in great danger of fainting and falling. The older the patient the longer and more marked this complication is, though it will occur in

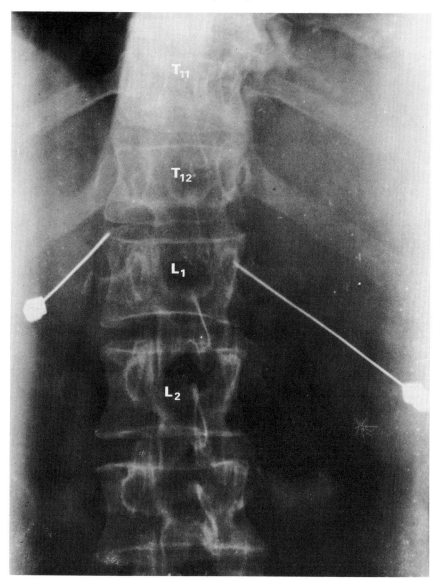

FIGURE 82. Antero-posterior X-ray view.

younger patients to some extent. The older patients may well feel dizzy
and faint merely on sitting up in bed.

It is wise, therefore, to take precautions after the coeliac plexus block to
mitigate the effects of hypotension. In this centre bilateral elastic stockings
are put on the patient routinely post-operatively. On return to the ward at

15-minute intervals for two hours the blood pressure is taken when lying flat, after sitting up for two minutes and, if these do not show a fall, after sitting up with the legs dependent over the edge of the bed for two minutes. If these are all normal nothing more is done until the following day when the process is repeated. If hypotension is absent or slight one elastic stocking is

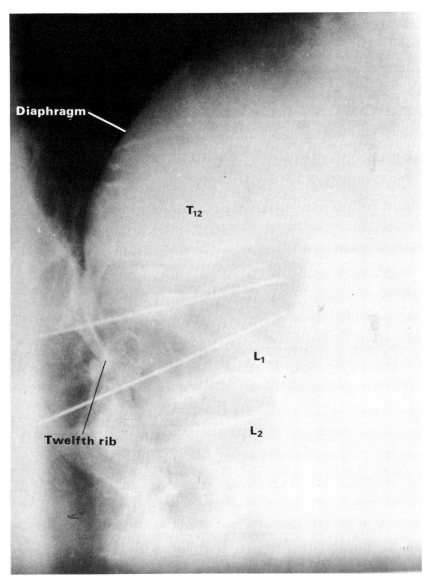

FIGURE 83. Lateral X-ray view. Both needles are 1 cm anterior to the L₁ vertebral body.

removed and the test repeated. If all is well the patient is allowed to walk about and if nothing untoward occurs the second stocking is removed.

If there is hypotension then the elastic stockings are left on and if it is marked then a tight abdominal binder is used as well. Oral vasoconstrictors such as Ephedrine can also be used. In time the hypotension becomes controlled by bodily adaptation and in most cases the constricting devices can be removed within a month or so. The younger patients below 45 adapt very rapidly, and the younger the quicker accordingly.

The indication for coeliac plexus block is in the relief of pain and this means principally the relief of the intractable pain of cancer.

TRIGEMINAL NERVE BLOCKS

These are carried out peripherally at branches (e.g. the infra-orbital) or at major trunks (such as the maxillary), or at the gasserian ganglion, or at the sensory root. The importance of the trigeminal nerve depends on it being the sensory nerve of the entire face except for the portion over the angle of the jaw which is supplied by the second cervical nerve. It is destroyed in the treatment of trigeminal neuralgia and the most satisfactory needle technique of treating this condition is by radio-frequency current heat coagulation of the sensory root. This method has been described elsewhere in this book. However, where this method is not available or when diagnostic blocks are required, methods of injecting the ganglion, or proximal or distal portions of the nerve are needed.

The anatomy of the trigeminal nerve is rather complicated in its intracranial portion. The sensory root arises from the bipolar cells in the gasserian ganglion and on entering the pons each fibre divides into an ascending and descending branch. The ascending fibre has its terminal nuclei in the upper sensory nucleus which lies in the dorsal part of the pons close to the trigeminal motor nucleus. The descending fibres terminate in the lower sensory nucleus which is an upward prolongation of the substantia gelatinosa. This nucleus can be traced as low as the level of the second cervical nerve. The descending sensory fibres, which constitute the spinal root of the trigeminal nerve, accompany the lower sensory nucleus terminating in it at difference levels. The arrangement of the fibres and cells in the spinal root is reversed and those associated with the ophthalmic region are at the lowest part of the root. Above these lie the maxillary fibres and highest of all the mandibular ones.

The trigeminal or gasserian ganglion lies in the gasserian impression on the upper part of the petrous temporal bone near the apex. It is semilunar in shape being convex in front and concave behind and measures about 1·25 cm antero-posteriorly. The sensory root becomes expanded at the posterior concave surface of the ganglion and its fibres become separated into fasciculi. The gasserian ganglion is invaginated into the dura in such a way that the anterior portion is closely covered by dura mater while the posterior part is in a recess of this covering called Meckel's cave. Medially is the cavernous sinus, and medially and inferiorly is the carotid artery. The small motor root is on the deep surface of the ganglion but remains separate. The motor root passes out through the foramen ovale where it joins the third division of the trigeminal nerve, the mandibular nerve.

The divisions of the gasserian ganglion are three and they arise from the anterior convex border. The upper first division, the ophthalmic, is the smallest. It lies in the outer wall of the cavernous sinus, and divides into its constituent branches as it approaches the superior orbital fissure.

The second division, the maxillary, arises below the first, and lies in the lateral wall of the cavernous sinus below the first division and after passing forward a short distance enters the foramen rotundum and the pterygo-palatine fossa.

The mandibular nerve is the third division and is the largest. It passes downwards into the foramen ovale.

Each of these three divisions provides the sensory fibres to a definite area of the face. The ophthalmic nerve supplies branches to the con-junctiva, lacrymal gland, and skin near the lateral canthus by means of the lacrimal nerve; to the mucous membrane of some of the anterior portion of the nasal cavity and to the skin of the nose; and by the supraorbital and supra-trochlear nerves the skin of the upper eyelid and forehead.

The maxillary nerve gives off various branches which supply the mucous membrane of the posterior and inferior portion of the nasal cavity, the upper molar teeth, the hard palate, and adjacent gum. The infra-orbital nerve supplies the anterior teeth and gums of the upper jaw and the area of skin between palpebral fissure, the side of the nose, and a line joining the lateral canthus of the eye and the corner of the mouth.

The mandibular nerve is a mixed nerve unlike the other two, which are entirely sensory. The motor root supplies all the muscles of mastication, while the sensory portion supplies the anterior two-thirds of the tongue, the mucous membrane of the oral cavity not already supplied by the second division, most of the temporal region and the skin over the mandible, and the mental region. It supplies the lower teeth. As previously mentioned there is a corner of the jaw of variable area supplied by C_2.

MANDIBULAR NERVE BLOCK

The mandibular nerve block can be approached from a number of directions, the most straightforward being through the foramen ovale. The most direct of these is by the same anterior approach that is used for the gasserian ganglion block except that the needle remains just in or outside the foramen so that only the mandibular division is anaesthetised. This will be discussed when the gasserian ganglion block is described. The lateral approach is the simplest of the approaches to the mandibular nerve, the needle being inserted from a lateral approach below the zygoma. From this aspect the foramen ovale faces slightly forward and slightly laterally, though the main direction is downwards (see Fig. 83*a*). This means that it is possible to insert the needle through the foramen ovale into the gasserian ganglion and

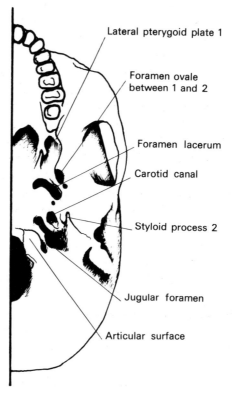

Lateral pterygoid plate 1

Foramen ovale
between 1 and 2

Foramen lacerum

Carotid canal

Styloid process 2

Jugular foramen

Articular surface

FIGURE 83*a*. Base of skull.

this is one of the techniques of performing the gasserian ganglion block that can be adopted. The expertise for the anterior gasserian ganglion block is more easily acquired as it is a more direct approach.

The lateral approach is made through a wheal raised under the mid-point of the zygomatic arch and a 8 cm 20- or 22-gauge needle with a depth marker is inserted perpendicular to the skin until it touches the lateral pterygoid plate at about 4 cm depth. A lateral X-ray view of the skull will facilitate this but recognising the various structures on the X-ray film requires some experience. If the needle tip does not touch the lateral pterygoid plate within 5 cm the needle is withdrawn and the direction changed. When contact is made the marker is set 1 cm from the skin and reinserted 1 cm posterior to the point of contact. The aim is to place the tip of the needle just below the foramen ovale, and at 5 cm depth paraesthesiae are often produced but by no means always. If a diagnostic block is required then 2–5 ml of 2 per cent Lignocaine can be injected and will produce a satisfactory block without previous paraesthesiae. If a semi–permanent block is needed with say pure alcohol, then paraesthesiae should be produced. If they are not produced then 1–2 ml of anaesthetic solution is injected and if good anaesthesia of the mandibular division alone develops then the injection of alcohol (2 ml or so) can go ahead. It is always necessary to perform a test block with local anaesthetic before the alcohol is injected in case the needle has entered the foramen ovale. Even if the needle has not penetrated as far as the ganglion alcohol may track up or around the mandibular nerve to it. If the needle is inserted 5·5 cm and no paraesthesiae have been obtained it should be withdrawn and another direction used.

Shortly below the skull the mandibular nerve splits up into its various branches. The three main sensory nerves are from before backwards, the long buccal nerve, the lingual nerve, and the inferior alveolar nerve. If paraesthesiae are obtained when the needle tip is not close to the skull some indication is given for the change in direction of the next insertion by the paraesthesiae produced—cheek, tongue, or lower jaw. Even when the needle tip penetrates the mandibular nerve trunk the paraesthesiae that are produced will be in one or other of these areas. If facilities are available for base of skull films taken in the submento-vertical position, the needle will be seen overlying or near the foramen ovale, and some idea of direction and depth can be obtained from this and from the lateral film (see Fig. 7). In the older patient extension of the head may be difficult and the full position may be impossible. The problem is that the lower jaw may cover the foramen ovale when there is not enough extension.

The complications of this block are common to all injections using this approach and are few in number. Haemorrhage shown by a haematoma is the most common but is not usually of any size in the mandibular block. If the needle is inserted too far posteriorly it may penetrate the Eustachian tube and the patient may report that there is pain in the ear. If a little local anaesthetic solution is injected some of the fluid will find its way into the mouth.

The indications for block of the mandibular nerve are for malignant conditions of the lower jaw and anterior tongue when pain is a feature; for diagnostic blocks when there is uncertainty as to the origin of pain; and in trigeminal neuralgia when pain is confined to all or part of the lower division.

MAXILLARY NERVE BLOCK

The approach advocated is essentially the same as that of the mandibular nerve. A wheal is made below the mid point of the zygomatic arch and the 8 cm 20- or 22-gauge needle inserted perpendicular to the skin until it touches the lateral pterygoid plate at about 4 cm depth. The depth marker is moved to 1 cm from the skin and the needle is withdrawn and reinserted 1 cm anterior and 1 cm above the first point of contact. This should place the needle point within the pterygopalatine fossa in close proximity to the maxillary nerve, its branches and the sphenopalatine ganglion. 2–4 ml of 2 per cent Lignocaine are injected and should produce anaesthesia in the second division of the trigeminal nerve.

As in the mandibular block when alcohol is to be used, paraesthesiae are necessary as the pterygopalatine fossa is close to the orbit. When carrying out this block the depth of needle insertion must be observed closely and this is most easily done by antero-posterior X-ray views seen on the image intensifier television screen. It is worthwhile moving the head into a little extension and then flexion to obtain the best position where the foramen rotundum can be seen clearly below the inner end of the inferior border of the orbit. Owing to the different levels of the foramen rotundum and the foramen ovale at the base of the skull and to the fairly solid bone masking the foramen ovale this antero-posterior view is of more value in the maxillary block than in the mandibular.

The anatomy of the pterygopalatine fossa is straightforward in that medially and above it at right angles lies the infraorbital fissure which leads into the orbit. Laterally is the pterygomaxillary fissure which opens into the infratemporal fossa. If the subzygomatic needle is inserted too deeply it can be very close to the infraorbital fissure and large volume injections may produce temporary proptosis. Similarly haemorrhage from the maxillary artery may produce the same result from a haematoma. Rarely there are bony abnormalities of this region making it impossible to place a needle in the correct position.

The indications for this block are the same as for the mandibular nerve except the areas of reference are to the maxillary nerve distribution.

GASSERIAN GANGLION BLOCK

The method of Härtel is the one recommended. It can be used for the mandibular nerve, for the gasserian ganglion, and for the trigeminal nerve roots. It makes use of the fact that the exit of the mandibular division of the trigeminal nerve, from the base of the skull is through a relatively large foramen. This foramen, the foramen ovale, is in constant position about 4·5 cm medial to the tubercle of the zygoma, and about 7 cm posterior to the pupil.

It is oval in shape with average diameters of about 8 mm and 4 mm. It is situated with the anterior pole more medially than the posterior. Behind it, in the same antero-posterior line, lies the foramen spinosum. This is a small round foramen and its position is constant so that the combination of the oval foramen ovale and the round foramen spinosum posterior to it, is an obvious feature seen in the base of skull X-ray. Anterior to the foramen ovale on the base of skull is the infra-temporal surface of the greater wing of the sphenoid bone. This surface is quite smooth and when a needle (inserted from the direction to be described shortly) hits this infra-temporal plate it can be felt as smooth. Posterior to the foramen ovale is the petrous portion of the temporal bone which is rough. This roughness can also be appreciated by the needle tip impinging on it. Thus with experience it is possible to appreciate whether the needle tip is anterior or posterior to the foramen without the use of check X-rays. Once again the author feels that the use of X-rays is of such benefit to accuracy that it should be used when available.

The image intensifier can be used satisfactorily in the lateral view but the penetration needed for the basal view is not at present available on these machines. A larger fixed machine has to be used and a skull table is an added advantage. Although there are two commonly used positions for carrying out the gasserian ganglion block, each operator usually develops their own variation. The first is with the patient in the sitting position and, in fact, some operators have the patient in a dental chair. There are advantages in this position as the height of the patient can be altered very easily, and it is possible to get a good 'sight' along the needle which is an advantage in choosing the correct direction. If X-rays are to be used in this position then special arrangements have to be made owing to the height at which the apparatus must work. The second position is the supine one and this is not as good for directing the needle along the correct line, but it is easier to use an image intensifier in the lateral view and to obtain the base view with other apparatus. The author advocates the supine position.

Certain skin markings are made with a skin pencil. These are:

(1) A curved line along the lower border of the zygoma. Cross lines are marked on this at the mid point of the zygomatic arch, and over the zygomatic tubercle which is just anterior to the articular surface of the temporo-mandibular joint. The line between the zygomatic tubercles passes through the foramen ovale, the line between the mid zygomatic points passes through the infra-temporal plates.

(2) Another line is drawn from the angle of the mouth posteriorly. A cross line is placed on this at the level of the second molar tooth, or 3 cm posteriorly to the corner, or a line is dropped from the lateral edge of the bony orbit on to it. All these various methods will give the same final position approximately. The skin wheal is raised at this junction point some 3 cm lateral to the corner of the mouth so that the needle direction is taken from this position. Two further lines are therefore drawn in before the block proper is carried out.

(3) One starts at the skin wheal position and is drawn on the face towards the pupil when the patient is gazing straight ahead.

(4) The second is usually drawn from the skin wheal to the mid point of the zygoma but as will be seen later the author uses instead a line drawn to the tubercle of the zygoma (see Fig. 84).

There are 'trigeminal needles' which are commercially available. They are about 10 cm long and are marked at 1-cm intervals and are reasonably stiff being about 18-gauge. There is an advantage in having a stiff needle as if it is held up on the edge of the foramen ovale its tip can be moved easily because of its rigidity. The author uses a 20-gauge disposable spinal needle in most straightforward cases and altering position usually means with-drawing it to the skin and reinsertion. It is possible with these fine, flexible needles to get a small amount of movement at the tip by pressing firmly on the shaft at skin level and moving it in and out rapidly a few millimetres with the other. These finer needles are not marked in centimetres.

The trigeminal needles are often used time after time and will be resharpened and therefore shortened. Before using them it is wise to count the number of markings and to observe whether the terminal section is a full centimetre long or only a portion. It is useful to have some idea of depth when carrying out the block and the markings are used for this purpose. Alternatively, the shaft length is measured with a rule beforehand.

Normally, the needle is inserted through the skin wheal and inserted so that when viewed from in front of the patient the needle is directed towards the pupil, and from the lateral view is directed towards the mid zygomatic point. The direction is thus upwards, medially and posteriorly. Insertion on this line will contact the infra-temporal plate (see Fig. 84). The distance inserted is variable depending on the exact point of penetration of the skin (this is not critical) and whether, for instance, the skull shape is dolicocephalic and prognathaus, but it should be measured and noted. This distance is usually given as 5 cm but experience has shown it to vary up to 7 cm. The depth marker, if used, is now set 1·5 cm from the skin and the needle is withdrawn to the superficial tissues and reinserted a little more posteriorly so that its point will pass through the foramen ovale. It is not easy to redirect a needle in this fashion.

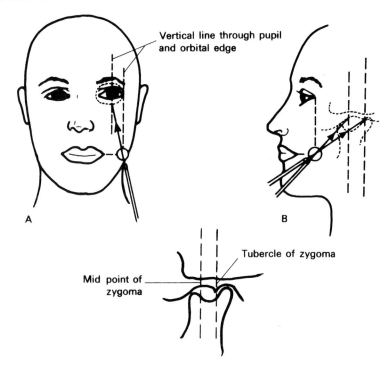

FIGURE 84. Skin markings for gasserian ganglion block.

A long needle seems to have a will of its own and to some extent the bevelled edge of the tip acts in the same way which ensures that the wedged end of a wood chisel moves in the direction of the wedge. Use can be made of this characteristic by turning the bevel. Repeated withdrawals and insertions must be made in this fashion until the foramen is entered. Damage to the vessels of the soft tissues is likely and haematoma formation can occur and can be massive. Paraesthesiae are often obtained when the needle passes through the foramen but the foramen is so large that it is possible to insert the needle through it without hitting the nerve. The needle is inserted up to the marker or its equivalent.

The above method does not make use of X-rays. Using the image intensifier in the lateral view is awkward as it is a cumbersome piece of equipment which gets in the way. The author's technique involves using a finer needle inserting it as above and aiming it directly at the foramen. In other words, looking at the needle from in front, it is directed to the pupil but in the lateral view is directed to the tubercle of the zygoma. The needle is inserted not more than 6·5 cm or stops when bone is touched. Lateral and base of skull X-rays are taken at this point and developed with rapid techniques. They are ready for viewing in a few minutes and then redirection as necessary is made. Using this method avoids the guesswork of deciding in which direction to alter the needle after the first insertion, and even avoids deciding whether the needle tip lies anterior against a smooth portion of bone or posterior against rough—a decision not easy without considerable experience.

The directions usually given to place the needle tip in the gasserian ganglion vary. For instance, when destruction of the first division or the first and second divisions is required a placement in the ganglion amongst these fibres is more likely when the needle tip is more medial than in the usual position obtained by aiming at the centre of the pupil. Thus, to obtain the upper division the insertion of the needle can be made 1·0 cm more laterally and the direction is to the inner canthus of the eye. So, an insertion made through the centre of the foramen ovale tends to be in the second and third divisions. An insertion through the lateral portion of the foramen tends to be in the third division or misses the ganglion entirely, while the insertion point is made nearer to the corner of the mouth.

The X-ray appearance of the two foramen ovales may be quite different, one having a less well-defined edge than the other. Sometimes improvement is made by another X-ray plate exposure with the head in a slightly different position but there may be a real difference in the bony contours of the two sides.

Very occasionally there is a bony ridge anterior to the front of the foramen which prevents the needle entering the foramen. It is not so much that it is impossible to enter the foramen as that the needle has to enter along a track which avoids the anterior edge altogether. The problem being that the ridge is part of the anterior edge itself. It may be necessary to change the usual point of entry of the needle through the skin.

Sometimes the foramen ovale which traverses the thickness of the bone at the base of the skull and is therefore about 5 mm long, is not a perfectly smooth canal. It may have a spur projecting into it, or there may be a narrow-ing of the canal at the outer end. This will mean that the needle is unable to penetrate through it into the deeper parts.

In this circumstance, an injection made at this point will certainly produce a mandibular nerve block, but occasionally the solution may track through the bony canal to the ganglion. It may track along the nerve tissue itself if the injection is made into the substance of the nerve and, in this way, not only will a mandibular block occur but a second division block as well.

There may be destruction of bone in the region of the foramen ovale from malignant processes, or there may be distortion of bone from such conditions as Paget's disease of bone. Trigeminal neuralgia is not uncommon in the latter bony condition and bulges and bosses on the bone may make it difficult to approach the foramen in the direction described above. As it is difficult to carry out surgical section of the nerve roots under these conditions because of gross haemorrhage from thickened vascular bone, any approach through the foramen that is available may need to be used. For instance, a needle can be inserted (under general anaesthesia) through the skin of the submental region and successively through the tongue and soft tissues of the mouth. Despite gross deformities of bone an approach can be found.

There are three blocks of peripheral branches of the trigeminal nerve that are often used. These are the supraorbital nerve; the infraorbital nerve; and the inferior dental nerve. There is a fourth that is always mentioned in textbooks, and that is the mental nerve block through the mental foramen but this is very rarely used in the Pain Relief Centre (I have seen it used once, but have never used it myself). It is a block that is used very regularly in dental practice.

THE SUPRAORBITAL NERVE

The supraorbital nerve and the supratrochlear nerve are terminal branches of the frontal nerve, which is one of the branches of the maxillary division. The supraorbital nerve usually divides into two branches after it reaches the edge of the orbit forming a medial and a lateral branch. It emerges over the superior edge of the orbit and can often be felt in or near the superior orbital notch, which is about 2·5 cm from the mid-line. Sometimes the superior orbital nerve divides into its two branches before it reaches the edge of the orbit and of the two, the lateral branch is the larger. The supra-trochlear nerve is medial to the supraorbital and lies at the superior medial angle of the orbit.

These two nerves supply the skin over the fronto-parietal region of the forehead and of the adjacent scalp.

Blocking these two nerves is very simple as the supratrochlear can be found at the angle between the upper and medial borders of the orbit, the injection being made at the adjacent root of the nose.

The supraorbital nerve is found at or near the supraorbital notch and an injection is made directly or in the vicinity of the notch. These methods are quite satisfactory when a diagnostic block is required, but if a permanent block with, say, alcohol is to be made then a fine 25-gauge needle is used to search for the nerves. Injection is not made until paraesthesiae are obtained. The amount of local anaesthetic solution needed is quite small for a direct injection—of the order of 0·25 ml. When a diagnostic block is made only 1–2 ml is required. Even small amounts such as these will produce oedema and swelling of the upper eyelid, and the patient should be warned about this. Swelling may be so great that it will be impossible to open the eye for several hours.

This block is useful to remove trigger zones in trigeminal neuralgia and in post-herpetic neuralgia.

THE INFRAORBITAL NERVE

This nerve is the continuation of the maxillary division and emerges on the face through the infraorbital foramen. There are two methods of blocking this nerve, the external and internal approach. The internal approach is the one normally used by dental surgeons but it is made through the mucosa of the mouth and therefore is potentially dangerous from the point of view of carrying infection into the deeper tissues. Many thousands of these injections are made in dental practice every day without infection resulting, so infection must be a remote occurrence.

The author uses the extraoral route exclusively (see Figs. 85 and 86). In this method a small 23-gauge, 2·5 cm needle is manœuvred about 1·5 cm inside the infraorbital canal. An injection of a 0·5 ml 2 per cent Lignocaine will produce anaesthesia in the infraorbital distribution. When a permanent block is required this injection is followed by 1–2 ml of absolute alcohol. When the nerve is not completely anaesthetised first there may be a severe but brief pain from the alcohol.

The special problems when injecting this nerve within the bony canal are: that the nerve can be damaged by pressure; that there may be intra-vascular injection through the corresponding artery or vein; that when the wall of the canal is not closed by bone between it and the maxillary antrum this can be penetrated and the injection made into the antrum.

The technique of this injection depends on the stoma of the infraorbital canal being found. This is 1–1·5 cm below the inferior orbital ridge and 3 cm from the mid-line, and can be palpated sometimes through the skin. Occasionally it is the nerve branches issuing from the foramen which can be felt. The direction of the canal is inwards and downwards and therefore any needle inserted into it will be directed upwards and outwards. The infra-orbital foramen is just above the canine fossa, and the angle of descent of the canal is about 45°. The point of insertion of the needle must allow for this angle and is about 1 cm lateral to the ala nasi which is about 2·5 cm from the mid-line (see Fig. 86). This point of insertion is usually shown in diagrams

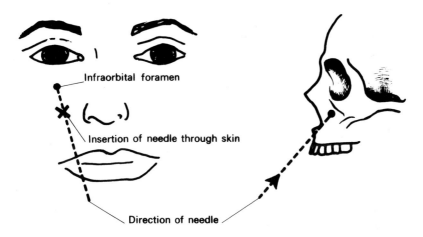

Infraorbital foramen

Insertion of needle through skin

Direction of needle

FIGURE 85. Infraorbital block.

as level with the lowest edge of the ala, and this is satisfactory if a diagnostic block is made at, or near, the orifice with a diffusible local anaesthetic. Entry into the orifice and on into the canal is easier if the insertion is made a little higher than this, at a mid position between the lower and upper edges of the ala. After insertion through the skin a search is made for the foramen aiming upwards and outwards and towards a point about 2 cm posterior to the inferior edge of the orbit. The slight hollow which is the foramen can often be found by using a search pattern over the small area of bone where it should be. At this position the patient will often describe paraesthesiae, and the needle is tried at different angles until it slips in. It should be inserted no more than 0·75 cm and the injection made as above. When alcohol is to be used it is wise to carry out a preliminary injection of local

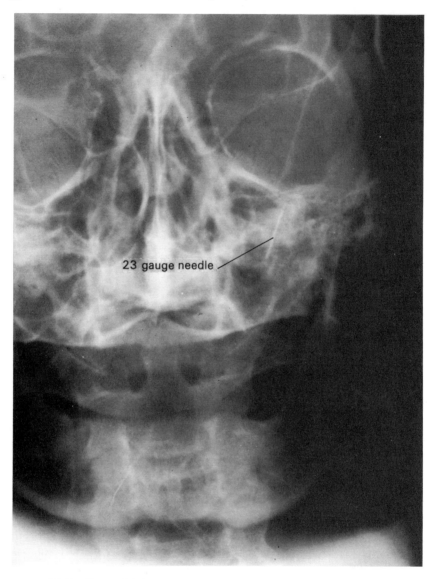

FIGURE 86. Needle in left infraorbital canal.

anaesthetic and test ocular movements and the presence of diplopia, as the
solution may track back into the orbit. The roof of the canal is deficient
posteriorly but may be absent over a longer stretch than normal anteriorly
and injection into the orbit may be easier than expected. Occasionally the
infraorbital canal is stenosed, or there may be multiple small foramina, and

if the canal cannot be entered then anaesthetic solution or alcohol can be deposited at the foraminal opening on the maxillary surface.

Trigeminal neuralgia is often present in the second division and usually has trigger points which are blocked off by this injection. The trigger points are commonly at the side of the nose, on the upper lip, or in the upper teeth. When the painful portion of the second division is more lateral than the infraorbital distribution an infraorbital block may not relieve the trigeminal neuralgia but a diagnostic block will make this clear.

THE INFERIOR DENTAL NERVE BLOCK

This is most commonly used in dental practice. The inferior dental nerve, sometimes called the inferior alveolar nerve, enters the bone of the lower jaw through the mandibular foramen. This is on the medial aspect of the ramus of the mandible, midway between the anterior and posterior borders of the ascending ramus and about 1 cm above the occlusal surface of the last molar tooth.

Various complicated methods of performing this block are described involving a 10-cm needle and 5-ml syringe, though a dental syringe is much handier and simpler to use in the normal oral approach. Behind the last molar tooth is a small triangular area and the initial insertion of the needle impinges on this area not more than 1 cm above the last molar tooth. The direction of the syringe and needle is such that it lies over the canine and first premolar tooth of the opposite side. It is then swung laterally parallel to the teeth on the side to be injected and inserted further until it slips off the bone medially to the ramus. It is then swung back again and inserted until the point lies approximately halfway between the two borders of the mandible (see Fig. 87). An injection of 2–3 ml of 2 per cent Lignocaine will give anaesthesia to all the lower teeth and mental region. Depending on how much solution diffuses on the lingual nerve, will decide whether or not the anterior two-thirds of the tongue is affected as well.

A simpler method is to place the thumb of the operator on the triangular area, the index finger behind the ramus of the mandible, and the remaining fingers resting on the angle of the jaw, or thereabouts. The syringe approaches from the direction of the incisor teeth and is inserted so that it finishes up midway between the thumb and first finger and 1 cm above the last molar tooth. The injection is made as before.

There is a very useful extra-oral approach which depends on the mandibular foramen being midway between the tip of the coronoid process and the angle of the mandible. This distance is measured and a marker placed on the needle at half this distance. The skin inferior and medial to the angle of the jaw is anaesthetised and the needle is inserted vertically upwards towards the coronoid process keeping close to bone. Whether or not paraesthesiae are obtained 2–3 ml of 2 per cent Lignocaine is injected. This

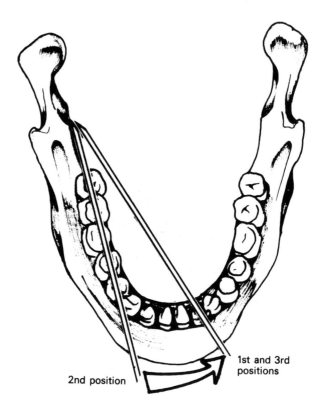

FIGURE 87. Inferior dental nerve block.

is a useful block when pain produces a trismus of the lower jaw, and also when intra-oral infection or an inability to open the mouth wide is present.

When a patient has trigeminal neuralgia confined to the lower jaw the simplest method of dealing with it actively is with a block of the inferior dental nerve. If alcohol is to be used at the mandibular foramen paraesthesiae must be obtained before the injection of alcohol. This procedure seems straightforward but in practice is difficult to put into effect.

BRACHIAL PLEXUS BLOCK

The brachial plexus is formed by the anterior primary rami of the 5th, 6th, 7th, 8th cervical, and 1st thoracic nerves, often receiving in addition, a small branch from cervical 4 and thoracic 2. It supplies all the motor and carries most of the sensation from the upper limb.

The various portions of the brachial plexus unite and separate in a complicated fashion. Between the anterior and middle scalene muscles, the anterior primary divisions of the nerves mentioned unite to form three trunks. The primary divisions of cervical 5 and 6 form the upper trunk, the

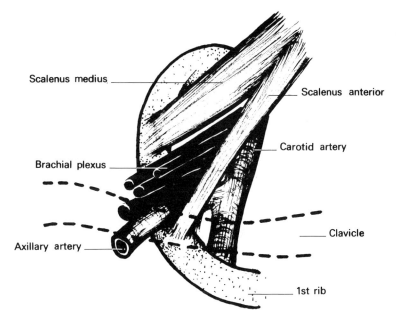

Scalenus medius

Scalenus anterior

Carotid artery

Brachial plexus

Clavicle

Axillary artery

1st rib

FIGURE 88. The brachial plexus anatomy (above first rib).

7th cervical nerve forms the middle trunk and the 8th cervical and 1st thoracic form the lower trunk.

These three trunks emerge from the lower and lateral border of the scalene muscles and continue antero-laterally and inferiorly until they lie on the upper border of the first rib lateral to the subclavian artery. At this point they are grouped very closely together and a single injection can block the whole plexus (see Fig. 88).

It should be particularly noted that the first rib descends so that its direction is from postero-superiorly to antero-inferiorly, running more or less up and down behind the clavicle with its anterior surface facing forwards.

At the lateral edge of the first rib each of the trunks divide into an anterior and posterior division and these pass underneath the clavicle and enter the axilla at its apex. The divisions unite again within the axilla to form three cords which are in relation to the axillary artery. The lateral cord formed by the anterior divisions of the upper and middle trunks contains fibres from the 5th, 6th, and 7th cervical nerves. The medial cord which is the continuation of the anterior division of the lower trunk contains fibres from the 8th cervical and 1st thoracic nerves. The posterior cord is formed from all the posterior divisions and thus has fibres from all the nerves involved in the brachial plexus.

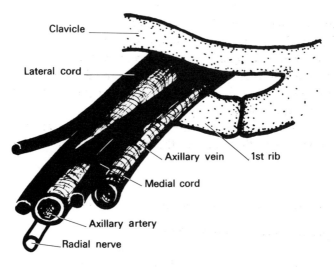

FIGURE 89. The brachial plexus anatomy (lateral to first rib).

It should be noted that there is a fascial compartment extending from the anterior and middle scalene muscles laterally which encloses the brachial plexus and the subclavian artery and local anaesthetic deposited in this relatively small compartment will anaesthetise the whole of the brachial plexus (see Fig. 89).

There are thus two methods of carrying out a brachial plexus block. First, there is the supra-clavicular method and secondly, the axillary approach.

The supra-clavicular brachial plexus block

The patient lies on his back with the head turned to the other side, a skin wheal being raised 1 cm above and lateral to the mid-point of the clavicle.

In thin individuals the first rib can often be palpated and the subclavian artery can always be felt pulsing. The brachial plexus is just lateral to the subclavian artery.

A 5 cm 20-gauge needle is inserted through the wheal and directed 1 cm lateral to the subclavian artery. It is important to contact the first rib which is quite superficial in the average patient at this level and the needle should not be pushed further on or the pleura may be penetrated.

As soon as the first rib is contacted and if paraesthesiae down the arm are obtained, then without moving the needle the aspiration test is performed and if negative 10 ml of 2 per cent Lignocaine is injected.

If paraesthesiae are not obtained then a search for the brachial plexus is made by 'walking' the needle along the first rib, bearing in mind that the direction of the first rib is antero-posteriorly facing the operator. Each time the first rib is contacted, a fan-wise injection of local solution is made as the needle is withdrawn. If only sensory block is required, then 1 or 1·5 per cent Lignocaine can be used but if motor block is required then 2 per cent Lignocaine should be used.

At this level the nerves have rather thick sheaths and are bulky structures and it will take a little time for the effect of the local anaesthetic to be produced.

Axillary approach, brachial plexus block

The only nerve which is not blocked by this approach to the brachial plexus is the musculo-cutaneous nerve which often leaves the brachial plexus high up in the axillary fossa. It may be left out of this brachial plexus block. It supplies sensory fibres to the radial portion of the forearm.

The patient lies on his back with the arm abducted at 90°. The axillary artery is palpated and a 5 cm 20-gauge needle inserted through the skin towards and slightly above the artery. It should be noted that at this point the plexus lies quite superficially around the artery and too deep an injection causes failure of the block.

Gentle care should be taken with this particular insertion of the needle as haematoma formation within the sheath may prevent good anaesthesia.

When the needle vibrates showing pulsation transmitted from the artery, it lies within the fascial compartment. The anaesthetic solution is then injected after the aspiration test, 20 ml of 1·5 per cent or 2 per cent Lignocaine can be injected and the dose is adjusted for size with larger males receiving 25–30 ml.

It is an advantage to place a tourniquet below the point of injection to block off the fascial compartment at this point so that the injected solution must spread upwards towards the scalene muscles.

Production of the block takes longer with this method than with the supra-clavicular technique and may take up to half an hour in adults.

The one great advantage of this particular technique is that there is no danger of pneumothorax.

SPINAL NERVE BLOCK

One of the most convenient places to block a spinal nerve is as it leaves the bony spine through the spinal foramina. The techniques of carrying this out are slightly different at the various spinal levels. Cervical, dorsal, lumbar, and sacral blocks are regularly used in the Centre for Pain Relief and are discussed in some detail here. It is seldom necessary to block a wide area in the pain clinic, usually a block of a few nerves in succession will resolve the problem of which nerves are transmitting painful stimuli. This, for instance, is why the C2 nerve block is mentioned separately from the cervical paravertebral block.

There are eight pairs of cervical nerves with the first emerging above the first vertebra and the eighth below the seventh vertebra. Each gives off a small meningeal branch, lies behind the vertebral artery, and divides into a posterior and anterior primary rami. The first does not divide in this fashion but remains as one motor nerve distributed to the muscles of the sub-occipital triangle. The posterior primary rami divides into medial sensory and lateral motor branches. The medial branches supply the skin of the posterior part of the neck and occipital scalp. The medial branches from the second and third nerves form the greater occipital nerve and the third occipital nerve. The lateral branches of the posterior primary rami supply the muscles of the posterior neck. The anterior primary divisions of the upper four cervical nerves form the cervical plexus, the lower four form the brachial plexus to which the 1st thoracic contributes.

Just lateral to the foramina the nerve and primary divisions lie posterior to the vertebral artery. They lie in a groove in the transverse processes which have anterior and posterior tubercles. The posterior tubercle is larger than the anterior, and thus it is easier to approach the nerves laterally than from a posterior approach. Also it is best to direct the injecting needle downwards on to the transverse processes as the needle cannot easily enter the theca with this approach.

CERVICAL PLEXUS BLOCK

The deep cervical plexus block is carried out paravertebrally using either the lateral or posterior approaches. For the reasons given above the lateral approach is best unless tumour tissue or an abcess is present.

The patient is supine and the head is placed a little posterior by a small pillow under the shoulders. The head is turned to the opposite side which throws the transverse processes into prominence. A line is drawn along them from the prominent sixth transverse process (Chassaignac's) to the mastoid process. The second transverse process is 1·5 cm below (caudad to) the mastoid process on this line, or slightly posterior to it. Even in thin people there may be difficulty in palpating this transverse process, the lower ones are not as difficult.

A wheal is made at this point with local anaesthetic and at two further points each 1·5 cm below the one above, and each on the line. These cover the third and fourth transverse processes. A fine 5-cm needle is inserted through each wheal and should contact the transverse process at a depth of about 3 cm. Paraesthesiae may be obtained. If bone is not contacted the needle should not be advanced to a depth of more than 4 cm or it may penetrate the vertebral artery or the subarachnoid space. Insertion of the needle slightly higher (cephalad) on the line than the distances mentioned will ensure that the approach is downwards and therefore safer. When all three needles are inserted they should be in line. The aspiration test is carried out and 2–3 ml of 2 per cent Lignocaine is injected down each. It is possible to feel the needle tip on the transverse process by moving it slightly.

Most of the difficulty in positioning the needles on the transverse processes can be obviated by using the image intensifier. This is particularly true when a C2 nerve block alone is to be made for pain in the occipital distribution. A preliminary diagnostic block is made and followed by alcohol. Paraesthesiae are a great help and they should be sought out.

In all cases when positioning the needles on the transverse processes, but particularly in the case of the C2 transverse process, parallax can be used. The image intensifier head starts in the lateral position but is moved in a small arc anteriorly and posteriorly round the neck while the position of the tip of the needle is seen on the television X-ray screen. Only when the needle actually rests on the transverse process will there be no gap between it and the transverse process in all positions. This is a very simple check to make.

The cervical plexus block produces anaesthesia of the occipital region, the neck and the 'cape' area. Complications are often due to intra-vascular injection, the neck having many large vessels. The most likely intravascular injection is into the vertebral artery and if small quantities are injected into it the patient will complain of dizziness. If the injection is of more than 1 or 2 ml unconsciousness results and lasts about five minutes. Oxygen and artificial support to the respirations will be required for this length of time until the large normal blood flow re-distributes the local anaesthetic.

The phrenic nerve normally takes its roots from C3, C4, and C5 and paralysis of the diaphragm on one side may result from diffusion of the solution. Similarly the recurrent laryngeal nerve can be affected producing a hoarse voice. A subarachnoid injection producing a total spinal anaesthetic is a possibility while a cervical sympathetic block will produce a Horner's syndrome.

GREATER OCCIPITAL NERVE BLOCK

This is useful in painful conditions affecting the posterior scalp. The nerve is blocked medial to the occipital artery which is palpated about 3 cm from the mid-line, i.e. lateral to the external occipital protuberance. If alcohol is to be used then paraesthesiae should be obtained before injection of 0·5–1·0 ml, but with local anaesthetics larger amounts can be used.

If the block is to be extended a little laterally then the lesser occipital nerve is blocked 2·5–3 cm lateral to that of the greater occipital nerve block. The third occipital nerve is just medial to the greater and is blocked with it.

SUPERFICIAL CERVICAL PLEXUS BLOCK

The patient is in the same position as for the deep cervical block. The nerves are blocked at the posterior border of the sternomastoid muscle. The skin wheal is made at the mid position along the posterior border which is about 2 cm or a little less above the point on the sternomastoid where the external jugular vein crosses it. A fine 5-cm needle is used to make injections in three directions. The first is inserted vertically through the wheal behind the muscle until the deep fascia is penetrated when 2·5–3 ml of 1 per cent Lignocaine is injected and the same amount subcutaneously. The second injection is made parallel to the posterior border, below the deep fascia and in a cephalad direction and over a 3–4 cm length 5 ml of anaesthetic solution is deposited. The third is similar except that it is caudad. Aspiration tests are performed with care during this block and the injections are best made during withdrawal of the needle. A total of 15 ml is used at least.

DORSAL AND LUMBAR PARAVERTEBRAL BLOCKS

The basic technique for these two blocks is essentially the same though the anatomy is a little different in the two regions. The needle is inserted a few centimetres lateral to the spine of one of the vertebrae until it touches the transverse process. It is then withdrawn and reinserted in a direction that takes it underneath and medial to that transverse process, and deeper. The final position places the tip of the needle close to the nerve as it exits from the intervertebral foramen. If the nerve is actually touched paraesthesiae are obtained, the needle is not inserted any further and the injection of local anaesthetic solution made immediately after aspiration. Anaesthesia in this case occurs very rapidly. If paraesthesiae are not obtained the needle is slowly advanced until it touches the body of the vertebra just anterior to the nerve. It is then withdrawn 1 cm, the aspiration test is carried out, and the injection is made.

PARAVERTEBRAL DORSAL BLOCK

Knowledge of the bony anatomy is essential in this region. The imbrication of the dorsal spinous processes is such that the tip of one spinous process is always at a lower level than that of its own transverse process. The spinous process is on the same plane as the intervertebral foramen of the next lowest vertebra and in the mid-thoracic region will probably be lower than this as it is in the same plane as the transverse process of the second vertebra below. For counting the dorsal vertebrae there are certain landmarks which are useful. The spine of C7 is the most prominent one at the base of the neck. Also when standing erect the line joining the spines of the scapulae passes through the D3 spine, and a line joining the inferior angles of the scapulae pass through the D7 spine.

It may be easier to count upwards from the lumbar vertebrae and a line joining the highest points of the iliac crests passes through the L4 spine, or the interspace between L4 and L5.

When an image intensifier is used it is quite simple to see the twelfth rib and count from there, or to count from the sacrum upwards. It must be remembered that not infrequently the lumbar vertebrae are actually or apparently increased in numbers by variations at the lumbosacral level.

For unilateral blocks the patient is in the lateral flexed position and having selected the nerves to be injected the spinous processes overlying the transverse processes of the selected nerves are marked and a skin wheal raised 3 cm lateral. An 8 cm 20- or 22-gauge needle is used and inserted vertically into the skin parallel to the mid-sagittal plane until it touches the transverse process. The marker is moved 2·5 cm from the skin and with-drawn to the superficial tissues and reinserted with the point going under-neath and medially to the transverse process to position the tip near the vertebral foramen. If paraesthesiae are obtained the injection is made at that point—after the aspiration test. The injection is 5 ml of 2 per cent Lignocaine. If none are obtained before the marker touches the skin the needle is with-drawn and reinserted in a slightly different direction. If bone is touched (at the postero-lateral vertebral body) the needle is withdrawn 1 cm and 5 ml of 2 per cent Lignocaine solution is injected.

If more than one nerve is to be injected the needles will form a line. When in the correct position, and after some 10 ml of solution has been injected filling up the paravertebral space, further injection down one needle may be accompanied by a slow flow of drops of solution out of the hubs of the others.

If skin analgesia is required in the thoracic region at least three adjacent nerves need to be injected owing to their overlapping sensory fields.

This paravertebral block will affect the somatic sensory nerves and the sympathetic vasoconstrictor fibres, but a large number of nerves have to be blocked before hypotension will occur. If it does occur it is most likely to appear in the older patients.

If the needle advances too far it can penetrate the pleura producing a pneumothorax. This usually settles without great problems but if the pneumothorax is large, or a tension pneumothorax develops, active measures must be instituted.

Whenever needles are inserted near the spinal column there is the danger of subarachnoid puncture and injection but they have to be considerably off line for this to happen. A possibility which is not as rare is for the needle to penetrate a paravertebral or intercostal vessel. This should be picked out by the aspiration test. There is also the possibility of subarachnoid injection by penetrating a long dural cuff exposed outside the intervertebral foramen.

When the image intensifier is used for this block (and also for the lumbar paravertebral block) there is no doubt as to the level that is being injected as this can be seen quite clearly. Both antero-posterior and lateral views are used as the former shows the transverse processes, while the latter is most useful showing the depth. Unfortunately, the lateral view cannot be obtained in the upper dorsal region as the shoulder joints and the scapulae are also in the X-ray beam. Nevertheless, an antero-posterior alone can be helpful.

In the upper dorsal spine the ribs are directed more laterally while in the lower dorsal region they are directed downwards to a greater degree and encroach on the space. Under ordinary circumstances this does not make the slightest difference to the injection, but in the occasional patient who has grossly sloping shoulders and a narrow chest, the ribs may slope very markedly. The space between one transverse process and the next can be reduced and this will make quite a difference to the ease of insertion. Conversely in the emphesematous patient, where the ribs are in a permanently raised position, the spaces tend to be widened and the insertion easier, but the lung is more vulnerable and production of a pneumothorax easier.

PARAVERTEBRAL LUMBAR BLOCK

The anterior primary rami of the upper four lumbar spinal nerves form the lumbar plexus, while part of the fourth joins the fifth to form the lumbosacral trunk. The lumbosacral trunk unites with the anterior primary rami of the upper three sacral nerves to form the sacral plexus.

The only difference in the lumbar paravertebral block compared to that of the dorsal paravertebral block is in the relationship of the lumbar spines to the transverse processes and the intervertebral foramina. The lower edge of the spinous process of a lumbar vertebra is at the same cross-sectional level as the intervertebral foramina and therefore the spinal nerve of the same vertebra. The upper border of the spinous process is at the same cross-sectional level as the transverse process of the same vertebra. As in the dorsal paravertebral block the patient is placed in the lateral flexed position, with the spinous processes brought to the same horizontal level by a pillow placed under the waist if necessary. The line joining the highest points on the iliac crests passes through the spine of the fourth lumbar vertebra, or the space between the fourth and fifth.

The technique is exactly similar to that of the dorsal paravertebral block with a few slight modifications due to the larger size of the lumbar vertebrae. Thus the wheal is raised 4 cm from the mid-line, and the transverse process is usually found at a depth of about 5 cm with the insertion level with the upper border of the spinous process. The depth marker is set at 3 cm and the needle directed downwards and inwards towards the intervertebral foramen and spinal nerve. Aspiration is carried out before injection of the local anaesthetic solution. The dangers and complications are similar to those of the dorsal paravertebral block, though it is easier to perform an inadvertent subarachnoid injection than in the dorsal region.

One point should be made clear and it applies to both the dorsal and the lumbar paravertebral blocks. There is no absolute necessity for the spinal nerve to be approached by first touching the transverse process. Sometimes because the skin wheal has been made too high, i.e. superior to the transverse process it may be easier to aim at the spinal nerve above—below the transverse process above. Also once one paravertebral needle has been inserted correctly others can be placed in position directly missing out the intermediate stages of touching the transverse process, withdrawing, re-directing, and so on. Of course the use of the image intensifier makes this quicker procedure even shorter, as the position of the transverse processes can be seen without difficulty. Certain branches of the dorsal and lumbar nerves are commonly involved in pain problems and knowledge of blocks for these nerves is useful.

INTERCOSTAL NERVE BLOCKS

The intercostal nerves run in the intercostal spaces below the corresponding rib and can be blocked anywhere along this length. However there are three positions where there are special anatomical reasons for a block at that point. First, the most prominent part of a rib is the posterior angle and even in obese patients where it may be 4 or 5 cm deep it is still the most accessible position. At this position blocking the nerve produces a block of the entire distal nerve. Secondly a block made at the posterior axillary line blocks all the nerve distal to it including the lateral cutaneous branch, and thirdly a block at the anterior axillary line does not include this lateral cutaneous branch.

There is no difficulty in carrying out a block at any of the points mentioned as long as care is taken to avoid producing a pneumothorax. This is done by using a fine needle no longer than is necessary to reach the rib surface and 1 cm or so beyond. This will vary with the obesity of the patient but in most cases a standard 23-gauge 2·5 cm needle is sufficient for the anterior and posterior axillary line blocks. The posterior angle block will usually be possible with this size of needle in the average patient but a longer one will be required when the patient is fat.

One hand holds the 5- or 10-ml syringe containing 2 per cent Lignocaine, while the other marks the selected rib. A preliminary wheal can be made but usually the needle is directly inserted into the skin until it hits the marked rib. It is then withdrawn a small amount and the skin and tissues slide downwards until a reinsertion of the needle will just glance past the lower border of the rib. The needle is allowed to go no more than 0·5 cm deeper to the lower border of the rib or a pneumothorax may result. Aspiration is made and not more than 5 ml of solution injected.

The position of the patient is important. When the injection is to be at the posterior angle the upper injection sites may be beneath the medial border of the scapula. These are uncovered by placing the patient in the lateral position with the side to be blocked uppermost and with the upper arm hanging over the side of the table. This will pull the scapula out of the way. If bilateral block is to be made the patient is placed prone, with a hard pillow under the chest to raise it so that both arms can hang over the edge of the table.

The position for the posterior and anterior axillary blocks is supine with the arms abducted out of the way. The anterior axillary line in the female cannot be used in the upper ribs, so any position lateral to the breasts is used to complete the block.

ILIOHYPOGASTRIC AND ILIOINGUINAL NERVE BLOCK

These two nerves arise from the anterior primary rami of the first lumbar nerve and supply the skin of the inguinal region except for that part of the scrotum and adjacent thigh supplied by the genito-femoral nerve. The iliohypogastric lies above the ilioinguinal but they can both be blocked at the anterior superior iliac spine. As they both arise from the first lumbar nerve a paravertebral block of this nerve would be effective.

The block at the anterior superior iliac spine is performed along a line joining this spine to the umbilicus. A skin wheal is made, three fingers breadth (5 cm) from the spine on this line and 20 ml 1 or 2 per cent Ligno-caine injected in fanwise fashion through all layers, cutaneous, fascial, and muscular, deep to the wheal and laterally as far as the anterior superior spine. Care should be taken not to penetrate the peritoneum. The addition of adrenaline 1 in 200,000 is an advantage in this block.

LATERAL FEMORAL CUTANEOUS NERVE BLOCK

This arises from the second and third lumbar primary rami. It supplies the lateral side of the thigh as far as the knee. It passes beneath the lateral end of the inguinal ligament about one finger's breadth medial to the anterior superior iliac spine and this is the usual situation where it is blocked. The nerve, as in the ilioinguinal and iliofemoral nerve block, cannot be picked off so a fanwise infiltration is made below the fascia lata where the nerve lies.

A skin wheal is made 2 cm medial to the anterior superior ilian spine and below the inguinal ligament. The fanwise injections are made in a direction parallel to the inguinal ligament. A 5 cm 22-gauge needle is inserted through the wheal perpendicularly and infiltration performed on withdrawal. The injection continues more laterally with each reinsertion and the needle will contact bone laterally. The complete fan is carried out if there are no paraesthesiae using 15 ml of 1 or 2 per cent Lignocaine with adrenaline 1 in 200,000, but if these are produced the needle is not moved further and 5 ml of 2 per cent Lignocaine is injected at that point.

This block is useful in the diagnosis and treatment of neuralgia parasthetica (neuralgia of the lateral cutaneous nerve of the thigh). In this condition there are paraesthesiae, pain, and numbness in the distribution of the nerve in the thigh. Treatment of the condition is by repeated blocks at the anterior superior iliac spine, and a steroid can be added to the solution. If a permanent block is to be performed then paraesthesiae must be obtained before injection of the neurolytic agent. A surgical section of this nerve is relatively simple and can usually be carried out under local anaesthesia. It is often preferred to the neurolytic block once the diagnostic block or blocks have confirmed the diagnosis.

LUMBAR PLEXUS BLOCK

This is particularly useful for patients suffering from intermittent claudication. In some patients with this condition reconstructive vascular surgery will remove one or more localised blocks in the vascular tree of the lower limb and thus relieve the claudication. But in many patients there is a generalised narrowing of these vessels so that reconstructive surgery is impossible and some other method must be used to provide relief.

It is important to realise why these patients cannot walk further than they do. It is rarely because there is insufficient blood supply to do this but usually because the products of metabolism accumulate and produce intense pain and the patient cannot walk because of this pain. Remove the pain and the patient is able to walk a further distance before pain recurs. It is obvious that no short-acting block will be of value here, since whatever technique is used must have a long-lasting effect. The technique advocated by Feldman seems to provide the answer. This involves spreading a long-lasting neurolytic agent, 7·5 per cent phenol in myodil, or 10 per cent aqueous phenol, over the lumbar plexus where it lies underneath the fascia of the psoas muscle. The solution used is of a strength which blocks the small C nerve fibres largely to the exclusion of others. These carry the stimuli which are interpreted as pain, and the injection does not normally affect power. This, however, depends on the relative size of the individual's nerve fibres.

The psoas muscle takes its origin from three parts. First, the inner portion of the anterior surface of the transverse processes of the lumbar vertebrae. Second, the lateral portions of the intervertebral disc, the adjacent lateral borders of the twelfth dorsal vertebra, and all the lumbar vertebrae. Thirdly from the fibrous arches which cross the lumbar vessels on the bodies of the lumbar vertebrae.

The lumbar plexus is situated deep in front of the transverse processes of the first, second, and third lumbar vertebrae. It lies in the substance of the psoas major, being mostly formed by the anterior primary rami of the first four lumbar nerves as previously mentioned. Thus any injection placed within the psoas major sheath will affect the lumbar plexus.

The technique of the lumbar plexus block depends on the use of an image intensifier and cannot be carried out easily without its use. It is possible to perform this block with ordinary X-ray films used in quantity, or better still by means of polaroid X-ray films but these methods are definitely second best. An 8 or 10 cm 20-gauge needle is used. If phenol in myodil is the agent to be injected this gauge of needle is a necessity but if an aqueous phenol solution is used then a smaller gauge could be selected. The needle is inserted as though for a paravertebral block at the L2 level but initially is not inserted much beyond the inner (anterior) border of the transverse process. A small injection of myodil radio-opaque material is made, and it can be seen on the image intensifier television screen whether the myodil is spreading in the muscle bundles of the psoas. If it is not then the needle is manœuvred in the origins of this muscle, by advancing it 0·25 cm or so, and a further injection made until the myodil is seen to progress downwards into the bulk of the muscle (see Figs. 90–93). Sometimes the initial injection tends to spread upwards and this may cause pain by encroaching on the crus of the diaphragm. Again a little movement of the needle will stop progression of the injection in this way (see Fig. 90). A total of 5–7 ml of 7·5 per cent phenol in myodil is used in divided doses while observing the steadily increasing spread of myodil within the psoas sheath by use of the image intensifier.

By the very nature of this type of injection there must be a limit to the length of time it will last. Feldman states that in a series of sixty-five patients 90 per cent doubled their claudication walking distance within twelve hours. At the end of twelve to eighteen months some 45 per cent of patients had maintained some degree of improvement. Thus it is likely that the block may need repeating in due course and there is no problem about this. However, if the operator does not like the accumulation of myodil in the tissues that will result when the standard method of carrying out the block is repeated, a variation can be made. After the initial injection of a small

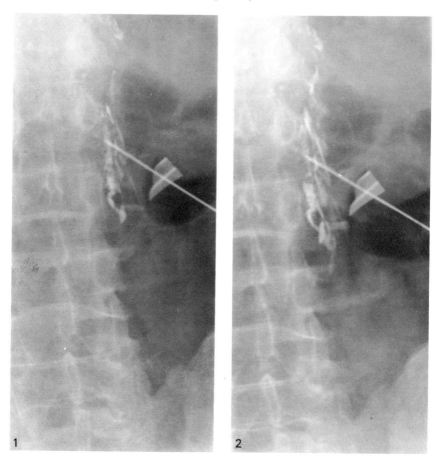

FIGURE 90.

FIGURES 90–93. Lumbar plexus, spread of myodil.

amount of myodil established that it was progressing along the psoas muscle correctly an aqueous solution can be used, or as the author prefers the injection continues with 5 per cent phenol in glycerine. From time to time during this injection a small quantity of myodil is injected from another syringe, 0·15–0·5 ml is sufficient, to show on the image intensifier whether the solution is behaving correctly or not. When using the 5 per cent phenol in glycerine solution a larger amount can be used as it is weaker than the $7\frac{1}{2}$ per cent recommended by Feldman. The weaker solution also has a lesser effect on motor nerve fibres. If a glycerine solution is used the ampoule containing it should be warmed before use to decrease the viscosity, and a 5 ml or even 2·5 ml syringe used to inject it.

LIMITED REGIONAL HIP BLOCK

This block is useful in relieving pain in chronic osteoarthritis of the hip. It is worth a trial in patients who are unable to have hip replacement surgery and in whom conservative measures do not relieve or mitigate the pain and the consequent immobility. Sometimes in the older patient where activity will be limited even after complete relief of the pain a percutaneous cordotomy can be considered instead.

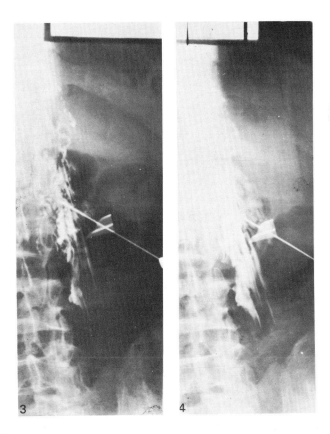

FIGURE 91.

There are a number of nerves contributing to the structures around the hip joint. These are the obturator, the femoral, the sciatic and sympathetic fibres from the lumbar sympathetic plexus, and the nerve to quadratus femoris. In about 30 per cent of patients there is also an accessory obturator nerve which has a course over the superior pubic ramus rather than through the obturator foramen with the main branch. All these nerves will give some

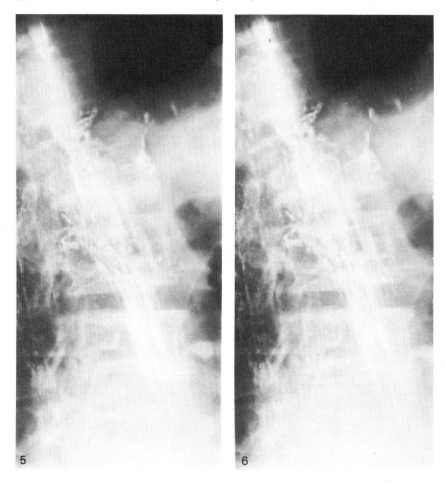

FIGURE 92.

nerve twigs to the joint capsule but the obturator nerve and the nerve to quadratus femoris are the most important.

The technique of these two blocks is not difficult though as the majority of patients treated are old, with a painful hip or hips, it may be difficult or even impossible to achieve the optimum position. For instance in the block of the obturator nerve it may be difficult to abduct the leg even slightly, or in the case of the nerve to quadratus femoris to rotate the hip externally. The use of an image intensifier may help though the views used may need to be improvised.

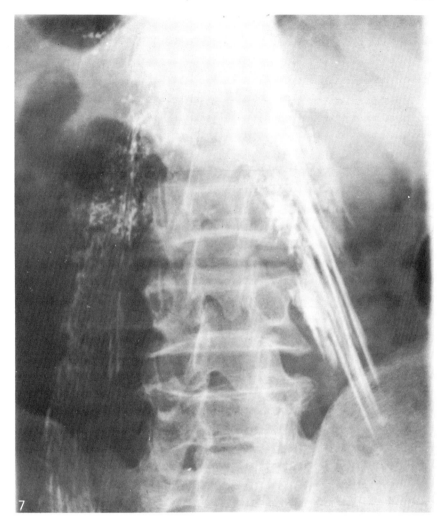

FIGURE 93. One week interval between sides.

OBTURATOR NERVE BLOCK

This nerve formed by the lumbar plexus from the second, third, and fourth lumbar nerves, lies on the pelvic brim above the obturator artery and enters the thigh through the obturator canal. The obturator membrane is attached to the entire circumference of the obturator foramen except superiorly. The obturator canal is a fibro-osseous canal whose upper boundary is formed by the obturator groove on the inferior surface of the superior pubic ramus and whose lower boundary is the upper border of the obturator membrane. The direction of the obturator groove is downwards, forwards, and inwards, and this is the direction of the obturator canal which contains the obturator nerve and the obturator vessels. In the obturator canal the obturator nerve divides into two divisions, anterior and posterior. The anterior gives off articular branches on to the hip joint within the obturator canal, while the posterior division passes through the obturator canal and gives an articular branch to the knee joint. The accessory obturator nerve, when present, does not pass through the obturator canal, it gives articular branches to the hip joint.

The obturator nerve is blocked by placing the patient supine, with the femur slightly abducted, and marking the mid-point between the pubic tubercle and the femoral artery. The superior pubic ramus is 2–3 cm below this mark, and as James remarks in his article on this block, 'it is often helpful in the more obese patients to draw up a fold of skin from the groin prior to the insertion of the needle'—a delightful understatement.

A 10 cm 18- or 20-gauge needle is inserted at right angles to the skin at the selected point to hit the superior pubic ramus. The needle is then manœuvred underneath this portion of the pubic ramus by turning it through 90° together with the portion of skin through which it is inserted with the needle almost parallel to the shaft of the femur, it can then be advanced upwards into the obturator foramen, to a depth of about 3 cm. The needle tip is kept in contact with the inferior and medial surfaces of the superior ramus of the pubis. Paraesthesiae are sometimes produced but this is by no means invariable.

There is the possibility of haematoma formation from the obturator vessels accompanying the nerve and aspiration must be performed before the injection. During the preliminary cleaning and sterilising of the pubic skin the genitalia should be protected.

BLOCK OF THE NERVE TO QUADRATUS FEMORIS

This nerve is formed from the fourth and fifth lumbar and the first sacral nerves, and passes through the inferior portion of the greater sacro-sciatic foramen. It lies below the pyriformis muscle in contact with the deep surface of the sciatic nerve. It passes downwards lying on the bone and enters deep to quadratus femoris. It supplies a branch to the gamellus inferior and to the hip joint.

The patient is placed in the prone position with the affected hip externally rotated as much as possible. As previously mentioned this is not always possible. A line is drawn between the posterior superior iliac spine and the sacro-coccygeal joint. The middle and lower third junction is marked. A wheal is raised 5 cm posterior to the greater trochanter of the femur, level with the lower portion of the sacrum. A long stiff needle 15 cm, gauge 16, is inserted at this point at an angle of 45° to the horizontal plane and advanced towards the point already marked. After the needle tip strikes bone it is worked medially, if possible, for a centimetre or so. This places it on the posterior surface of the body of the ischium very close to the sciatic nerve, and thus to the nerve to the quadratus femoris which lies between the bone and the sciatic nerve. 20 ml of 1 per cent Lignocaine is injected. It diffuses along the surface of the bone but will also block the sciatic nerve to a greater or lesser degree, so that there may be a transient motor paralysis.

The use of an image intensifier is helpful though a number of views will need to be tried to obtain a reasonable view of the ischial bone near the ischial spine. A stiff needle is required to 'walk' the tip along the bone but if this is not used then a finer needle say a 20-gauge can be used, but must be placed accurately.

These two blocks benefit patients with osteoarthritis, or spastic conditions of muscle. When used for these conditions the pain relief is not absolute but it will produce good relief for a few months in about 60 per cent of patients with osteoarthritis, and in about 30 per cent of spastic conditions. Pain relief may be sufficient in some patients who have become bedridden to become mobile again.

TRANSSACRAL NERVE BLOCK

The vertebrae of the sacrum are fused but paravertebral nerve block of the sacral nerves can be produced by inserting a needle through the posterior sacral foramina and injecting anaesthetic solution. The foramina represent spaces left in the fused portion of the transverse processes of the sacral vertebrae. It should be remembered that the anterior foramina are directly anterior to the posterior ones so that a needle may be inserted through the posterior one and exit into the pelvis through the anterior one. The thickness of the sacrum diminishes towards the coccyx.

The sacrum forms the roof and part of the posterior wall of the pelvis. The pelvic cavity is not a downwards continuation of the abdominal one but is a large posterior extension from the inferior portion of it. As the sacral vertebrae decrease in size from above downwards, the sacral bone is triangular with the base upwards and anterior. Thus when the patient is lying prone, preliminary to a transsacral block, the most superficial part of the bone is the lower portion in the region of the sacro-coccygeal junction. The upper portion of the bone, in the region of the first sacral foramina, is somewhat deeper but it runs in a sloping fashion into the back of the patient. This direction, if projected, would go through the table on which the patient is lying. It is worth spending a little time considering the position of the bone before attempting a transsacral block.

Not only does the sacral bone lie in the line mentioned above but its outer surface is convex. Thus needles inserted in succession through the posterior foramen at right angles to the skin are not parallel but spread out like a fan. The posterior sacral foramina are narrower than the corresponding anterior ones, and the bone of the posterior surface is rough and irregular. Down the centre of the sacrum on its outer surface is the sacral crest. This sacral crest is usually formed by four distinct ridges which represent the spinous processes of the vertebrae which are fused together to form the sacrum. Sometimes the crest is complete forming a continuous ridge. The spinous process of the fifth sacral vertebra is absent and thus there is a triangular opening at the inferior end of the sacral crest. This opening is the outlet of the sacral canal. Lateral to the crest is a groove formed by the fused laminae, and lateral to this groove is a row of four foramina which decrease in size from above downwards. Medial to the posterior foramina and encroaching over them is a small projection which is the developmental remains of the articular processes of the sacral vertebrae. The lower pair of projections belonging to the fifth sacral articular processes are expanded to form enlargements called the sacral cornua. They correspond to similar cornua on the first coccygeal vertebra. These two pairs of cornua are connected by ligaments and the space that is bridged over on each side forms the fifth sacral foramina. The fifth sacral nerve passes through this foramina.

Lateral to each foramina is a tubercle which represents the transverse process of that sacral vertebra. These four tubercles rest on an area of solid bone lateral to the foramina which is the lateral mass of the sacrum.

The sacral canal lies posterior to the fused bodies of the upper four sacral vertebrae, being triangular in its upper part and crescentic in the lower. There are four intervertebral foramina through which pass the sacral spinal nerves. Each opens on to the surfaces of the sacrum by anterior and posterior sacral foramina. These arise a little way from the origin of the intervertebral foramina. They thus have the shape of a wide 'V' with the point of the 'V' at the intervertebral foramen. But as has already been mentioned a needle can be passed from the superficial surface of a posterior foramen through the deep surface of the anterior foramen, thus knowledge of the thickness between the outer surface of the posterior foramen and the inner surface of the anterior must be used, otherwise an injecting needle may be inserted too deep and the injection deposited outside the ligament closing the anterior foramen. As there is another ligament closing off the superficial surface of the posterior foramen an injection deposited between them will bathe the nerve roots.

The sacral foramina lie in two straight lines. These lines are not parallel but follow the general triangular shape of the sacrum and thus become closer together as they become inferior. The first sacral foramina lies 2 cm from the mid-line, the second and third foraminae lie on the line between the first and the fourth, and the fourth is 1·5 cm from the mid-line. The straight line connecting the foramina passes 1·0 cm, medial to the posterior superior iliac crest above, and also through the corresponding sacral cornua. The thickness of the sacrum is 2·5 cm at the first transsacral canal, 2·0 cm at the second, 1·5 cm at the third and 1·0 cm at the fourth. These depths are approximations as there are individual variations, depending on the thickness of the sacrum.

TECHNIQUE

This block is best carried out with the patient in the prone position and with the buttocks elevated by firm pillows placed under the hips and upper thighs. If a theatre table is used it can be broken in addition. The skin is prepared, sterilised, and towelled up, and the landmarks are then marked in by a sterile skin pencil or marking solution.

The posterior superior iliac spine is identified and marked, and the point 1·0 cm medial and 1·0 cm inferior to it is also marked. This mark overlies the second sacral foramen. The sacral cornua is identified and a mark made 1·0 cm inferior and lateral to it. This mark lies over the fifth posterior sacral foramen. A line is drawn between these two marks, and it is divided into three equal portions by two more marks. These overlie the third and fourth posterior sacral foramina. The first foramen is on this line 2·0 cm above the first mark. The marks overlying the various foramina should form a straight line more or less parallel to the mid-line. 8-cm needles are used for injecting the first and second sacral nerves and 5 cm needles for the lower ones. In thin patients the 5-cm needle will be sufficient for all patients. It is useful to have depth markers on the needles and in turn a wheal is raised over each mark and a needle inserted into the foramen. The first sacral foramen insertion is usually performed first and the direction is not perpendicular to the skin but is slightly medially and inferiorly. However, it is important to appreciate where the posterior surface of the sacrum is, and therefore it is wise to touch this surface quite deliberately on the first pass. The depth marker is then placed 1·5 cm from the skin and the needle withdrawn and reinserted in fan-wise fashion until it passes through the foramen. It is inserted to the depth of the marker or its advance is stopped before this point is reached if para-esthesia are obtained. The procedure is repeated for the other foramina bearing in mind that the depth of insertion reduces as one descends. The needle for the second sacral paravertebral block is advanced 1 cm, while in the third, fourth, and fifth paravertebral blocks the needles are inserted between 0·5 and 0·75 cm.

The volumes of anaesthetic solution required are 5 ml for the first and second, 4 ml for the third and fourth, and 3 ml for the fifth. The usual aspiration test is carried out before each injection to ensure that the needle is not placed intravascularly or that there is no abnormality of development of the sacrum and dura and that cerebrospinal fluid has not been obtained.

CAUDAL BLOCK

The caudal block is an epidural block carried out through the sacral hiatus. Normally, the spinous process of the fifth sacral vertebra is not fused and there is an arched opening, the sacral hiatus, with an easily palpable sacral cornua on each side. The sacral hiatus is closed by a firm membrane.

Ventrally, the caudal canal is closed by the fused bodies of the sacral vertebrae and the anterior sacral foramina open into its space. Dorsally, the sacral canal is normally closed by the fused sacral spinous processes but there are minor variations of the upper border of the sacral hiatus and in a small percentage of cases there is a complete failure of all the laminae of the sacral vertebrae to fuse. Careful palpation and, if necessary, radiological investigation will determine this.

The epidural space in the caudal canal is continuous with the epidural space around the rest of the dura in the spinal cord extending right up to the foramen magnum. The epidural space contains the nerves of the cauda equina and blood vessels. Usually, the caudal dura mater ends at the level of the second sacral vertebra but it can extend lower. Similarly, the lower end of the spinal cord can on occasion descend lower than L2 but it is unlikely that it will be damaged provided reasonable care is used. Before injecting any solutions on to the caudal canal the aspiration test for blood and cerebrospinal fluid must be carried out.

The position of the patient is very similar to that used in the trans-sacral method with the legs separated and the heels rotated outwards. The blocks described in this section are those used in pain relief work but it should be mentioned here that if a caudal block is to be provided for anaesthesia for obstetrics then the position mentioned would never be used, the patient being placed in the lateral position instead.

Usually, the simplest method of deliniating the caudal hiatus is to feel the sacral spines with the ball of the thumb and gradually move it downwards until a triangular region is felt with the sacral cornua on either side. In fat patients the posterior superior iliac spines are marked and an equilateral triangle drawn using this distance for the sides, the apex pointing caudally. The apex of this triangle will be situated very close to the sacral hiatus.

The direction of the epidural space in this region is along the length of the body but to penetrate the ligament over the sacral hiatus the initial insertion is perpendicular to the sacral hiatus and as soon as the needle penetrates it it is swung through an angle of about 40° and inserted about 0·5 cm. There are great differences in the shape of the sacral canal at this level some being very easy to enter and others being flattened, narrow, and difficult. If the point of the needle after insertion touches the anterior wall of the sacral canal it should be withdrawn slightly before rotating into the position mentioned above.

There are special caudal needles available, some quite large as when a catheter for continuous epidural block is to be inserted, but normally a 21-gauge needle or thereabouts is adequate and is inserted through a small skin wheal. Anaesthetic solution is not injected if cerebrospinal fluid is obtained and if blood is aspirated injection is not carried out until it is known that the needle does not lie within a blood vessel.

15–20 ml of 1 per cent Lignocaine will give a saddle block at least, and 25 ml will produce a block to the level of T12 or thereabouts. There are individual variations and some operators use solutions with adrenaline.

Large volumes of fluid can be injected if required, although the author does not usually do this as he is extremely cautious with all injections around the spinal cord, but up to 50 ml of local anaesthetic solution with a long-acting steroid is often used in low back pain and painful post-operative lumbar laminectomy conditions.

EPIDURAL BLOCK

The caudal block already mentioned is a special case of an injection being made into the epidural space. In the case of the caudal block it is made into the lowermost portion of the epidural space which extends between the two layers of the dura mater and the whole length of the spinal cord from its junction at the edge of the foramen magnum down to the sacral hiatus.

Injection into this space cannot therefore extend higher than the foramen magnum.

The space contains venous plexuses as well as fat and connective tissue. Laterally, the epidural space is in communication with the paravertebral spaces through the intervertebral foramina. In the lumbar region the paravertebral space is triangular in shape and the apex dorsally. As the spinal cord ends between L1 and L3 in this region in the majority of patients most epidural blocks are carried out below this level.

At other levels the extent of the space varies depending on the expansions of the spinal cord. Thus it is large above the level of the third cervical vertebra where the cervico-thoracic enlargement of the spinal cord begins and this enlargement continues to about T4 so that the epidural space increases below this level.

The identification of the epidural space is carried out by a number of techniques but they all depend on the fact that there is a reduced pressure in the epidural space. Usually, there is a negative pressure in the epidural space and when a needle enters it, any fluid or air in the needle tends to be sucked inwards. The simplest method is to exert manual pressure on the plunger of a syringe containing saline solution which is attached to the spinal needle as it is slowly inserted in the selected space. As soon as it enters the epidural space there is a loss of resistance and solution begins to be injected into the space.

The syringe can be dispensed with and a drop of saline is placed on the hub of the needle and is observed very carefully as the needle is advanced. When the epidural space is entered the hanging drop is sucked into the needle. The method the author favours is the Mackintosh balloon which is attached to the spinal needle after it has been inserted through the superficial tissues, and inflated with a few ml of sterile air. As soon as the tip of the needle enters the epidural space the balloon deflates.

Epidural blocks can be carried out by a single dose method, or a Tuohy needle, or one of the recent adaptations of this needle can be used and a catheter inserted through it so that a continuous epidural anaesthetic is provided.

In pain relief work the author has found this technique most useful for placing stimulating electrodes in the epidural canal at various levels of the spinal cord so that stimulation studies can be carried out. These are exceedingly useful when a trial method of electrical stimulation is to be made with the future prospect of implanting a dorsal column stimulator if this and the other tests are satisfactory.

The electrode can be implanted at any level of the spinal cord as will be seen from the X-rays (see Chapter 9). Usually the electrode will run quite easily in the required direction but sometimes this does not happen and much time is spent coaxing it into the correct position.

Because the epidural space contains a venous plexus there is an ever-present danger of haemorrhage when needles, catheters, or electrodes are passed. Usually this is of no consequence but if haemorrhage continues paraplegia can result. Any report that a patient is unable to move the lower limbs after such a procedure should be treated most seriously and urgently. It is never wise to believe it is hysterical (as it may be) until all other possibilities are urgently examined. The treatment of paraplegia from haemorrhage will be speedy decompression by laminectomy.

SUBARACHNOID DIFFERENTIAL BLOCK

This is a most useful technique when there are problems in deciding whether the pain a patient has is of psychogenic origin, is travelling over sympathetic fibres, or over the normal sensory fibres. It is particularly useful for pain in the lumbar region and lower limbs when the patient is placed in the lateral position and a subarachnoid spinal tap made at a convenient level. Initially, 5 ml of saline is injected and the patient will appreciate that something has been injected into his back. A wait of five minutes and an enquiry is made as to the level of the patient's pain. Improvement of the pain at this stage is due either to a placebo effect or to a psychological cause. The next injection is 5 ml of 0·25 per cent procaine which will block sympathetic fibres and after a five-minute interval it is followed by 5 ml of 0·5 per cent Procaine which will block sensory nerves. Finally, it is followed up by injection of sufficient solution and sufficient strength to produce complete motor and sensory block.

After each injection, as in the case of the saline, enquiry is made as to the patient's pain. If pain is relieved after sympathetic fibres are blocked then this indicates the direction the treatment should follow. If pain is relieved after sensory block then this demonstrates quite adequately that the patient has organic pain. If the pain is still present after complete motor and sensory block then again treatment can be developed accordingly.

SCIATIC NERVE BLOCK

The sciatic nerve can be blocked by an anterior or a posterior approach with the patient lying either on his back for the anterior approach or on his side for the posterior approach.

The description here is of the posterior approach and if knowledge of the anterior approach is required, one of the specialist books on local blocks should be consulted.

Posterior sciatic nerve block

The sciatic nerve is usually blocked between the ischial tuberosity and the greater trochanter of the femur where it is just posterior to the ischium. This is its position just after leaving the pelvis through the greater sciatic foramen where it lies below the piriformis muscle. It then descends towards the posterior thigh and comes to lie in a hollow between the tuberosity of the ischium and the greater trochanter of the femur. This position lies on the junction of the middle and medial thirds of the line connecting these two points.

Essentially, the technique consists of placing the patient in such a position that the surface markings of the sciatic nerve can be properly worked out. There are two methods of doing this and in each case the patient lies on the side which is not to be blocked with the knee bent and the body tilted about 40° anteriorly. The superior border of the greater trochanter is marked, this being the point of insertion of the piriformis muscle and another is made over the posterior superior iliac spine. A line is drawn connecting these two points and the position of the femur adjusted until the long axis of the femur is a continuation of this line. The mid-point of this line is marked and another line is drawn at right angles in a caudal direction. The insertion of the needle is made 4–5 cm along this second line, which is the surface marking of the sciatic nerve emerging from the greater sciatic foramen.

Subcutaneous intramuscular infiltration with a 20-gauge spinal needle, 10–12 cm long is used, and contact should be made with the bone. A depth marker is moved 1 cm from the skin. If paraesthesiae are obtained before bone is reached, then the needle has penetrated the nerve and 5–10 ml of 1 per cent Lignocaine are injected.

If paraesthesiae are not obtained then a series of fan-wise insertions of the needle are made in a direction at right angles to the sciatic nerve until paraesthesiae are obtained. If no paraesthesiae are obtained, and this is rare, 15–20 ml of 1 per cent Lignocaine are injected in various fan-wise directions down to, but no further than, the depth marker.

When the needle enters the sciatic nerve the patient will experience marked discomfort from pain and paraesthesiae and should be warned beforehand that this might happen, so that they will not move too much.

The second method of obtaining the landmarks of the sciatic nerve is to identify the ischial tuberosity and greater trochanter of the femur. A line is drawn between them. At the junction of the medial and middle thirds, a wheal is raised and the needle inserted through this perpendicular to the skin. It is advanced until paraesthesiae are obtained in the same way as previously. Again, if paraesthesiae are not obtained in the first few fan-wise insertions, local anaesthetic can be deposited during withdrawal of the needle through the tissues and after a negative aspiration test has been obtained.

This method of obtaining the position of the sciatic nerve gives a position slightly inferior on the thigh than the first method.

FURTHER READING

ARTICLES

APPLEGATE W.V. (1972) Abdominal cutaneous nerve entrapment syndrome. *Surgery*, **71**, 118.

BONNEY G.L.W. (1973) Causalgia. *Br. J. Hosp. Med.* **9**, 593–596.

BRIDENBAUGH L.D., MOORE D.C. & CAMPBELL D.D. (1964) Management of upper abdominal cancer pain. *J.A.M.A.* **190**, 10, 877.

BURN J.M.B. & LANGDON L. (1970) Lumbar epidural injection for the treatment of chronic sciatica. *Rheum. and Physical Med.* **10**, 368.

CHAPMAN G.M. (1972) Regional nerve block with the aid of a nerve stimulator. *Anaesthesia*, **27**, 185.

DAM W. & LARSEN J.J.V. (1974) Peripheral nerve blocks in relief of intractable pain. In *Relief of Intractable Pain*. Chapter 6. Ed. M. Swerdlow. Excerpta Medica, Amsterdam.

FELDMAN S.A. (1974) Lumbar sympathetic block. In *The Treatment of Chronic Pain*. Chapter 6. Ed. F. D. Hart, M.T.P. Co., Lancaster, Great Britain.

GREENBLATT G.M. & DENSON J.S. (1962) Needle nerve stimulator-locator. Nerve blocks with a new instrument for locating nerves. *Anesth. Analg. Curr. Res.* **41**, 599.

HALPERN D. & MEELHUYSEN F.E. (1966) Phenol motor point block in the management of muscular hypertonia. *Arch. Phys. Med.* **47**, 659.

HANNINGTON-KIFF J.G. (1974) Intravenous regional sympathetic block. In *Pain Relief*, p. 69. Heinemann, London.

HITCHCOCK E. & PRANDIDINI M.N. (1973) Hypertonic saline in management of intractable pain. *Lancet*, **1**, 310.

JAMES C.D.T. & LITTLE T.F. (1976) Regional hip blockade. *Anaesthesia*, **31**, 8, 1060–1067.

LLOYD J.W., HUGHES J.T. & DAVIES-JONES G.A.B. (1972) Relief of severe intractable pain by barbotage of cerebrospinal fluid. *Lancet*, **1**, 354.

MAGORG F., ROZIN R., BEN-MENACHEN Y. & MAGORA A. (1969) Obturator nerve block. An evaluation of technique. *Br. J. Anaesth.* **41**, 695.

MONTGOMERY W. & COUSINS M.J. (1972) Aspects of management of chronic pain illustrated by ninth nerve block. *Br. J. Anaesth.* **44**, 383.

RANGER I., MEHTA M. & PENNINGTON M. (1971) Abdominal wall pain due to nerve entrapment. *Practitioner*, **206**, 791.

REID W., WATT J.K. & GRAY T.G. (1970) Phenol injection of the sympathetic chain. *Br. J. Surg.* **57**, 45.

REVILL S. I., ROBINSON J.O., ROSEN M. & HOGG, M.I.J. (1976) The reliability of a linear analogue for evaluating pain. *Anaesthesia*, **31**, 9, 1191–1198.

SMITH D.W. (1951) Stellate ganglion block. *Am. J. Surg.* **82**, 344.

WINNIE A.P. & COLLINS V.J. (1968) The pain clinic. 1. Differential neurone blockade in pain syndromes of questionable etiology. *Medical Clinics of North America*, **52**, 123.

BOOKS

Illustrated Handbook in Local Anaesthesia (1969) Ed. E. Eriksson. Copyright by A. B. Astra, Ltd. I. C. Sorensen & Co., Copenhagen.

Intractable Pain (1973) Ed. M. Mehta. Saunders, London.

Persistent Pain (1977) Vol. 1. Ed. S. Lipton. Academic Press, London and New York.

Regional Block (1965) 4th Edition. Ed. D. C. Moore. Thomas, Springfield, Illinois.

The Management of Pain (1953) Ed. J.J. Bonica. Kimpton, London.

Index